Managing Clinical Processes in Health Services

Managing
Clinical Processes
in Health Services

Roslyn Sorensen

Rick Iedema

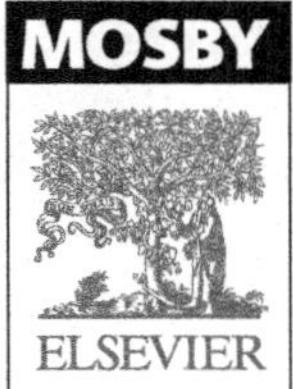

MOSBY

ELSEVIER

Sydney   Edinburgh   London   New York
Philadelphia   St Louis   Toronto

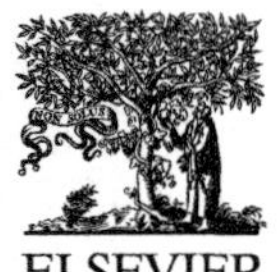

ELSEVIER

Mosby is an imprint of Elsevier

Elsevier Australia. ACN 001 002 357
(a division of Reed International Books Australia Pty Ltd)
Tower 1, 475 Victoria Avenue, Chatswood, NSW 2067

Every attempt has been made to trace and acknowledge copyright, but in some
cases this may not have been possible. The publisher apologises for any accidental
infringement and would welcome any information to redress the situation.

This publication has been carefully reviewed and checked to ensure that the content is as
accurate and current as possible at time of publication. We would recommend, however, that
the reader verify any procedures, treatments, drug dosages or legal content described in this
book. Neither the author, the contributors, nor the publisher assume any liability for injury
and/or damage to persons or property arising from any error in or omission from this publication.

National Library of Australia Cataloguing-in-Publication data

Sorensen, Roslyn

Managing clinical processes in health services / Roslyn Sorensen ; Rick Iedema.

Chatswood, NSW: Elsevier, 2008.

ISBN: 9780729538251 (pbk.)

Includes index.
Bibliography.

Health services administration--Australia.
Medical care--Evaluation.
Health facilities--Australia--Administration.
Medical protocols--Australia.
Total quality management--Australia.
Reengineering (Management)--Australia.
Organizational change--Australia.

Iedema, Rick.

362.10680994

Publisher: Luisa Cecotti
Publishing Services Manager: Helena Klijn
Edited by Matt Davies
Proofread by Tim Learner
Internal and cover design by Toni Darben
Index by Master Indexing
Typeset by TnQ
Printed by Ligare

Contents

Preface

Health services worldwide are under pressure to perform and expectations are strengthening about what they can and should deliver. Patients, consumers and communities expect health services to meet standards of service quality, responsiveness and accountability; clinicians expect to have a strong voice in decisions about the healthcare system; and policymakers expect health services to meet standards of cost effectiveness. Even though these key stakeholders don't necessarily agree about health services' goals, the demand for health services grows, costs continue to escalate and high-profile failures in quality of care mount raising concerns about the safety of the system and whether it can deliver value for money. Taken together, these pressures bring an urgency to improving the underlying systems on which good care is based.

Strategies to respond to these expectations range from top-down managerial approaches that often uncritically apply generic private sector performance-improvement principles to the public health sector, to isolated technical interventions at the individual patient level in clinical workplaces. These levels of the organisation work largely independently, and for health service performance to improve, the two domains must integrate. This book is positioned between these two domains, that is, between the abstract performance focus of corporate management and the clinical particularities of individual patient care. It is not specifically intended for 'managers' or 'clinicians' but for all those who seek to understand how health services work, or could work better.

The book takes an international perspective. In doing so, we take account of the health systems of developed countries to acknowledge the international influence on healthcare and health systems improvement, and to compare key points across countries with similar health systems.

What this book offers

Clinical process management is an emerging field of study. This book attempts to set a foundation for what is known about the topic based on evidence from the literature and related research. Methods of clinical process management are described and discussed and, where available, supported by evidence. Significant points are highlighted throughout the chapters in captions titled *Implications for practice*. Although clinical process management is becoming a separate field of study, it critically links policy, managerial and clinical activity as an integrated entity. The book also addresses what is not yet known, and presents this information as a series of questions titled *Points for reflection*.

Each contributor to the book is a specialist in their field. Through their contributions, their expertise is directed to understanding the way health services work and the context in which healthcare is delivered, and applying this knowledge to managing clinical processes in health services. Each chapter is set out using major themes as content headings. The content is designed to apply equally to public and private health services and to tertiary, secondary and primary healthcare sectors. We believe that the types of clinical processes that need to be managed to achieve the objectives of healthcare are common across all health services, and differ in degree rather than kind.

Rationale

The book is intended to provide clinicians, clinical managers and corporate managers with a practical guide to transforming health services by managing clinical processes and, in doing so, to link theory to practice. The need for such a text is supported by the growing awareness of the limitations that increasing specialisation of clinical work can bring and the importance of coordinating complex clinical and administrative healthcare processes, as multidisciplinary clinicians and managers care for populations of acutely ill people with multiple comorbidities and care needs. It is intended to consolidate new knowledge as clinical and administrative processes integrate vertically and horizontally within the organisation, so as to overcome the fragmentation of knowledge located in clinical specialties and management units.

The structure of the book

The book is structured in three parts. The first part addresses the environment within which health services are delivered and managed. The second part describes the operational aspects of managing clinical processes. The third part considers issues of accountability for health service outcomes.

In Part 1, we outline the scope of the book and describe the objectives, evidence and context for managing clinical processes. Leggat introduces the fundamentals of operations management as a means of gaining value in terms of outputs and outcomes from health service inputs. Stanton discusses the politics of healthcare, the challenges and opportunities involved in managing the healthcare workforce, and the strategic opportunities for health service improvement that can arise from managing human resources.

In Part 2 Claridge & Cook conceptualise the health system as a production process, and delineate the tools and rules needed to transform health into a process-oriented sector. Kerosuo considers the place of the patient in healthcare and mechanisms to incorporate the patient into decision-making processes about their care. Willis and colleagues analyse healthcare as a collectivity, specifically the role of multidisciplinary teams in engaging with patients and families in sharing decisions about care outcomes and treatment processes. We join Jorm & Piper to extend this collectivity, to explore the co-productive nature of healthcare. Berg et al reconsider the organisation of complex health services and propose care programs as a way of integrating these critical clinical and organisational elements to achieve performance outcomes.

In Part 3 Boaden & Harvey discuss the types of organisation needed in health services to improve quality and patient safety. Merry takes this issue to the level of clinical units to delineate the types of issues, processes and outcomes clinicians and managers need to engage in to manage risk and to ensure patient safety. Jorm et al analyse policy approaches to health improvement, and show the extent of change in policymaking by comparing policy developed in 1990 with that of today. Mooney advocates for the place of the community in healthcare decision making, including citizens' juries through which community values can become known and used as the basis for prioritisation and resource allocation.

Finally, we bring these building blocks together to consider the implications for practice. We conclude that health services need strategic, operational and communicative space to begin to understand, reorient and redesign health services that are sustainable and responsive to need and that are patient and community centred. Recognising that this is a new and emerging field, and also that many people in many countries are tackling the task of transforming healthcare, Berding has compiled a range of resources for readers to continue their interest in how to manage clinical processes in health services. Hopefully, through this book, many more such resources can be added to the list.

Roslyn Sorensen & Rick Iedema
Sydney 2008

Contributors

Margaret Banks holds a science degree, a postgraduate diploma in physiotherapy and a master's degree in health administration and has been a practising physiotherapist. She has been involved in policy development projects for state and federal governments and two national bodies: the Australian Health Workforce Advisory Committee and the Australian Government's national peak body on safety and quality. Margaret sits on the NSW Australian College of Health Service Executives council and coordinates the NSW Fellowship Program on behalf of the college.

Friederike Berding holds a four-year degree in international business (German Diplom) from the International School of Management (ISM) in Dortmund, Germany, and she is on track to complete a Master of Health Services Management at the University of Technology, Sydney (UTS). She has worked in hospital quality management in Germany, the scope of her Diplom-thesis, and has a strong interest in clinical process management.

Marc Berg has a medical background, holds a PhD, is a partner at Plexus Medical Group (a fast-growing healthcare consultancy agency), and is affiliated with the Institute of Health Policy and Management, Erasmus University Medical Center in the Netherlands. His main interests are the generation and organisation of high-quality and low-cost healthcare practices, both at the level of the healthcare practice itself and at the system level. He teaches and consults with executive leaders and policymakers to improve healthcare systems, both at the national (policy) level and at the healthcare organisation level.

Cé Bergen has a medical background and is an independent consultant. He has helped introduce the principles of care programs in many hospitals. His main focus is the interrelation of the re-organisation of healthcare work and the introduction of process-supporting information and communication technology (ICT) systems.

Ruth Boaden is Professor of Service Operations Management at Manchester Business School, University of Manchester, UK. She carries out a wide range of health service research that includes empirical work on patient flow, case management, quality and improvement, performance and patient safety. She has a focus on knowledge transfer arising from good research, to ensure that the findings are accessible and applicable to practice. She has published widely in academic and applied areas. She was director of the 'Leadership through effective people management' development program for NHS human resource directors and deputies from 2001 to 2006 and has directed a research centre concerned with the organisation of health services.

Tanya Claridge has a nursing background. She is a member of the School of Psychological Sciences and Stockport NHS Foundation Trust, University of Manchester.

Gary Cook has a medical and legal background. He is a member of the Clinical Effectiveness Unit, Stockport NHS Foundation Trust.

Sandra Dunn is Professor of Nursing – Clinical Practice in Charles Darwin University Graduate School of Health Practice. Her role includes multidisciplinary professional development and education; research with a strong clinical focus; curriculum development and quality assurance; and postgraduate supervision.

Judith Dwyer is head of the Department of Health Management at the Flinders University School of Medicine. She is a former CEO of Southern Health Care Network in Melbourne, and of Flinders Medical Centre in Adelaide. She has worked in the Australian health system for more than 20 years in a broad range of community, hospital and government settings. Judith's research and consulting work is focused on leadership and governance of the healthcare system, and on primary healthcare services for Aboriginal and Torres Strait Islander communities. She was the inaugural president of Women's Hospitals Australasia and founding chair of the Australian Resource Centre for Healthcare Innovation.

Gill Harvey is Senior Lecturer in Healthcare and Public Sector Management at the Centre for Public Policy and Management (CPPM), part of the Manchester Business School at the University of Manchester. She has a professional background in nursing and prior to taking up her post at CPPM, worked for nine years as the director of the Royal College of Nursing's Quality Improvement Programme. Gill's research interests are focused on two main areas: organisational failure and turnaround; and evaluative research around issues of implementation and facilitating quality improvement in practice. She is a past co-chair of the European Forum for Quality Improvement in Health Care and for several years was an associate editor of the *Quality and Safety in Healthcare* journal.

Rick Iedema is Professor of Organisational Communication and Associate Dean (Research), Faculty of Humanities and Social Sciences, University of Technology, Sydney. His work centres on discourse, analytical and ethnographic investigations into the organisation and enactment of healthcare provision through which he has a strong national and international publishing record. His research interests include (as a co-investigator on projects with health departmental bodies such as the NSW Health Department Quality Branch, and the NSW Clinical Excellence Commission) the shift in clinical work from paper-based towards electronic information and communication media; hospital accreditation; a 'video-ethnographic' project focusing on clinicians' identity as it is 'performed' in situated clinical interactions; and an organisational change project that investigates whether and how clinicians learn from adverse events.

Christine Jorm is an adjunct professor at UTS Sydney and she is the Senior Medical Advisor at the Australian Commission on Safety and Quality in Health Care. Christine practised as a clinical anaesthetist before moving into the area of safety and quality. She has an MD in neuropharmacology and a sociology PhD.

Hannele Kerosuo is a research associate at the Center for Activity Theory and Developmental Work Research, University of Helsinki, Finland. Her doctoral dissertation investigated the boundary dynamics of development, learning and change in healthcare organisations. Her work has focused on the development of 'negotiated care' and 'knot-working' in healthcare organisations. Currently, she is involved in research on stabilisation and diffusion of innovative forms of working and learning at work. She has a professional background in social and healthcare administration. Hannele has published and co-authored articles in *Culture and Organisation; Management and Learning;* and *Outlines: Critical Social Studies.* She has also edited volumes in the area of management studies and health communication. Recently, she has co-edited the activity–theoretical special issue of the *Journal of Workplace Learning* with Professor Yrjö Engeström.

Sandra Leggat is Professor of Health Services Management and Head of School at the La Trobe University School of Public Health in Melbourne. She has Australian and international experience in health system policy, organisation and management. She is editor of *Australian Health Review*, the leading Australian journal in healthcare policy and management, and is a member of the Northern Health Board of Directors. Sandra is a physiotherapist and has had substantial experience in health service management with the Inner & Eastern Health Care Network, The Toronto Hospital (now University Health Network), Baycrest Centre for Geriatric Care and the Health Station Community Health Service. Her research is focused on improving people and performance in healthcare.

Alan Merry is Professor of Anaesthesiology at the University of Auckland. He chairs the Quality and Safety Committee of the World Federation of Societies of Anaesthesiologists, is a councillor of the Australian and New Zealand College of Anaesthetists, and chairs the college's Quality and Safety Committee. He has co-chaired the New Zealand Medical Law Reform Group, has been President of the Auckland Medico-Legal Society and founded Safer Sleep Ltd. He is co-author of *Errors, Medicine and the Law* (with Alexander McCall Smith), *Essential Perioperative Transoesophageal Echocardiography* (with David Sidebotham & Malcolm Legget) and *Safety and Ethics in Healthcare – A Guide to Getting it Right* (with Bill Runciman & Merrilyn Walton).

Gavin Mooney is Director of the Social and Public Health Economics Research Group (SPHERe), Professor of Health Economics at Curtin University in Perth and Visiting Professor at the Centre for Health and Humanity at Aarhus University (Denmark) and at the Health Economics Unit at the University of Cape Town. He was the founding director of the Health Economics Research Unit at the University of Aberdeen in Scotland. He has built an international reputation as a health economist over the past 30 years, first in the UK, then Denmark and in the past 14 years in Australia. He has a strong interest in equity in healthcare, particularly with respect to Aboriginal health, and in the economics of the social determinants of health, and publishes and presents in this area. In recent years he has become particularly interested in communitarianism and using this philosophy in the economics of health, especially with respect to equity.

Donella Piper has a legal background and is a PhD candidate at the Faculty of Humanities & Social Science at the University of Technology, Sydney researching 'The Role of Legislation in Facilitating Community Participation in Healthcare Governance: NSW Health a Case-study'. She was a Director of the New England Area Health Service (NEAHS) from 2002 to 2004. During the term of her appointment she was chair of the NEAHS Clinical Ethics Committee and a member of the NEAHS Medical and Dental Appointments Committee. She lectures in law and related subjects.

Wim Schellekens has a medical background and is Head Inspector for Hospital and General Practice Care in the Dutch healthcare sector. Prior to this, he was the CEO of the Dutch Quality Institute, the CBO. In both roles, he has been at the forefront of quality improvement efforts in the Netherlands. In 2004 Wim initiated the largest Dutch hospital improvement project to date, 'Sneller Beter' (Better Faster), in which 25% of all Dutch hospitals participated. The development of care programs was a vital element of this work.

Roslyn Sorensen is Senior Lecturer in the Faculty of Nursing, Midwifery & Health and researcher in the Centre for Health Services Management at the University of Technology, Sydney. She teaches in a range of subjects related to health service organisation and management. Her research interests and activities lie in health policy development and implementation, health service governance and accountability, managing clinical processes in clinical workplaces and health service organisations, and understanding the personal and professional dynamics in managing change. She has worked at the federal level of government developing policy to support health service change and publishes and presents in this field.

Pauline Stanton is an associate professor in the Graduate School of Management at Melbourne's La Trobe University where she specialises in human resource management. She is an active researcher with a strong national and international publishing record in her field. Pauline currently works with a team of researchers exploring the links between people management and organisational performance in healthcare. She has previously worked in and with a variety of industries and organisations in both Australia and the UK in the public and private sectors. She has been a CEO of a community-based women's health service, an education and training consultant and has extensive experience in industrial relations and project management.

Sara Twohill completed a Bachelor of Social Science at the University of New South Wales in 2004 and was awarded first class honours in 2005. She has held research positions at Sydney West Area Health Service where she worked in the drug and alcohol area and more recently as a policy officer with the Commonwealth Government's national peak body on safety and quality, the Australian Council on Safety & Quality in Health Care.

Rebecca Warburton is Professor at the Michael Smith Foundation for Health Research and Scholar at the University of Victoria, British Columbia, Canada. She is a health economist and conducts research into the costs and benefits of patient safety and quality improvement initiatives at the Vancouver Island Health Authority. Her interests lie in the use of research evidence to inform public policy and improve the delivery of healthcare and other government services. She joined the University of Victoria's School of Public Administration in 1999, prior to which she worked for the British Columbia provincial government. Her government experience included two years at the Treasury Board and 13 years at the Ministry of Health, working in both policy and research positions.

Eileen Willis is an associate professor in the School of Medicine at Flinders University. Her research interests include the health professions and health sector work, industrial relations and the management of change. She has a particular interest in the impact of working time and the impact of healthcare reform on the management of caring work.

Reviewers

Laurie Grealish Dip Nurs, MNurs, Cert Oncology Nurs, Grad Dip Nurs Studies
Senior Lecturer, Discipline of Nursing, School of Health Sciences, University
of Canberra, ACT

Marilyn Orrock RN, RM, DNE, BA, MHA, FRCNA
Senior Lecturer, Health Services Administration, Faculty of Nursing and Midwifery,
University of Sydney, NSW

Maria Fedoruk Grad Cert Higher Ed, PhD, MHlthAdmin, Grad Dip Mgt, BSci,
Dip App Sci, RN, Crit Care Cert, JP
Lecturer, School of Nursing and Midwifery, Division of Health Sciences, University
of South Australia, SA

Lynne Slater RN, RM, Grad Dip HSc (PHC), MMs
Director, Clinical Education, School of Nursing and Midwifery, Faculty of Health,
University of Newcastle, NSW

PART 1

Setting the context

Health and healthcare are important not only to patients, clinicians, managers and policymakers, they are also important to governments who continually strive to improve the health of populations and the cost effectiveness of health services. In doing so, governments recognise the finite nature of resources and strive to balance investment in healthcare with investment in other equally deserving portfolio areas. But who decides where investment for health improvement should be made is a contested issue. In this part, we consider the environment within which governments attempt to improve the health of their populations, the pressures that are brought to bear and the ways in which these pressures are being managed.

Ensuring value for money is a concern for governments and for health service managers. Achieving value is not necessarily a straightforward task in complex and diverse settings such as health. Operations management techniques are a set of practices drawn from the manufacturing industry and applied in the public sector. They are an essential and important step forward in understanding and responding logically and rationally to managing complex systems, and their relevance to managing clinical processes is to find out what works and applying it. The uptake of operations management in health is in its infancy but there is potential to use its models and methods to transform the manner of healthcare delivery by systematising and standardising care, not just for individual patients, although this is important, but crucially for populations of patients with similar conditions as the demand for healthcare continues to rise. Pertinent questions here are: To what extent can generic tools and method from private sector manufacturing be applied to the public health sector; and, What types of changes are needed to adapt private sector models to the unique characteristics of public healthcare and to local health services?

Most investment in healthcare is in the healthcare workforce. Developing the skills to manage people is therefore an essential part of good health service management. Human resource management has been relatively neglected in the past, assumed to concern only bureaucratic administrative functions. But managing people is strategically important to patient outcomes, organisational outcomes and clinician wellbeing. What type of a strategic role can and should human resource management take in managing clinical processes?

In the chapters following we give a broad overview of the main elements of health sector reform and clinical process management, consider the models and methods for transforming health services and discuss the industrial relations climate within which health services operate.

Chapter 1

Managing clinical processes: objectives, evidence and context

Roslyn Sorensen & Rick Iedema

Introduction

Good health is important to individuals and to national economies (Suhrcke et al 2006). Without good health, economic prosperity and the wellbeing of individuals suffer. Consequently, health is an important responsibility for governments, and is often the biggest and most politically sensitive of portfolios, especially in countries where healthcare is predominantly publicly funded. Governments actively manage the main indicator of a population's health, health status, and their success in doing so is evident in their ranking on health outcome measures relative to their peers. To maintain their performance standing, governments must manage pressure on resources to balance the demands for healthcare with those of other portfolios, such as defence, education, and law and order. Making the best use of resources is therefore an important objective for all health systems.

The use of resources can be maximised by optimising the quality of care. Care provided in the right way the first time that produces expected outcomes will be less expensive than poor-quality care that has to be repeated. While the quality of care in most developed countries is good, it is not as good as it could be. Quality is being scrutinised and judged as deficient, based on findings that the level of adverse events in the health services of many developed countries is high. This is despite generally good health outcomes overall and patient satisfaction with the system. But optimising the quality of healthcare and maximising resource use, i.e. producing cost effective care, is difficult. Healthcare is complex: multiple caregivers from diverse backgrounds who are often geographically dispersed in independent services deliver a range of services that need to be coordinated. Healthcare is expensive: the rapidly advancing technologies of health are costly and the demand for them is potentially insatiable.

Hence, cost effectiveness will depend on how well those who manage health services and those who deliver them agree on the goals of care, understand the methods for their achievement and cooperate to do so.

Healthcare goals are generally not well integrated at either the policy or service level. Emphasising any single goal to the exclusion of others can be detrimental to achieving comprehensive health service outcomes. Policymakers commonly use budgeting and service downsizing to contain the cost of care; clinicians commonly call for more funding as the answer to quality problems. But containing costs without attention to other equally important goals may have unintended effects on quality and safety, and increasing funding without reference to available resources or accounting for those consumed may jeopardise service sustainability. Hence, the overriding aim for all health systems should be to achieve good quality care without risk to patient safety while maximising resource use. Achieving this aim will mean simultaneously managing the three main elements of healthcare, namely quality, risk and resources, at the point at which care is produced, that is, in health services. Doing so will mean moving beyond just managing the clinical particularities of individual patients or the organisational abstractions of performance targets, to redesigning systems so as to link these two ends coherently, productively and practically. To discuss how this can be done, this introductory chapter:

- outlines the objectives of managing clinical processes in health services
- provides evidence for the importance of managing seemingly conflicting objectives simultaneously
- discusses the context within which clinical process management takes place.

The objectives of managing clinical processes

The relationship between health outcomes and health services

Health status is an indicator of the state of a nation's health. Most OECD countries achieve similar levels of performance on key indicators of health status, particularly life expectancy (OECD 2005). Most countries seek to protect their ranking and actively manage this measure. However, while health status outcomes are impressive for non-Indigenous populations, those for Indigenous populations are often much lower (Bramley et al 2004) and the gap may be widening (Freemantle et al 2007). Table 1.1 below sets out selected indicators of performance on health status for selected peer countries. The data show overall performance and performance on specific life-expectancy measures for the four leading countries in 2004, compared with those of other selected OECD peers.

Health targets, such as health status measures, are important because, theoretically, they focus the system on the effectiveness as well as the efficiency of care. However, the extent to which health status outcomes are linked to health service effectiveness and efficiency is not clear. For instance, the proportion of funds spent on health is not necessarily an indicator of performance on health status outcomes. As an example, Japan has one of the lowest proportions of GDP spent on health (8% in 2003) but a high overall life expectancy (81.8 years), while the US spends a relatively high proportion of its GDP on health (15.2% in 2003) but has a lower overall life expectancy (77.5 years) (OECD 2006b). If health status outcomes are not necessarily linked to the size of health budgets, other factors must explain the difference. Knowing what factors 'produce' health and understanding how budgets are spent is therefore important in understanding such differences. But health reform policy and programs aimed at

Table 1.1 Overall performance – selected indicators, selected countries[1]

Performance statistics	Switzerland	Sweden	Spain	France	Australia	Canada	New Zealand
Overall performance of the health system[2]	1st	2nd	3rd	3rd	8th	13th	14th
Life expectancy at birth – males	77.2	77.15	76.1	75.6	76.6	76.7	75.7
Life expectancy at birth – females	82.8	82.1	83	83.1	82	82	80.0

Source: The Conference Board of Canada 2004

[1] The seven countries featured here were those featured in the Conference Board's report.
[2] Overall performance was determined by a benchmarking analysis using 24 indictors organised in three broad categories: health status (seven indicators), non-medical factors (seven indicators), and health outcomes (11 indicators). Health status included: life expectancy males/females, disability-free life expectancy males/females, self-reported health status, infant mortality rate, low birth weight; non-medical factors included: body weight, tobacco consumption, alcohol consumption, road traffic accidents, sulphur oxide emissions, immunization-DTP (diphtheria, tetanus and polio), immunization for influenza; health outcomes included: lung cancer mortality rates males/females, acute myocardial infarction mortality rates males/females, stroke mortality rates males/females, PYLL* due to suicide-males, PYLL due to lung cancer males/females, PYLL due to breast cancer.
*PYLL = potential years of life lost.

improving health service performance appear to be largely separated from the policies and programs that underpin health status outcomes. Busse & Wismar (2002) describe health targets as the 'forgotten corner', because of their separation from the main agenda of health services reform. A comparative study of national and regional health target programs among OECD peers, including the European Union, Australia, Canada, New Zealand and the US, showed that Australia alone linked health targets to health services performance (Busse & Wismar 2002).

Busse & Wismar offer a number of reasons for this separation. Firstly, the policies and programs that support health targets tend to be top-down and the involvement of the general public or their elected parliamentary officials is limited. This means that policy may not contain strategies to encourage grassroots alliances to mobilise health improvement activities in the community and in health services. Secondly, and consequently, there are few incentives for local and professional individuals and groups to be involved. This is important because getting the agreement and commitment of those who produce and co-produce health is a significant factor in improving health outcomes. Yet the evidence is clear that integrating community and professional groups in decisions that affect them is effective. Communities can make difficult decisions about prioritising health services in the face of scarce resources. This is evidenced by the Oregon experiment in the US that sought to involve communities in rationing decisions that took into account the health of vulnerable groups, and the New Zealand experience where professional groups assisted government to develop rationing criteria for elective surgery (Hadorn & Holmes 1997, Klein et al 1996). Importantly, Wiseman et al's Australian study found that the public overwhelmingly want their preferences to inform decisions about priority-setting and funding allocation (Wiseman et al 2003) (see Mooney, Chapter 13).

> **Pause for reflection**
>
> Communities can participate meaningfully in decisions about setting priorities and allocating resources in health, and community values can become a criterion for decision making. How might governments take community capacity and values into account?

For governments, a constant priority is managing the gap between the supply of health services and the demand for them. Governments tend to use the blunt levers of economic policy to contain costs to manage the gap, in preference to more organic processes that involve communities in such decisions. The European Union, Australia, New Zealand and Canada all use economic policy in this way, as do the US and Japan (Abel-Smith & Mossialos 1994, Fujii & Reich 1988, Malcolm 1990, Segal 1998, Dickey 1997, Byrne & Rathwell 2005). Economic policy is a useful lever for governments to manage health services, because it allows control over resource allocation at the macro level at which government decision makers operate. Moreover, the pressures on the health system are likely to continue, hence the pressures on governments to manage the gap between service supply and demand will also continue. Managing the resource consumption of health services will remain an important strategy to contain public spending on health to within manageable levels as populations in developed countries age, the demand for expensive advanced medical technology rises and consumer expectations about choice, access, quality and accountability increase.

Pressures on the health system

These pressures on the health system need to be taken into account when assessing how well they perform. Health service performance is affected by the rising cost of care, the increasing demand for services, the levels of risk to patient safety and the overall quality of care. Each of these pressures is discussed briefly in turn.

First, in terms of the rising cost of care, health services consume a sizable portion of a nation's resources. Table 1.2 below compares the total expenditure on health as a percentage of GDP (gross domestic product) for selected OECD peers from 1960 to 2004. The expenditure of these countries (Australia, Canada, New Zealand and the UK) is compared with that of countries with relatively low and high expenditure (Japan and the US respectively). The data show that for the six countries selected, all experienced substantial rises in the percentage of GDP spent on health over the 44-year period. National budgets are finite, and as health spending rises, the proportion of GDP spent in other areas of need reduces. Consequently, most governments actively manage their expenditure on health. The high level of public funding facilitates such

Table 1.2 Total expenditure on health – percentage of gross domestic product

Country Year	Australia	Canada	NZ	UK	Japan	US
1960	4.0	5.4	5.1 (1970)[3]	3.9	3.0	5.1
2004	9.6	9.9	8.4	8.3	8.0	15.3

Source: OECD 2006

---

[3] OECD data for New Zealand GDP spent on health began in 1970.

management, although countries such as the US experience more difficulty, presumably because of a dominant private sector (OECD 2006a) less amenable to centralised cost containment objectives.

Second, the demand for health services is rising, and is likely to continue to rise in line with the ageing of the population in developed countries. As an example, Figure 1.1 below shows the increase in admitted patients in Australian hospitals from 1998–99 to 2004–05.

Governments and health services must manage this increasing demand, and health resources must be rationed to manage it within allocated budgets. Reducing bed numbers and patients' lengths of stay are common strategies to contain costs within budget limits while maintaining patient throughput. Table 1.3 below shows data for seven selected countries, as in Table 1.1, for 2004 on three key indicators of efficiency, namely waiting times for health services, average lengths of stay and proportion of hospital beds per 1000 population. The data vary widely. Of the two countries with lower lengths of stay (Sweden and New Zealand) and bed ratios (Sweden), each experiences waiting times for rationed hospital services to contain the proportion of GDP spent on health: for Sweden to 9.1%; for New Zealand to 8.4% (OECD 2006b). The two countries that report no waiting times for hospital services (Switzerland and France) also have the highest proportion of beds, and in the case of Switzerland, the highest average length of stay. Thus, the trade-off for maintaining access to health services with no waiting times appears to be a higher proportion of GDP spent: for Switzerland 11.6% in 2004; for France 10.5% (OECD 2006b).

The extent to which reducing bed numbers is a sustainable strategy to manage throughput and cost emerges in Figure 1.2 overleaf. The data show that as an example the consistent reduction in bed numbers in Australia from 1998–99 to 2002–03 was not sustainable, with bed numbers rising again from 2003–04.

Third, risks to patient safety have become a priority for many health services in developed countries (see Warburton, Chapter 9 and Merry, Chapter 11). The methodology to quantify adverse events developed in the 1990s has revealed a pattern of patient risk

Figure 1.1 Expected demand for admitted patients: Australian hospitals 1998–99 to 2004–05

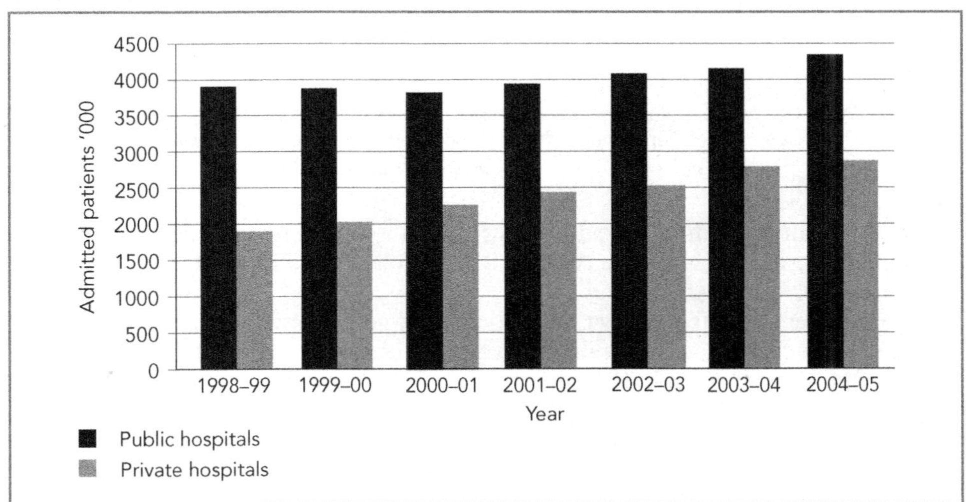

Source: Australian Government Department of Health and Ageing, *Australian Health Care Agreement* data reported by the states and territories

Table 1.3 Hospital performance – selected indicators, selected countries

Performance statistics	Switzerland	Sweden	Spain	France	Australia	Canada	New Zealand
Are there waiting times at hospitals for health services?	No	Yes	Yes	No	Yes	Yes	Yes
Average length of stay in hospital – days	9.2	5.0	7.5	5.5	6.2	7.2	3.3
Hospital beds/1000	3.9	2.4	3.2	8.4	3.8	3.2	6

Source: The Conference Board of Canada 2004

Figure 1.2 Bed numbers: Australian hospitals 1998–99 to 2004–05

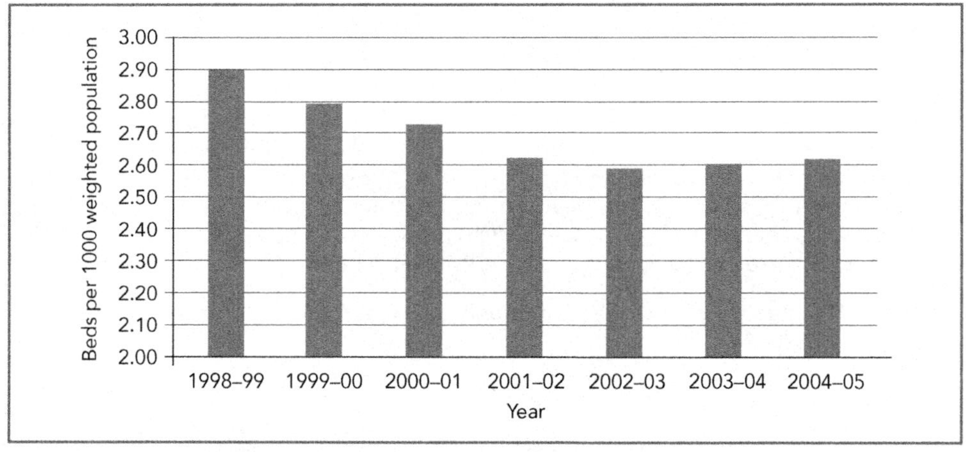

Source: Australian Institute of Health and Welfare (AIHW) 2004, *Australian Hospital Statistics 2002–03*; Australian Government Department of Health and Ageing, *Australian Health Care Agreement* data reported by the states and territories (2003–04, 2004–05)

associated with acute inpatient admissions within a relatively consistent range across selected countries for which data are available, from 7.5% in Canada to 17.7% in the US, as Table 1.4 shows.

Three issues arise from these data. First, a large majority of the adverse events reported caused significant disability or death and were considered highly preventable: 57% in the Australian study (Wilson et al 1995). Second, the cost of adverse events was high, estimated to be in excess of $800 million per annum, again in the Australian case. This represents a significant proportion of the health budget that potentially could be directed to meeting the supply–demand gap. Third, these figures raise questions about their cause, whether individual clinicians are at fault, or inadequate systems. This issue is important when decisions about health service priorities and funding for improvements are being considered.

Table 1.4 Levels of adverse events associated with hospital admissions[4]

Country	Percentage of admissions associated with an adverse event	Focus of study
Australia	16.6	Acute hospital admissions
United States	17.7	Acute hospital admissions
United Kingdom	10.0	Emergency department
Canada	7.5	Acute hospital admissions
New Zealand	12.9	Acute hospital admissions
Denmark	9.0	Acute hospital admissions

Sources: Baker et al 2004, Andrews et al 1997, Davis et al 2001, Vincent et al 2001, Wilson et al 1995, Schioler et al 2001

[4] Similar protocols were used so that comparisons can be made across studies (Baker et al 2004).

Errors occur in all health and hospital services and must be managed as routine. For instance, Cullen compared adverse drug events in ICUs with events in non-ICUs (Cullen et al 1997) and when adjusted for volume, the rates were found to be comparable. This study is significant, because it revealed that preventable and potential adverse drug events occurred in units that functioned normally, involving caregivers working under reasonably normal circumstances and not necessarily or not only in units at the extremes of workload and stress, such as ICUs. Cullen's estimate of cost of between $5.6 and $2.8 million in a 700-bed teaching hospital suggests that eliminating error is not only good for patients, it is also good for budgets.

In addressing the issue of cause, Baker et al believes that poorly designed systems are at fault. This view notwithstanding

> [H]ealth care organisations have historically focused on identifying and disciplining clinicians who were closest to incidents. However, experts suggest that the greatest gains in improving patient safety will come from modifying the work environment of healthcare professionals, creating better defences for averting adverse events and mitigating their effects.

(Baker et al 2004:1678)

The implications of this for managing clinical processes arise in terms of the types of solutions devised to address adverse events, and whether they should focus on improving the skills and competencies of individual clinicians, or rectifying underlying systems problems.

Fourth, the overall quality of health services has concerned policymakers, health service managers, clinicians and patients, and it had done so well before the high levels of adverse events came to light. The problems with quality are serious and extensive. Chassin (1998) maintains that they arise from treatment underuse (failure to provide a treatment when needed), overuse (when harm exceeds the benefit of a treatment) and misuse (when complications occur from the treatment). He maintains that the need for rapid change in health services is urgent because

> [O]ur present efforts resemble a team of engineers trying to break the sound barrier by tinkering with a Model T Ford. We need a new vehicle or, perhaps, many new vehicles.

(Chassin 1998:1005)

Strategies to improve performance

Policymakers and health service managers have generally responded to the problems in overall quality with broad quality improvement programs such as continuous quality improvement (CQI). Just how effective such programs are is uncertain, because of a paucity of evaluation. Some clinicians believe that the quality of care has actually deteriorated in the countries where they have been implemented (Ferlie & Shortell 2001). A possible reason for this is that the broad scope of programs is too ambitious as they attempt to cover the myriad systems that appear to impact on quality. Thus, the links between cause and effect have been difficult to establish. What these programs do reveal is further evidence of wide variations in the processes and outcomes of care in technologically advanced systems.

Ferlie & Shortell (2001) suggest that organisation-wide quality improvement programs may serve a ritualistic purpose – as a habitual response to the institutional demands of accreditation and government bodies. The programs are criticised because they often lack a consistent external driver, adequate information systems, clinician involvement and senior management leadership and support. Further, the difficulty of adapting private sector principles and practices (on which such programs are generally based) in the public health sector raises questions about their appropriateness. What these criticisms illustrate is that the particular environment of public health services is a critical factor in trying to change them, and that the underlying and more conventional and circumscribed ways of organisational working are influential. Concepts such as 'the learning organisation' have become popular in fostering attitude change and in initiating skills and practices to generate and manage knowledge around attributes such as culture, leadership, teamwork, communication and technology. Yet despite repeated recommendations that urgent attention be given to these underlying system connections, comprehensive action has yet to occur (Hindle et al 2006).

Efforts to remake these connections to improve quality are often hampered by a lack of clinically relevant information. Central administrators favour tools such as business process reengineering, lean thinking, six sigma,[5] root cause analysis and statistical process control. But when applied from the corporate level of the organisation, these tools can fail to provide meaningful information to operational clinicians and managers. Applying such tools in the public sector in the same way as they are applied in the private sector will not necessarily achieve expected results, especially if management commitment is not sustained, expectations are unrealistic or change is resisted in the workplace (Vakola 2000). Expectations, for instance, that '(t)he fundamental rethinking and radical redesign of business processes (will) … achieve dramatic improvements in critical, contemporary measures of performance, such as cost, quality, service and speed' (Hammer & Champy 1993:32) suggest that a fashion is being followed rather than a sustainable strategy being adopted to address the difficult, complex, and *different*, problems in the public health sector.

---

[5] Six sigma is one of a number of performance improvement tools. Chassin (1998) defines it as 'a statistical measure of variation... (A)dopting the goal of Six Sigma quality means setting tolerance limits for defective products at such high levels that fewer than 3.4 defects occur per million units (or opportunities)' (Chassin 1998:566).

Nonetheless, the type of tools described above could potentially produce clinically relevant data for decision making if applied at clinical unit level. An example is developing and prioritising workplace strategies to detect errors and prevent adverse events.In this respect, while the systems origin of error is largely accepted, there is contention about where the responsibility for remedy should lie. Clinical governance policies place the main responsibility for practice change on clinicians, particularly doctors, but the voluntary uptake of clinical governance initiatives means they are variable and sporadic. Initiatives such as clinical incident monitoring do appear to have positively influenced clinicians' critical reflection about their performance and practice, albeit in isolated pockets (Iedema et al 2006a), but as presently structured, clinical governance policies are not sufficient to comprehensively implement formal systems to routinely monitor performance in clinical workplaces and to integrate performance across the organisation. While this may suggest that the immediate responsibility for implementing risk management strategies should lie with hospital managers, the task is well beyond the capacities and resources of individual hospitals and of individual hospital managers.

Pause for reflection

Clinically relevant data is essential to providing clinicians and clinical managers with meaningful information with which to identify problems and generate workable solutions. How should this data be produced, who should do it and how can it be applied?

Yet managerial strategies to improve clinical performance are common in public health services – think of efficiency, downsizing, performance indicators, clinical targets and practice reform guidelines. These strategies have an advantage in shifting the focus of change to the health service itself, although centrally managed health service objectives can have unforeseen consequences. One critique is indicator proliferation. In the case of the UK National Health Service (NHS), indicators of performance on which managers were required to report rose to 2500 in 1989 (Carter et al 1995). Centralising health service management to this degree is neither feasible nor desirable, nor is it a coherent, constructive or sustainable strategy. The NHS, for example,

> … is a confusing ant heap of frenetic, but frequently uncoordinated sets of unrelated activities, which somehow add up to the delivery of healthcare to the entire population. Not only is it the largest organisation in Britain; it is the only one whose services are used by almost every woman, man and child every year (with) … about 250 million contacts annually between the NHS and consumers.

(Carter et al 1995:102)

Such centralised objective setting and performance management is not popular with clinicians or with health service managers. In the view of clinicians, instrumental top-down management methods have contributed to the erosion of quality of care and public confidence in the system (Hornick et al 1997). In the view of managers, health service delivery is over-administered and under-managed (Hunter 1996). Neither clinicians nor managers have faith in the application of market-based private sector principles to public sector problems. Where objectives are in conflict or contradictory, bottom-up strategies may be more suitable to manage problems and implement realistic solutions. Top-down strategies that seek to separately micromanage single performance goals are unlikely to make a significant impact on the type of health system activity that Carter et al describe above. Rather, organic strategies are more likely to work if developed

> **Pause for reflection**
>
> Organically derived performance improvement strategies and associated performance indicators are needed to drive change from the bottom up, and capable of being incorporated within a comprehensive framework of service planning and performance evaluation. How might this occur?

incrementally, are grounded in the social reality of clinical care, involve frontline staff in their design and implementation, and are capable of being incorporated within a comprehensive framework of service planning and performance evaluation.

Planning and evaluation frameworks are important to bring a sense of purpose and cohesion to complex systems, especially when they are in rapid transformation. Ideally, centrally developed frameworks would be limited to setting broad objectives and performance targets for national priorities (Ham 2005). Deciding on the particular strategies through which to implement these broad national targets should lie with health organisations themselves. Hence, decentralising decision making assumes a shift of power away from over-centralised strategies and micromanaged problems to more autonomous health services to tailor performance improvement strategies to local need, local conditions and local cultures.

> Only in this way will the enterprise of managers and clinicians at the local level be released to deliver the further improvements in performances set out in (a) new planning framework.
>
> (Ham 2005:107)

Thus, improvement is more likely to occur from knowing how clinical work is done and managing the clinical processes through which healthcare is evidence based and planned, organised, evaluated and managed by multidisciplinary teams around high-demand, high-cost, high-risk clinical treatments, than from generic, derivative, instrumental approaches. This will be the case especially if those who make the decisions about clinical treatment and hence resource use, namely clinicians and clinical managers, have the knowledge, resources, skills, enthusiasm and organisational authority to do so. As demand and resource containment intensifies in the public health sector, so too will pressure on clinicians and clinical work. This will further intensify with concerns about unsafe practices and inadequate systems. Thus, understanding the detail of clinical work and clinical systems is doubly critical to managing it. Yet the focus on managing inputs remains strong at the central policy level even though central scrutiny and surveillance has not significantly improved service access, cost, risk and quality.

Evidence for managing clinical processes

The technical dimension of clinical work is the one most often targeted for performance improvement. There is a view that implementing technically best practice models of care will reduce practice variations and eliminate unanticipated outcomes. It is generally not well recognised that this technical element is just one factor among others in successful organisational change (Iedema et al 2006b). Social factors also affect the way people relate to each other and communicate to produce complex and diverse care that is delivered by myriad clinicians in geographically dispersed locations (Muir Gray 1997). Hence, the social dimension of managing clinical work is emerging as an important element in organisational change (Harteloh 2003). However, social factors are not routinely included in change programs, especially in organisations where scientific paradigms dominate. Similarly, organisational factors that affect what is done, by whom, when, in what sequence, with what outcomes and purpose are also often neglected.

> **Box 1.1** Implications for practice – Setting the objectives of healthcare
>
> A framework of health system objectives and health service performance is essential to prioritise improvement strategies, to coordinate and align actions and to evaluate outcomes. Who should set objectives and monitor performance and how can policy development be dynamically linked with strategy implementation?
>
> Pressures on health services come from the rising cost of care, the increasing demand for services and consumer expectations of quality. If good health outcomes are important to individual people and national economies, how can the focus of performance be redirected from managing costs to managing cost effectiveness?
>
> Cost effectiveness means managing quality, risk and resource use simultaneously. How can these three elements unite within a comprehensive method of clinical process management and how will the connections be made between those who make health policy, those who organise health services, those who deliver them and those who consume them?

Awareness of the significant variations in technical care across practitioners has brought forth a plethora of guidelines that enunciate and promote evidence. The range of guidelines developed in the diverse areas of medical, nursing and allied health attests to the potential of guidelines to improve quality, outcomes, service and resource use in a wide range of clinical conditions (see Claridge & Cook, Chapter 4 and Berding, Resources). The technical importance of guidelines has been well established to the point that guideline proliferation has become a problem. Our intention is not to go over this well-trodden ground but to consider how guidelines can be implemented and whether their use can be sustained. While technical–rational knowledge is essential in acquiring and appropriately applying clinical practice skills, it is just one facet of clinical practice improvement. Achieving evidence-based practice is a multifaceted endeavour that includes social, organisational and technical factors (Grol 2001).

> **Pause for reflection**
>
> Improving health service performance comprises technical, social and organisational factors integrated within a comprehensive strategy of organisational change. Why is this so?

In the case of guidelines for acute coronary syndrome (ACS) boxed below, implementing evidence-based models of practice requires not only technical skills, but also political, social and organisational ones (Gibler et al 2005).

Gibler (2005) identifies the predictors of successful guideline implementation as being strong clinical champions who have the necessary communication skills to influence others and a general willingness to collaborate. This implies that forging collaborative and collective approaches to managing care for populations of patients among clinicians socialised within traditional, individualistic professional cultures is a precondition to achieving the technical objectives of care. It appears that the scepticism of unprepared senior clinicians can alienate others and discourage their participation in improvement activities. Thus the social dimension of change is critical

… because organizations are composed of people who react or fail to react to perceived changes in the environment [;] it is the activities of people that determine how organizations become structured.

(Barley & Kunda 2001:79)

> **Box 1.2** Case study – Barriers to guideline implementation
>
> *Practical implementation of the guidelines for unstable angina/non–ST-segment elevation myocardial infarction in the emergency department*
>
> A variety of barriers to guideline implementation are experienced in the emergency setting. Delays in receiving cardiac biomarker data because of slow laboratory turnaround, high patient volume in the ED (emergency department), decreasing throughput, and a lack of standardised diagnostic and treatment approaches are only some of the barriers that can inhibit providing appropriate care to patients. Specialties other than cardiology provide inpatient care to individuals with ACS. Making all physicians who care for these patients aware of the 2002 ACC/AHA UA/NSTEMI guidelines is a significant challenge in any hospital setting. Finally, multiple cardiology groups at an institution can make an agreement on specific diagnostic and treatment regimens for patients with ACS difficult to achieve.
>
> Source: Gibler et al 2005[6]

[6]Source: Circulation 111:2699-2710 doi: 10.1161/01.CIR.0000165556.44271.BE

Thus, collaboration and cooperation is the key to the way clinical work is done in health, specifically between doctors and nurses, clinicians and managers, and with patients and their families. But such collaboration is fraught with difficulty. People hold different perceptions about the meaning of collaboration and the extent to which it actually exists. Doctors report high levels of collaboration with nurses and other doctors; nurses report lower levels of collaboration than do doctors (Surgenor et al 2003). Further, nurses, and patients, are often excluded from participating in care planning and decision making that affects them (Bryan-Brown & Dracup 2002). An associated difficulty is the effect of cost containment policies on nursing numbers and the loss of morale, enthusiasm, corporate knowledge and organisational cohesion that this entails (Finlayson et al 2002). Moreover, collaboration between medical sub-specialists about patient care cannot be assumed (Sorensen & Iedema 2006) and the multidisciplinary treatment of patients within clinical units and the flow of patients between clinical units is often sub-optimal (McQuillan et al 1998).

Pause for reflection

Collaborating to achieve good patient care is based on values such as being an inclusive team member, pooling information and sharing decision making. What types of social skills will clinicians and managers require to become good team members?

The social capacity of clinicians and managers to communicate effectively is important to the organisation of care, specifically in generating, integrating and managing knowledge within and between clinical workplaces, between clinical and managerial domains and between different healthcare sectors. Assumptions are often made that clinicians and managers know what to do and how to do it. This is not always the case (Iedema et al 2004).

To illustrate this point, consider Table 1.5 below, which presents research findings from 12 acute clinical settings and details the number of multidisciplinary clinical caregivers who treated patients undergoing an elective caesarean section, a relatively routine procedure (Sorensen et al 2003). The data show that in a random sample of patients (between 32 and 46 patients across settings), the average number of clinicians caring for

Table 1.5 Frequency of clinician involvement with and location of patient sample

| Setting | Patients | No. of wards | Nursing | | Medicine | | Allied health | | Total setting | Total over 10 patients |
			Nurses	No. of nurses over 10 patients	Doctors	No. of doctors over 10 patients	Allied health	No. of AH over 10 patients		
1	35	4	165	6	75	5	2	0	242	11
2	46	5	160	13	67	8	6	2	233	23
3	43	3	148	3	50	8	8	0	206	11
4	43	6	177	4	74	8	5	1	256	13
5	41	10	219	6	92	2	14	3	325	11
6	39	3	161	13	80	5	25	0	266	18
7	39	2	124	5	54	9	8	1	186	15
8	38	1	146	15	46	8	13	0	205	23
9	42	4	178	14	63	7	4	0	245	21
10	32	4	196	2	108	3	3	0	307	5
11	38	2	160	25	80	7	1	0	241	32
12	38	4	221	8	73	13	11	1	305	22
Total	474	50	2055	114	862	83	100	8	3017	205

Source: Sorensen et al 2003

these patients ranged from 4.3 to 9.6. Of these, only 6.8% treated more than 10 patients in each setting, and patients were located in as many as 10 different wards. These findings suggest that bed management policies do not mandate the collocation of patients with similar conditions and that multiple caregivers with varying levels of knowledge, skills, confidence and expertise deliver and manage patient care. Hence, ward-based clinicians may be relatively inexperienced in managing the wide mix of patient care needs that confront them, including relatively routine treatment as well as complex care.

These data further suggest that caregivers manage patient care across differences in knowledge, experience, time and space. To overcome such differences clinical pathways are being promoted as a means to limit clinical complexity (Hindle & Yazbeck 2005), although their use is not without problems. Little research has been done into the links between pathways, patient outcomes and resource use (Dy et al 2006); they are often perceived as limiting or prejudicing medical autonomy (Hindle & Yazbeck 2005) and often regarded by clinicians as little more than a management efficiency tool (Sorensen et al 2003). Clearly, not all care can be systematised and standardised in pathways (Lillrank & Liukko 2004). Some patients will need to be case managed, especially where extensive comorbidities exist and the services they require are complex and exceptional. Managing clinical processes therefore will mean identifying the conditions and procedures that lend themselves to systematisation and standardisation, and those that do not, and flexibly managing patient care needs.

> **Box 1.3** Implications for practice – Managing clinical processes
>
> High-demand, high-risk, high-cost treatments should be planned, organised and evaluated around evidence of what works; diverse multidisciplinary geographically dispersed clinicians must collaborate to standardise routine treatment for patient populations and to tailor care for individual patients with complex needs. How can health services transform to manage these two modes of patient care in parallel?
>
> The expectations of clinicians and managers must be reoriented to recognise and accept that clinical work is delivered and managed by teams of multidisciplinary clinicians who collaborate to co-produce healthcare. How might this reorientation occur in professions that seek to guard their autonomy?
>
> Social and organisational skills are needed to deliver and manage routine and complex healthcare between multiple caregivers from diverse disciplines located in dispersed, independent services. What characterises the relationships between those who provide care and those who manage it, and the environments that support clinical process management?

The context of clinical process management

Health organisations are complex entities and the detail of how they work is not well understood. Management texts often conceptualise organisations as amalgams of generic elements and this tendency reinforces a view that studying the detail of work is not necessary to understanding organisational effectiveness. In this event, organisational change is hampered by a lack of knowledge about how work is done and who does it. Studies of work tend to be ignored or marginalised, even though work and organising

> … are bound in dynamic tension because organizational structures are, by definition, descriptions of and templates for ongoing patterns of action.

(Barley & Kunda 2001:76)

Thus, top-down management strategies can have far-reaching and unintended effects, particularly if they remain uninformed about local practice. By imposing new organisational structures

> … the patterns of work are invariably altered, and there is a risk that when the nature of work changes, for example because of technologies, the organizational structures either adapt or become misaligned with the activities they organise.

(Barley & Kunda 2001:76)

> **Pause for reflection**
>
> Uninformed organisational restructures can fail to produce expected efficiency gains and can add to the stress and chaos of clinical work. How can this be overcome?

However, resources are finite, patient safety is a concern, and healthcare services must respond to these realities to remain efficient and effective. Improving the way care is managed in large organisations can be overwhelming for both clinicians and managers. Thus, understanding the context in which clinical practice improvement takes place will aid the process, specifically understanding the real and complex world of clinical decision making and the difficult and uncertain conditions within which many clinical decisions are made. Yet, in the case of healthcare, clinical practice improvement must also take into account the limited amount of care that is evidence based. For instance,

> (a)ccepting that the 'dominant medical paradigm of scientific truth and certainty' is to a large extent a fiction, or at best an exaggeration, has profound implications for the way in which we think about the management of scarce resources.
>
> (Klein et al 1996:93)

Hence, understanding the limits of existing approaches to researching and improving care and focusing our attention on the details of the clinical work to see what solutions can be derived ground-up will help shift healthcare from being constituted by cultures of top-down management and measurement, to cultures of participation and self-directed learning. Incompetence and unsafe practices cannot be condoned, and the capacity of individual clinicians to do their job will always be paramount in service effectiveness. However, the ability of health services as a system to provide a safe environment is also at issue. Inadequate systems of care exist within units, between units, within healthcare teams and between clinical and management domains. Within units, medical clinicians can be faced with daunting decisions often taken within a context of uncertainty and experimentation (Harvey 1996); between units, the lack of routine structured processes to coordinate patient planning, transfer and treatment is an impediment to effectiveness (McQuillan et al 1998). However, the strategies that clinicians devise and promote (Wachter 1999) to cut through the conflict, complexity and inadequacy of modern modes of acute healthcare delivery may be limited, specifically if they miss the very deep-seated structural, personal, professional and cultural problems that exist.

Pause for reflection

Quick-fix solutions, devised and promoted by consultant gurus, central managers or clinicians will fail if they do not address and actively manage the very deep-seated structural, personal, professional and cultural problems that exist in public healthcare. How might these problems be otherwise overcome?

The environment in which healthcare is delivered is changing rapidly. Environmental factors affect not only the context in which clinicians and managers work, but also the way they work, and the way they work together. Changes in social and demographic trends, a rise in chronic diseases and increasing consumer expectations are leading to a demand for evidence-based and patient-focussed healthcare in both hospitals and the community. The skills and responsibilities of caregiving groups is changing accordingly, and the traditional map of the healthcare professions may not align with a reorganising workforce (Barley & Kunda 2001). Hence, the pressures to reconfigure clinical care will intensify as each occupational group tries to justify its place in the healthcare team and in the healthcare environment. These workforce pressures will further intensify with the shift in employment patterns from 'tight' to 'loose' coupling, increasing contract employment and outsourcing, the rapidly changing technological environment that includes computerisation, expectations of service transparency and accountability, the shift of clinical work organisation from individual clinicians to multidisciplinary teams and the recognition that healthcare is a collective and social process. Hence, organisational change necessitates not just good clinical skills, but also good social skills, a high level of awareness of oneself and of others, and a knowledge of how healthcare organisations actually work.

Traditional skills will not be sufficient in this new system. Boundary crossing, teamwork, knowledge management and collaboration will be de rigueur. New competencies will initiate changes in recruitment, skill mix and gender divisions; resource allocation will acknowledge the changing patterns of disease and illness from acute to long-term chronic conditions and from cure to prevention; and advanced health technologies will alter the way work is conceived of and executed. Within this new system different mindsets will be needed to reorient a managerial emphasis from a preoccupation with resources and costs, to health outcomes and patient satisfaction. New processes are needed through which the expertise and values of clinicians can be heard, acknowledged and incorporated with those of managers, policymakers and consumers. The language of healthcare must likewise evolve to describe, negotiate and organise the complex and rapidly changing environment of this new system. In this way new approaches are emerging to reshape the way work is organised and managed and the words used to describe it.

> **Box 1.4** Implications for practice – The changing context of healthcare
>
> How might studies of work be used to reorient and redesign systems to align with the changing objectives and expectations of healthcare? Who should undertake these studies? Who should initiate and participate in systems redesign?
>
> What are the characteristics of environments that will be receptive to and supportive of the shift from cultures of blame to cultures of learning in which both active and latent errors can be admitted, explored and rectified?
>
> What types of new processes will ensure that people with appropriate skills are available and employed to meet changing needs and what competencies will enable them to cross boundaries, work in teams and collaborate in a transformed health system?

Conclusion

The emphasis of health service management on the clinical care of individual patients and on meeting corporate performance targets is not sufficient to manage modern expensive, complex, dispersed and diverse healthcare. Between these two ends, healthcare occurs as a complex collection of services delivered by myriad caregivers, many of whom practice individually and autonomously. Understanding what healthcare entails and how to manage it is an emerging field of study and practice, demanding a new set of knowledge, attitudes, practices and values. This book is pitched at developing this understanding, so that clinicians, managers and policymakers can engage with the technical, social and organisational implications of producing cost effective healthcare. This will mean learning to simultaneously manage the increasing demand for health services, containing their costs, managing their risks and improving their quality.

The pressures on the health system and on health services to improve health outcomes are likely to increase and responding to them meaningfully is essential to ensure that health services are sustainable and the wellbeing of those who work in them is maintained. New skills and new roles are needed to reorient priorities and to redesign systems to connect the quality of individual patient care with organisational effectiveness coherently, productively and practically. Equally, new ways of researching health services are needed to illuminate the specifics of clinical work, and to use that knowledge for the redesign of services (Iedema & Jorm forthcoming). Developing such new knowledge, skills and motivation to design and manage clinical processes in the health services is central to this endeavour.

References

Abel-Smith B, Mossialos E 1994 Cost containment and health reform: a study of the European Union. Health Policy 28:89–132

Andrews L B, Stocking C, Krizek T 1997 An alternative strategy for studying adverse events in medical care. Lancet 349(9048):309–313

Baker G R, Norton P G, Flintoft V et al 2004 The Canadian Adverse Events Study: The incidence of adverse events among hospital patients in Canada. CMAJ, 170(11):1678–1686

Barley S R, Kunda G 2001 Bringing Work Back In. Organization Science 12:76–95

Bramley D, Hebert P, Jackson R et al 2004 Indigenous disparities in disease-specific mortality, a cross-country comparison: New Zealand, Australia, Canada, and the United States. The New Zealand Medical Journal 117:1215–1231

Brennan T A, Leape L L, Laird N 1991 Incidence of adverse events and negligence in hospitalised patients: Results of the Harvard Medical Practice study. New England Journal of Medicine 324:377–384

Bryan-Brown C W, Dracup K 2002 Keeping the turf (wars) trimmed. American Journal of Critical Care 11:408–410

Busse R, Wismar M 2002 Health target programmes and healthcare services – any link? A conceptual and comparative study (Part 1). Health Policy 59:209–221

Byrne J M, Rathwell R 2005 Medical savings accounts and the Canada health act: complimentary or contradictory? Health Policy 72:367–379

Carter N, Klein R, Day P 1995 How organisations measure success. Routledge, London

Chassin M R 1998 The urgent need to improve quality. JAMA 280:1000–1005

Cullen D J, Sweitzer B J, Bates D W et al 1997 Preventable adverse drug events in hospitalized patients: A comparative study of intensive care and general care units. Critical Care Medicine 25:1289–1297

Davis P, Lay-Yee R, Briant R et al 2001 Adverse events in New Zealand public hospitals: Principal findings from a national survey. NZ Ministry of Health, Wellington

Dickey B 1997 Assessing cost and utilization in managed mental healthcare in the United States. Health Policy 41:S163–S174

Dy S, Garg P, Nyberg D et al 2006 Critical pathway effectiveness: Assessing the impact of patient, hospital care and pathway characteristics using qualitative comparative analysis. Health Services Research 40:499–507

Ferlie E, Shortell S 2001 Improving the Quality of Healthcare in the United Kingdom and the United States: A Framework for Change. Milbank Quarterly 79:281–315

Finlayson B, Dixon J, Meadows S et al 2002 Mind the gap: the extent of the NHS nursing shortage. British Medical Journal 325:538–541

Freemantle J, Officer K, McCullay D et al 2007 Australian Indigenous Health – Within an International Context. Darwin, NT, Cooperative Research Centre for Aboriginal Health

Fujii M, Reich M 1988 Rising medical costs and the reform of Japan's health insurance system. Health Policy 9:9–24

Gibler W, Cannon C, Blomkalns A et al 2005 Practical Implementation of the Guidelines for Unstable Angina/Non-ST–Segment Elevation Myocardial Infarction in the Emergency Department. Circulation 111:2699–2710

Grol R 2001 Successes and Failures in the Implementation of Evidence-Based Guidelines for Clinical Practice. Medical Care 39:S46–S54

Hadorn D, Holmes A 1997 The New Zealand priority criteria project, Part 1: Overview. British Medical Journal 314:131–134

Ham C 2005 From targets to standards: but not just yet. British Medical Journal 330:106–107

Hammer M, Champy J 1993 Reengineering the Corporation. Harper Business, New York

Harteloh P 2003 Quality systems in healthcare: a sociotechnical approach. Health Policy 64:391–398

Harvey J 1996 Achieving the indeterminate: accomplishing degrees of certainty in life and death situations. The Sociological Review 44:78–98

Hindle D, Braithwaite J, Travaglia J et al 2006 Patient Safety: a comparative of eight inquiries in six countries. Centre for Clinical Governance Research in Health, Sydney

Hindle D, Yazbeck A-M 2005 Clinical pathways in 17 European Union countries: a purposive survey. Australian Health Review 29:94–104

Hornick P, Hornick C, Taylor K et al 1997 Should business management training be part of medical education? Annals of Royal College of Surgical Eng (supp) 79:200–201

Hunter D J 1996 The changing roles of healthcare personnel in health and healthcare management. Social Science & Medicine 43:799–808

Iedema R, Jorm C, Long D et al 2006a Turning the medical gaze in upon itself: Root cause analysis and the investigation of clinical error. Social Science & Medicine 62:1605–1615

Iedema R, Long D, Forsyth R et al 2006b Visibilizing clinical work: Video ethnography in the contemporary hospital. Health Sociology Review 15:156–168

Iedema R, Degeling P, Braithwaite J et al 2004 It's an Interesting Conversation I'm Hearing: The Doctor as Manager. Organization Studies 25:15–34

Iedema R, Jorm C forthcoming. Researching Patient Safety and Intervening in Clinical Practice: Interventionist Research as Social Entanglement. In: Patient Safety: critical perspectives. Waring J, Finn R, Rowley E (eds) Cornell University Press, Ithaca, New York

Klein R, Day P, Redmayne S 1996 Managing scarcity: priority setting and rationing in the National Health Service. In: Ham C (ed) State of Health Series. Buckingham. Open University Press, UK

Lillrank P, Liukko M 2004 Standard, routine and non-routine processes in health care. International Journal of Health Care Quality Assurance 17:39–46

Malcolm L 1990 Service management: New Zealand's model of resource management. Health Policy 16:255–263

McQuillan P, Pilkinton S, Allan A, Taylor B, Short A, Mortan G, Nielsen M, Barrett D, Smith G 1998 Confidential inquiry into quality of care before admission to intensive care. British Medical Journal 316:1853–1858

Muir Gray J A 1997 Evidence-Based Healthcare. Churchill Livingstone, Edinburgh

OECD 2005 Health at a Glance – OECD Indicators 2005

OECD 2006a OECD Health Data 2006 – statistics and indicators for 30 countries

OECD 2006b OECD Health Data 2006 – Frequently Requested Data

Schioler T, Lipczah J H, Pedersen B L et al 2001 Danish Adverse Event Study. Ugeskr Laeger 163(39):5370–78

Segal L 1998 The importance of patient empowerment in health systems reform. Health Policy 44:31–44

Sorensen R, Iedema R 2008 Redefining accountability: managing the plurality of medical interests in end-of-life care. Health: An Interdisciplinary Journal for the Social Study of Health, Illness and Medicine 12(1): doi.org/10.1177/1363459307083699

Sorensen R, Maxwell S, Coyle B et al 2003 Systematising care in Elective Caesarian section – controlling costs or quality? Centre for Clinical Governance Research: The University of New South Wales, Sydney

Suhrcke M, McKee M, Stuckler D et al 2006 The contribution of health to the economy in the European Union. Public Health 120:994–1001

Surgenor S D, Bilike G T, Corwin H W 2003 Teamwork and collaboration in critical care; Lessons from the cockpit. Critical Care Medicine 31:992–993

The Conference Board of Canada 2004 Challenging healthcare system sustainability. Understanding health system performance of leading countries, Ottawa

Vakola M 2000 Exploring the relationship between the use of evaluation in business process re-engineering and organisational learning and innovation. Journal of Management Development 19:812–835

Vincent C, Neale G, Woloshynowych M 2001 Adverse events in British hospitals: preliminary retrospective record review. British Medical Journal 322:517–519

Wachter R M 1999 An introduction to the hospitalist model. Annals of Internal Medicine 130:338–342

Wilson R, Runciman W, Gibberd R et al 1995 The Quality in Australian Healthcare Study. The Medical Journal of Australia 163:458–471

Wiseman V, Mooney G, Berry G et al 2003 Involving the general public in priority setting: experiences from Australia. Social Science & Medicine 56:1001–1012

Operations management: the search for value in healthcare organisation and performance

Sandra Leggat

Introduction

> If corporations have glass ceilings, then hospitals have concrete floors. What happens above in the general management seems awfully disconnected – in activity if not quite in consequences – from what happens below in clinical operations.
>
> (Mintzberg 2002:197)

In most organisations a set of activities creates value by transforming inputs into outputs. The outputs are products or services. Operations management, broadly defined as the planning, management and control of these activities ('the operations'), is a fundamental component of management practice. Operations research, management science or industrial engineering apply mathematical or statistical models to operating issues to guide management practice and improve operations. In many industries operations management has been key to productivity and quality improvements.

Effective management of clinical care processes, which are the fundamental operations of a healthcare organisation, is essential for a well-functioning healthcare system. Yet it is only recently that the healthcare sector has recognised the relevance of operations management. Well-established operations management approaches, such as six sigma; lean thinking; root cause analysis; failure mode and effect analysis; queuing theory; modelling and simulation; and supply chain logistics, have become recent additions to the health services management repertoire (see Warburton, Chapter 9).

This chapter provides the context for taking up operations management in managing clinical processes in healthcare. 'Traditional' clinical and managerial processes have been accepted as the basis for healthcare service planning, delivery and evaluation. But, as outlined in Chapter 1, healthcare systems throughout the world are experiencing pressure to change – consumer influence, competition, changes in public policy, and advances in technology and clinical practice require review of traditional processes. Effective clinical process management requires understanding of those variables that have the power to significantly improve healthcare processes, and ultimately the performance of the healthcare system. This chapter explores the reasons why process management is difficult in healthcare and suggests future directions to improve clinical care processes.

Operations management – a sound management discipline

Operations management originated with the industrial revolution in the 1700s. Up until this time consumers received their products and services from individual crafts-people. While the individual form of craft production is still evident today, the industrial revolution facilitated the widespread production of consumer goods. This mass production was based on inventions ranging from the division of labour, Eli Whitney's introduction of standardised parts in 1790, the principles of scientific management and the invention of the computer, which allowed complex analysis and modelling. These foundations of mass production enabled significant savings through economies of scale, largely achieved through standardising tasks to shorten production time and reduce variation and human error.

Unfortunately mass production also created problems in defining, measuring and ensuring quality. No longer was one craftsperson accountable for, and in control of, the product quality throughout the production process. Early approaches to quality control focused on finding defects and removing them at the end of the production process. As knowledge of production processes improved, scholars suggested that this inspection-based approach could be replaced with error prevention. In the early 1920s statistical process control was introduced to manufacturing processes to reduce errors. W Edward Deming used statistical process control and his knowledge of management to improve production in the US during World War II, and then introduced statistical control to Japanese manufacturers. Joseph Juran added a human dimension to quality control, suggesting the need for managers to be trained in quality methods. This requirement of training was not accepted in the US and Juran became known for his success in improving Japanese quality control after the war (see also Boaden & Harvey, Chapter 10).

The next wave of operations management innovation focused on lean manufacturing with just-in-time systems and processes. This meant that producers no longer had to store large inventories and products were 'pulled' through only those processes that added value, based on customer demand (Bowen & Youngdahl 1998). Efficiencies were achieved by grouping inputs with similar process requirements and by reducing set-up times. Importantly, lean structures shifted the responsibility for quality control from inspectors and quality departments to individual workers and teams (Bowen & Youngdahl 1998). These advances in operations management illustrate an ongoing cycle where a product is introduced and then continuously improved until a 'final' ultimate product is achieved. Once the preferred design has been identified, the focus of innovation moves to the production processes. In comparison with manufacturing, the health service sector has not found either the perfect design or the most appropriate processes.

Operations management – necessary, but insufficient in healthcare

Although operations management has been around since the industrial revolution, in healthcare we have been slow to capitalise on the analysis techniques and improvement methods of this discipline to manage clinical operations. There are some examples: In the late 1990s American hospitals advanced clinical process improvement and innovation (CPI) to decrease costs and improve quality (Savitz 2000) and by 1995 over 60% of US hospitals reported use of clinical process management (Walston et al 2000). But in comparison with other industries, where processes are designed to operate correctly 98–99% of the time, in healthcare studies have shown that clinical care processes may be defective 50% of the time (Resar 2006, Scott et al 2004, Runciman et al 2006). While healthcare has assumed some aspects of effective operations management, it is patchy and sub-optimal in comparison with other industries. Specialisation and standardisation are two principles that have transformed the operations of many industries but which have had mixed success in healthcare. Each is discussed briefly in the context of healthcare.

Specialisation in healthcare

There is an over-abundance of specialisation in workforce inputs in healthcare. Specialisation, or division of labour, defines the extent to which tasks in an organisation are subdivided into separate jobs. In healthcare, this is commonly based on professional expertise and clinical specialties. More than one hundred health professions can be identified, and within only one of these professions there are over 130 medical specialties. In Australia, while we continue to support this abundance of specialists, we have difficulty maintaining adequate numbers of practitioners within many individual specialties. The increasing specialisation of healthcare has required mechanisms to facilitate interdependence among the workers involved in a patient's care. The boundaries of these professional groups and an individual's hierarchical rank reduce information sharing (Edmondson 1996) making it difficult to manage care processes effectively. This has led to the hospital being referred to as the 'key battleground for the various forces arrayed in the division of labour in healthcare' (Dingwall et al 1988:228). While it is acknowledged that 'quality comes from improving processes, which invariably cut across professional and functional boundaries' (Buck 1998:752), the organisation of healthcare has not kept pace. The necessary inter-disciplinary and inter-departmental coordination are neither encouraged, nor rewarded.

In other industries specialisation has been effective in improving production processes, with a focus on ensuring specialisation of inputs other than the workforce, as well as specialisation of processes and outputs. While there is abundance of specialisation among healthcare providers, researchers have commented that unlike other industries, specialisation in other inputs (such as equipment, facilities, and even patients) has not been seen to be linked to improved clinical outcomes (Ramanujami & Rousseau 2006:823). Most recently 'lean thinking' approaches have been adapted from car manufacturers to healthcare settings and have resulted in an increasing focus on structuring service delivery to increase specialisation among patient inputs (Ben-Tovim et al 2007, Kelly et al 2007). The concept of the hospital as a 'focused factory', with highly specialised services consolidated in a relatively small number of sites, and with greater differentiation of patient types between emergency-driven hospitals and elective care (Leung 1999), is a good example of how specialisation of manufacturing production process can be adapted to the hospital setting.

Standardisation in healthcare

Standardisation has offered savings through efficiencies in many industries. Standardisation is broadly defined as the process of establishing agreed technical standards to achieve benefits for an organisation or industry. Standardisation can be applied to all parts of production – the inputs, the production processes and the outputs – and defines the specifications of the components in these parts, that is, the desired technical standards. In healthcare, like specialisation, standardisation is primarily directed to the competencies of health professionals (Glouberman & Mintzberg 2001b), with professional colleges and registration bodies structured to ensure standards of practice. While this aim has ensured standardisation of the largest proportion of the inputs, standardisation of other inputs (such as equipment and supplies) has not reached the levels achieved in other industries that have enabled efficient operations. Recently, standardisation of other inputs in healthcare has increased patient safety, as well as contributing to efficiency. For example, standardising medical supplies has enabled staff to rationalise their knowledge of the application of a wide variety of similar supplies, thereby assisting to improve error-free use. Standardising medical supplies also improves purchasing power.

Care pathways and clinical guidelines are examples of standardisation of the production processes ('the work') (see Claridge & Cook, Chapter 4). Recent initiatives, such as the UK National Health Service's (NHS) Map of Medicine, employ process management techniques, almost by stealth, to introduce greater standardisation in the craft-process relationship between clinician and patient. However, doctors relish their individual independence and reject standarisation of care (Degeling et al 2001). Thus, while there is evidence that the standardisation offered through pathways and guidelines improves quality of care (Caminiti et al 2005, Vikoren et al 2006) there has been mixed success in implementation and consistent use, with recent studies identifying substantial barriers. Within healthcare, the difficulties in standardising work reflect the

> … insoluble paradox between the need for consistent and evidence-based standards of care and the unique predicament, context, priorities, and choices of the individual patient.

> (Plsek & Greenhalgh 2001:627)

This paradox distinguishes health service management from management in other industries, as health is characterised by:

- complex decision making at the patient care level that is negotiated between the patient and healthcare professional
- serious consequences of errors in decision making that may result in death or injury
- an uncertain external environment, with the combination of public and private financing and delivery schemes making it difficult to navigate
- goals of service delivery, which are often ambiguous and potentially conflicting (Leatt & Porter 2003).

While these factors might suggest that healthcare by definition will have high variation, studies consistently confirm that the variation caused by the organisation of the delivery system outweighs the variation caused by the random arrivals of patients with their 'unique' needs (Haraden & Resar 2004). The need to balance standards of care with patient individuality may also explain the fact that in comparison with other industries, there has been little emphasis on standardisation of outputs in healthcare (Glouberman & Mintzberg 2001b). The reduction in anaesthesia deaths in the US from rates of 25 to 50 deaths per million in the 1970s and 1980s (Ross & Tinker 1994) to current rates of less than 5 per million (Eichhorn 1989) and the development of diagnosis-related groups are two examples of the standardisation of outputs, although it is difficult to find others.

Operations management – the obstacles in healthcare

Three hypotheses are proposed to explain why operations management has not permeated the healthcare industry and are discussed further below:

1. the influence of craft production in a mass production environment
2. the difficulties in applying production management concepts to services
3. the emphasis on inputs in public administration.

The influence of craft production in a mass production environment

Healthcare has tended to be craft-based production – a trained healthcare professional provides his or her craft for individual patients, with little need for management. But as healthcare has moved from service delivery primarily in the community (that is, in the patient's home or the doctor's local surgery) to institutions such as hospitals, aspects of mass production have been introduced.

The organisation and operation of the hospital illustrates the difficulties transferring craft production to a setting that requires teamwork, coordination and integrated production. Hospitals display a fundamental inconsistency in that they are organised in formal managerial and clinical hierarchies that are based on scientific management principles, yet they try to maintain a commitment to professional autonomy for clinicians (Leggat & Dwyer 2005). The complex multifaceted production processes in hospitals are managed with a craft production mentality. This has resulted in an emphasis on managing (through the hierarchies) those aspects of operations that don't interfere with the craft production relationship between clinician and patient. This was demonstrated by a review of management decisions in the NHS which found little managerial control over medicine (Harrison & Lim 2003), and by an Australian study that found that clinician managers focused on financial management, people management, organisational management and customer orientation (Braithwaite 2004). Clinical management was not identified as a primary pursuit of this group of managers. Instead, process, quality and data management – key components of clinical management – were only found in the secondary pursuits, where the clinician managers reported spending less time and effort (Braithwaite 2004). A more recent study of Australian public health managers found similar results (Braithwaite et al 2007).

Avoiding management of the clinician–patient relationship has resulted in independent, and largely inefficient, craft production. Instead of an effective interdisciplinary care delivery model, hospital organisation and hierarchy reinforces parallel care processes that only occasionally intersect. In addition, the healthcare professions have differing views on the evidence for effective practice, and the education, training and work practices of our health workers provide limited opportunities for the multidisciplinary evidence sharing and debate necessary to achieve consensus on clinical processes (Dopson et al 2002). When care is delivered through multiple clinical processes that are based on different clinical evidence and that only occasionally intersect, management of the processes to achieve efficient, consistent and high-quality care is difficult.

The healthcare craft production model depends on the staff involved to deliver error-free service. Quality control is largely focused on post-process audit. Other industries have realised that human beings cannot consistently maintain the required high performance levels and therefore create systems to reduce variation within processes. These systems anticipate and compensate for the likely errors that normal humans make (Resar 2006).

> **Pause for reflection**
>
> Why do healthcare managers in many countries struggle to find an appropriate operating structure that can influence service quality in a craft production environment? Why, as a result, is the healthcare industry characterised by a tension between craft production and mass production operation and quality control principles?

The difficulties in applying production management concepts to services

Services and products are different. Because operations management has evolved from production processes it has taken time to see how the concepts might translate to service provision, such as healthcare. While General Electric (GE) was able to quickly use a six sigma strategy to set reliability goals for manufactured products, it took much longer to apply the same concepts to the GE service-oriented businesses. Unlike manufacturing, service production and consumption take place simultaneously with high customer interaction, but the operations management concepts are the same. For example, while production control in other industries is concerned with the movement of materials, in healthcare the flows of the patients are critical to the process (Vissers & Beech 2005).

Evidence from the Institute for Healthcare Improvement suggests that improving patient flow can enhance clinical outcomes, address patient safety, increase patient and staff satisfaction and reduce operating costs (Haraden & Resar 2004). Yet application of process management to improve patient flow (from the perspective of both the patient and the providers) has been difficult, as no one has responsibility for the patient throughout their entire journey. As described by Glouberman & Mintzberg, within a hospital the medical staff tend to have discrete interventional relationships with patients, while the nursing and allied health staff play a more continuous part in the production process (Glouberman & Mintzberg 2001a). However, the nurses and allied health practitioners 'are functionally subordinate to the physicians' (Glouberman & Mintzberg 2001a:61) and are therefore unable to exert much control over the patient care processes.

Further, while manufacturers can provide detailed specifications of products, services have intangible outputs, with quality often perceived differently by different consumers. In healthcare, the outputs are often not fully known, are subjective and vague (Vissers & Beech 2005), and quality is difficult to measure (Peabody et al 2000). This leads to the next issue – inputs are much easier to measure, analyse and control than the service outputs or outcomes.

The emphasis on inputs in public administration

In both product and service systems, inputs (such as raw materials) are transformed through a process to outputs (such as services) as shown in Figure 2.1. Because the clinical outputs and outcomes are difficult to specify in healthcare, we have traditionally focused on measuring, monitoring and improving inputs. Policymakers and managers have largely been concerned with the number of patients accessing services and costs of the staff and facilities mobilised to provide the services. Despite the assertion that 'no provider should be allowed to practice medicine without measuring and reporting results' (Davidson & Randall 2006:49), in many jurisdictions the funders of public healthcare services require performance reporting on inputs and not clinical outcomes.

For example, a study on performance indicators in the Victorian public health sector found an overemphasis on financial and volume indicators at the expense of indicators of the outcomes of the clinical processes (Leggat et al 2005). The financial inputs (the costs) tend to be the easiest to measure. Because the outputs (the benefits) are difficult to define and measure 'analysts race around cutting the costs with no *measurable* effect on the benefits' (Glouberman & Mintzberg 2001b:74).

Figure 2.1 The main components of a production system

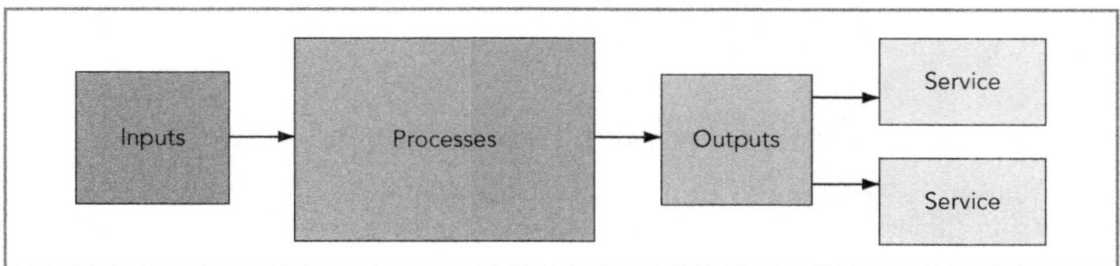

As discussed above, the healthcare service system is characterised by parallel care processes with sturdy walls between health professional disciplines, between service components and between organisations. One reason these boundaries have been allowed to develop is that health service performance indicators have traditionally focused on an individual service. Clinicians receive feedback on their part of the process. The underdeveloped information systems and lack of clear ownership of the end-to-end clinical process have made it difficult to track the throughputs and outputs of the care process as a whole. In most healthcare organisations the budgets and resulting reporting structures are departmentally organised. Traditional financial indicators were devised from cost accounting systems designed for an environment of mass production of a few standardised items, and not for the complexity of the healthcare processes and outcomes. The information systems supporting these indicators are optimised for managing transactions within departmental 'silos'. This means that few healthcare organisations have information systems that can effectively track care processes from beginning to end (Leggat et al 2005) and while clinicians appear to accept standardisation when they are provided with objective measures to review their performance, the existing measures perpetuate the system boundaries.

Although there is growing evidence of the effectiveness of information management in improving hospital care (Committee on Quality of Healthcare in America 2001, Institute of Medicine 2000), hospitals and health service organisations are judged to be at least 10 years behind in information investment in comparison with organisations in other industries of comparable size and complexity (Ferlie & Shortell 2001). At present there are few health organisations with information systems that can effectively link and integrate financial and clinical data and the information base to support evidence-based practice is quite limited (Kane & Mosser 2007). Ferlie & Shortell (2001:297) argue that information technology represents a 'powerful untapped force for changes that can improve the quality of care'. Berg (2005) suggests that information technology implementation is often only considered a technical project, and that this results in limited ability to access the information required to understand and improve processes (Berg et al 2005). The healthcare industry is only just realising the information that is required to understand and manage clinical processes. Hence, it will be some time before the process and outcome data that are used effectively in operations management in other industries are readily available in public healthcare.

> **Pause for reflection**
>
> Process and operations management are well-supported management disciplines that have been shown to improve efficiency and effectiveness in many industries. Aspects of operations management are visible in healthcare organisations, but there has been little application to the clinical care processes. Why is the craft production mode in healthcare hypothesised to constrain clinical process management? How are specialisation and standardisation applicable to the inputs, processes and outputs of healthcare delivery? What data are required to increase our understanding of clinical processes?

Operations management – value for healthcare

As discussed in Chapter 1, over the past decade healthcare has been perceived as an increasing financial burden, with less than the expected impact on improving population health. Consumers expect higher quality services, more information about treatment options that enable full participation in treatment decisions, and more visible accountability for the operation and outcomes of their health services. Stephen Duckett wrote in 1994 that, with the advent of casemix, Australian healthcare had entered a new era of accountability (Duckett 1994). Yet we continue to see public and professional concerns about the quality of care, and the healthcare sector has been under increasing scrutiny, with a strong push to improve the responsiveness, quality and safety of the services provided. In this search for value, there is increasing realisation that health system management must move beyond the existing emphasis on managing the inputs, to more effective management of the processes and the outputs. Improving outcomes requires management of those processes that transform the health system inputs.

Clinical, administrative and ancillary processes are used to deliver healthcare services. Clinical processes focus on the planning, design, delivery and control of the steps necessary to provide a service for a healthcare consumer (Vissers & Beech 2005). Management processes support the clinical processes, while the ancillary processes support the general functioning of the organisation, comprising functions such as cleaning and maintenance. Processes have been described as 'invisible economic assets and liabilities' (Keen & Knapp 1996), suggesting that a focus on effective process management is of financial benefit to the organisation.

One of the reasons that operations management has been effective in improving the production of products and services is the understanding of the customer that its principles and practices require. Michael Hammer, a strong proponent of business process re-engineering, originally considered a process to be solely the conversion of input to outputs. However, more recently, in partnership with Grady, Hammer suggested that a process was not just this transformation, but also included the stakeholders who interacted to achieve the desired results (Nwabueze 2000). This approach to understanding processes is critical in healthcare – the nature of the industry and its consumers and workforce must drive clinical process management as shown in Figure 2.2.

In healthcare delivery there are two principal customer groups that need to be included in the management of clinical processes: the consumers of healthcare (the patients, clients and their families) and the individuals who bring their craft to the hospital, home or community health centre (the health professionals). There is substantial evidence that improving the operations and outcomes of the healthcare system requires a consumer focus and high staff involvement (Committee on Quality of Healthcare in America 2001).

Figure 2.2 Co-producing health outcomes

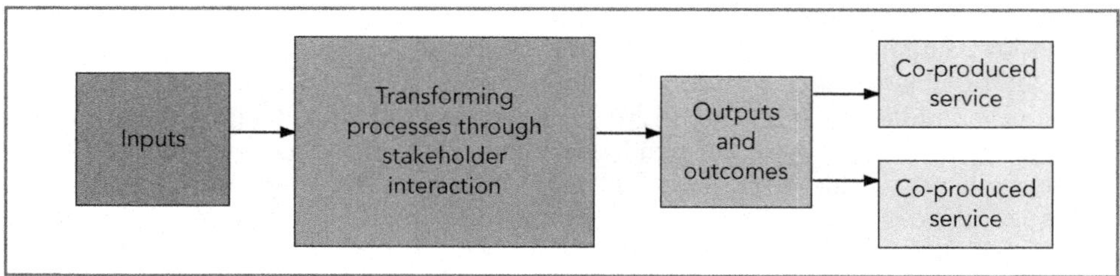

Consumer-focused care

Healthcare systems have been typically organised around the values of clinicians (Committee on Quality of Healthcare in America 2001), but recent evidence stresses that understanding how healthcare works for patients is essential to improving clinical outcomes (Batalden 1998, Committee on Quality of Healthcare in America 2001, Nicholson 1995). Advocates for applying operations management techniques in healthcare stress that enhancing the healthcare system requires an understanding of value that can only be defined by the customer (Womack & Jones 2003). While there is strong rhetoric around reorientation to a patient or consumer focus in most healthcare systems, healthcare professionals have yet to fully embrace consumer values. One has only to attend an emergency or outpatient department to see processes organised for health professionals and not for patients and families.

A 2006 literature review of hospital process improvement studies published between 1989 and 2004 found that the promise of 7428 titles and abstracts only resulted in 88 articles describing 86 process improvement studies in hospital care that had a robust method and sufficient information to evaluate the intervention (Elkhuizen et al 2006). The important finding of this review was that the studies were predominantly focused on cost reduction and resource utilisation; parameters related to the patient experience and patient values were rarely used (Elkhuizen et al 2006). This is consistent with the evolution of process management within other industries. A review of 33 organisations from seven industries with process re-engineering experience found that as organisations matured in process management, the focus shifted from an emphasis only on improving costs, to more strategic and consumer-focused aims of improving service delivery (Maull et al 2003). More recent operations management initiatives, such as lean thinking, have further progressed the focus on understanding and responding to consumer value (Hines et al 2004).

Because of the complexities of the healthcare system, many process activities have focused on a ward, unit or department. The organisation of the workforce has led to fragmentation of healthcare processes (Leggat 2007), and while patients travel through the system, it is difficult to examine the processes across the system. While there may be local successes in improving processes, these often lead to problems elsewhere in the organisation or broader system. The evidence is unequivocal that single-process projects are not as effective as a strategic system approach (Balle & Regnier 2007, Nwabueze 2000). Yet the complexity, visibility and high levels of regulation of the healthcare system make attempts at change more difficult than in other industries (Berwick 2002).

Further, societies are fiercely protective and have strong expectations for their healthcare systems. The media play a strong role in public debate and opinion about healthcare, often with direct impact on the careers of health professionals and politicians. These factors push for small-scale incremental changes, at the expense of the necessary strategic systemic approach. Drawing from the experience of other industries, key drivers of improved performance in quality and safety include an orientation to customer satisfaction that is supported throughout the organisation, an organisational configuration that ensures seamless interaction by the consumer, and information about customer relationships (Day 2004). Yet, there is strong evidence that patient involvement in the healthcare system 'is, in reality, constrained by organisational, clinical or economic factors' (Salmon & Hall 2004:53). A strong focus of operations management is the definition of customer value. The healthcare sector needs to increase understanding of customer value and incorporate it into the management of clinical processes to facilitate achievement of consumer-focused policy objectives.

> **Pause for reflection**
>
> Although characterised as having a primary focus on the operations of a business or organisation, a key aspect of operations management is the development of a strong understanding of customer value that is meant to influence all operating decisions. Why might this be so?

Fostering high commitment

Everything points to one central fact: Clinical activities cannot be coordinated by managerial interventions— not by outside bosses or coordinators, not by administrative systems, not by discussions of 'quality' disconnected from the delivery of it, not by all that constant reorganizing.

(Glouberman & Mintzberg 2001b:76)

The message has been consistent that clinicians need to be involved in managing clinical processes. Donald Berwick stressed that clinical operations needed to be effected by the 'managed', not by the managers (Berwick 1994), and there is increasing evidence that successful clinical process management is based on clinicians adopting a leadership role and championing the process (Hyett et al 2007) (see Stanton, Chapter 3; Warburton, Chapter 9; and Berding, Resources).

While essential, motivating clinicians has not been easy as the 'old boys' medical networks have largely made process control unworkable (Braithwaite 2004). While it is thought that clinicians should welcome any assistance that improves clinical care processes, professional autonomy continues to create barriers to clinical process management (Degeling et al 2001, Panella et al 2003). In addition, the different cultures that exist among the specialised health professional groups makes it difficult to find an approach to involvement that satisfies all (Degeling et al 2001). This has led to the suggestion that health professional education must move from the current content-oriented learning to process-oriented learning methods (Fraser & Greenhalgh 2001). If there is an expectation that clinicians and managers will manage clinical processes there is a need to ensure training in processes.

Finally, process management must be supported by integrated performance management (Maull et al 2003). Currently the health sector does not hold care teams accountable for achieving outcomes that are valued by consumers. For example, ancient Chinese palace doctors could be put to death if the emperor died. This resulted in very clear performance expectations with direct linking of expected outcomes and rewards. Although the airline and healthcare industries are often compared as complicated high-risk industries, the fact that pilots can lose their life in a plane crash (which also sets up clear performance expectations for pilots) is often jokingly cited as a major difference between the two industries. It has been suggested that the airline industry has demonstrated better success in process enhancement to improve customer quality and safety than the healthcare industry.

There is considerable general evidence to support effective performance management in improving organisational outcomes (Huselid 1995), and there is specific evidence relating performance appraisal to better clinical outcomes (West et al 2002). However there is much to be done to improve performance monitoring and management in healthcare (Bartram et al 2007, Leggat et al 2005, Leggat & Dwyer 2005). Process and performance are inextricably linked through operations management. Use of operations management to improve the management of clinical processes, by definition, requires establishing performance management expectations for providers that are responsive to consumer values.

> **Pause for reflection**
>
> How could operations management be used to encourage greater clinician participation in managing clinical processes? What operations management principles are particularly relevant?

Conclusion

The health sector has been slower than other industries to embrace operations management. The traditional organisation, production modes, availability of information and performance monitoring in healthcare have created considerable obstacles to effective operations management. Recognising that healthcare delivery processes may be defective a large proportion of the time has led to consideration of the applicability of tools and techniques from other industries, with the conclusion that health system improvements will only be achieved with a refocusing from the management of system inputs to effective management of clinical processes and resulting outputs – that is, operations management.

References

Balle M, Regnier A 2007 Lean as a learning system in a hospital ward. Leadership in Health Services 20:33–41

Bartram T, Stanton P, Leggat S G et al 2007 Lost in translation: making the link between HRM and performance in healthcare. Human Resource Management Journal 17:21–41

Batalden P 1998 Collaboration in improving care for patients: how can we find out what we haven't been able to figure out yet? Journal of Quality Improvement 24:609–18

Ben-Tovim D I, Bassham J E, Bolch D et al 2007 Lean thinking across a hospital: redesigning care at the Flinders Medical Centre. Australian Health Review 31:10–15

Berg M, Schellekens W, Bergeni C 2005 Bridging the quality chasm: integrating professional and organizational approaches to quality. International Journal for Quality in Healthcare 17:75–82

Berwick D M 1994 Eleven worthy aims for clinical leadership of healthcare reform. Journal of the American Medical Association 272:797–802

Berwick D M 2002 A user's manual for the IOMs 'Quality Chasm' report. Health Affairs 21:80

Bowen D E, Youngdahl W E 1998 'Lean' service: in defense of a production-line approach. International Journal of Service Industry Management 9(3)207–225

Braithwaite J 2004 An empirically-based model for clinician-managers' behavioural routines. Journal of Health Organization and Management Decision 18:240–61

Braithwaite J, Luft S, Bender W et al 2007 The hierarchy of work pursuits of public health managers. Health Services Management Research 20:71–83

Buck C R J 1998 Healthcare through a six sigma lens. The Milbank Quarterly 76:749–753

Caminiti C, Scoditti U, Diodati F et al 2005 How to promote, improve and test adherence to scientific evidence in clinical practice. BMC Health Services Research 19:62

Committee on Quality of Healthcare in America 2001 Crossing the Quality Chasm. A New Health System for the 21st Century. National Academy Press, Washington DC

Davidson A, Randall R M 2006 Michael Porter and Elizabeth Teisberg on redefining value in healthcare: an interview. Strategy & Leadership 34:48–50

Day G 2004 Winning the competition for customer relationships. Sloan Management Review

Degeling P, Kennedy J, Hill M 2001 Mediating the cultural boundaries between medicine, nursing and management – the central challenge in hospital reform. Health Services Management Research 14:36–48

Dingwall R, Rafferty A M, Webster C 1988 An Introduction to the Social History of Nursing. Routledge, London

Dopson S, Fitzgerald L, Ferlie E B et al 2002 No magic targets! Changing clinical practice to become more evidence based. Health Care Management Review, Special Issue 27:35–47

Duckett S J 1994 Hospital and departmental management in the era of accountability: addressing the new management challenges. Australian Health Review 17:116–31

Edmondson A 1996 Learning from mistakes is easier said than done: group and organizational influences on the detection and correction of human error. Journal of Applied Behavioral Science 32:5–28

Eichhorn J H 1989 Prevention of intraoperative anesthesia accidents and related severe injury through safety monitoring. Anesthesiology 70:572–7

Elkhuizen S G, Limburg M, Bakker P J M et al 2006 Evidence-based re-engineering: re-engineering the evidence. International Journal of Healthcare Quality Assurance 19:477–99

Ferlie E B, Shortell S M 2001 Improving the quality of healthcare in the United Kingdom and the United States: A framework for change. The Milbank Quarterly 79:281–315

Fraser S W, Greenhalgh T 2001 Coping with complexity: educating for capability. British Medical Journal 323:799–803

Glouberman S, Mintzberg H 2001a Managing the care of health and the cure of disease – Part 1: Differentiation. Healthcare Management Review 21:56–69

Glouberman S, Mintzberg H 2001b Managing the care of health and the cure of disease – Part 2: Integration. Healthcare Management Review 21:70–84

Haraden C, Resar R 2004 Patient flow in hospitals: understanding and controlling it better. Frontiers of Health Services Management 20:3–15

Harrison S, Lim J N W 2003 The frontier of control: doctors and managers in the NHS 1966 to 1997. Clinical Governance: An International Journal 8:13–8

Hines P, Holwe M, Rich N 2004 Learning to evolve: a review of contemporary lean thinking. International Journal of Operations & Production Management 24:994–1012

Huselid M 1995 The impact of human resource management practices on turnover, productivity and corporate financial performance. Academy of Management Journal 38:635–72

Hyett K L, Podosky M, Santamaria N et al 2007 Valuing variance: the importance of variance analysis in clinical pathways utilisation. Australian Health Review 31

Institute of Medicine 2000 To Err is Human: Building a Safer Healthcare System. National Academy Press, Washington

Kane R L, Mosser G 2007 The challenge of explaining why quality improvement has not done better. International Journal for Quality in Healthcare 19:8–10

Keen P G, Knapp E M 1996 Every Manager's Guide to Business Processes. Harvard Business School Press, Boston

Kelly A-M, Bryant M, Cox L, Jolley D 2007 Improving emergency department efficiency by patient streaming to outcomes-based teams. Australian Health Review 31:16–21

Leatt P, Porter J 2003 Where are the healthcare leaders? The need for investment in leadership development. Healthcare Papers 4:14–31

Leggat S G 2007 Health professional education; perpetuating obsolescence? Australian Health Review 31(3):325–26

Leggat S G, Bartram T, Stanton P 2005 Performance monitoring in the Victorian healthcare system: an exploratory study. Australian Health Review 29:17–24

Leggat S G, Dwyer J 2005 Improving hospital performance: culture change is not the answer. Healthcare Quarterly 8:60–6

Leung G M 1999 Hospitals must become 'focused factories'. British Medical Journal 320:942

Maull R S, Tranfield D R, Maull W 2003 Factors characterising the maturity of BOR programmes. International Journal of Operations and Production Management 23:596–624

Mintzberg H 2002 Managing care and cure – up and down, in and out. Health Services Management Research 15:193–206

Nicholson J 1995 Patient focused care and its role in hospital process re-engineering. International Journal of Healthcare Quality Assurance 8:23–6

Nwabueze U 2000 In and out of vogue: the case of BPR in the NHS. Managerial Accounting Journal 15:459–463

Panella M, Marchisio S, Di Stansilao F 2003 Reducing clinical variations with clinical pathways: do pathways work? International Journal for Quality in Healthcare 15:509–21

Peabody J W, Luck J, Glassman P et al 2000 Comparison of Vignettes, Standardized Patients, and Chart Abstraction. Journal of the American Medical Association, 283:1715–1722

Plsek P E, Greenhalgh T 2001 Complexity science. The challenge of complexity in healthcare. British Medical Journal 323:625–8

Ramanujami R, Rousseau D M 2006 The challenges are organizational not just clinical. Journal of Organizational Behavior 27:811–27

Resar R 2006 Making noncatastrophic healthcare processes reliable: learning to walk before running in creating high-reliability organizations. Health Services Research 41:1677–89

Ross A F, Tinker J H 1994 Anesthesia risk. In: Miller R D (ed) Anesthesia. 4th ed. Churchill-Livingston, New York

Runciman W B, Williamson J A H, Deakin A et al 2006 An integrated framework for safety, quality and risk management: an information and incident management system based on a universal patient safety classification. Quality and Safety in Healthcare 15:82–90

Salmon P, Hall G M 2004 Patient empowerment or the emperor's new clothes. Journal of the Royal Society of Medicine 97:53–56

Savitz L A 2000 Assessing the implementation of clinical process innovations: a cross-case comparison. Journal of Healthcare Management 45:366–379

Scott I A, Denaro C P, Bennett C J 2004 Achieving better in-hospital and after-hospital care of patients with acute cardiac disease. Medical Journal of Australia 180:S83–8

Vikoren T H, Musser R C, Tcheng J E et al 2006 From clinical pathways to CPOE: challenges and opportunities in standardization and computerization of postoperative orders for total joint replacement. Journal of Surgical Advances 15:195–200

Vissers J, Beech R 2005 Health Operations Management. Patient Flow Logistics in Healthcare. Routledge, London

Walston S L, Burns L R, Kimberley J R 2000 Does reengineering really work? An examination of the context and outcomes of hospital reengineering initiatives. Health Services Research 34:1363–1388

West M A, Borrill C, Dawson J F et al 2002 The link between the management of employees and patient mortality in acute hospitals. International Journal of Human Resource Management 13:1299–1310

Womack J P, Jones D T 2003 Lean Thinking. Simon & Schuster, London

Chapter 3

The politics of healthcare: managing the healthcare workforce

Pauline Stanton

Introduction

The healthcare workforce accounts for the largest proportion of all health service costs, and is recognised internationally as playing a key role in providing efficient and effective health services and improving health outcomes. In recent years health policy-makers, governments, practitioners and academics have given greater attention to the importance of human resources management (HRM) to health service performance (Bach 2001, Kabene et al 2006). Some of this interest is a reaction to the years of neglect of human resource factors in health sector reform despite the profound effect that such reforms have had on the work of managers and clinicians (Bach 2001, Rigoli & Dussault 2003). Current research suggests that effective HRM strategies are essential in improving health outcomes (Buchan 2004, Kabene et al 2006). Nonetheless, there is no agreement on exactly what effective human resource strategies might look like, and it is easy to ignore the powerful structural constraints and influences in the healthcare sector that detract from such agreement. Of particular note here is the role of government in providing direction to and managing health services. Another factor is the composition of the healthcare workforce itself, organised as it is around tradition-orientated disciplines often described as being rigid and reluctant to change, tribal and self-serving, as well as being strongly unionised with powerful professional associations.

This chapter explores the politics of healthcare and the potential for change. It outlines the nature of the healthcare workforce and identifies key stakeholders and their attitudes to change. The chapter also examines health sector employment relations, outlines the major health sector reform policies impacting on the workforce over the past two decades and charts the reaction of the workforce to those policies and explores the impact of these changes on the organisation including work intensification, workplace change and the greater control and scrutiny of clinicians.

The chapter concludes by arguing that the policies of health sector reform have often exacerbated the underlying problems and issues facing the sector and outlines an approach to creating a sustainable and responsive workforce that engages clinicians and managers in the process of change rather than forcing change on them. Key features of this approach to managing people in healthcare include the importance of leadership at all levels incorporating government, organisations, managers and clinicians; building people management skills; creating collaborative and committed team-based working environments through employee participation and engagement; and understanding and valuing high-performance practices.

Understanding the healthcare workforce

Healthcare is a labour-intensive industry with labour costs accounting for between 65 and 80% of total costs. The health workforce in many countries has expanded substantially over the past three decades. It is constituted by different professions and occupational groups each with their own history, culture and specialisations (Duckett 2005, Kabene et al 2006). The main features of professions are the long years of training, specialised knowledge, clinical autonomy and labour mobility (Gunderson 1982: 30–31). Health professionals often have a greater allegiance to their profession than to their employers and the professional bodies representing them are often powerful and well organised. They play an important role in the registration and regulation of their members and the definition of standards of practice. They participate both formally in the process of defining legal and administrative standards in healthcare and informally through lobbying governments (Bach 2001, Rigoli & Dussault 2003). Hence the professions are influential within both the industry and the community at large, with nurses and doctors in particular being held in high esteem. At the same time the health professions have a history of competition between each other over resources, prestige and control, and are often described as having a 'tribal mentality' (Hunter 1996).

Medical practitioners and medical specialists are generally regarded as the most powerful group in the healthcare sector as they make important resource decisions and largely control the production process. Wilson & Goldschmidt (1995) argue that doctors are trained to be independent, self-reliant and individualistic, to rely on their own judgment and to be accountable to their profession, only sharing their decision-making processes with colleagues in a non-judgmental way. They are at the apex of a hierarchical division of labour in healthcare (Freidson 1970). They decide who enters, who leaves and what treatment they receive. Hence, clinical autonomy, independence and judgment are at the heart of work practice reform in the health sector, although scrutiny of clinical practice is often seen as a challenge to clinicians' judgment. Yet if employers are to have some control over labour utilisation they must have some control over the production process. This can lead to a direct challenge to the medical profession and to a conflict between allegiance to the profession or to the organisation (Gunderson 1982, Harrison & Pollitt 1994, Hunter 1996). Governments internationally have made various attempts to challenge this autonomy by incorporating clinicians into management and into decision making around the allocation of resources and the management of change, albeit with varying levels of success (Harrison & Pollit 1994, Perkins et al 1997).

In many countries doctors are organised into powerful professions with considerable political clout. While they do not often take industrial action, their strong standing in the community and their control over the production process gives them latent power, which they often threaten to use and occasionally do (Stanton 2006). This means that the actions of doctors can be an obstacle to change. At the micro level, for example, doctors can resist the substitution of labour by blocking the delegation of tasks to other professional groups. At the macro level the organised opposition of doctors in the US through the American Medical Association 'contributed to the failure of reforms introducing managed care competition in healthcare in 1993' (Rigoli & Dussault 2003:10).

While doctors are the most powerful group, nursing is one of the largest occupational groups. In Australia nurses make up over two-thirds of the professional workforce allowing a certain amount of power through sheer numbers. They are represented by the Australian Nursing Federation which acts as both a professional association and a trade union with its membership increasing significantly at a time when internationally many trade unions have suffered dramatic membership decline (Bartram et al 2007a). Nurses have demonstrated that they are able and willing when necessary to support their union and exercise their industrial strength to protect their interests and the interests of the patient and the community. Nursing in Australia has had a long and at times bitter history as nurses have had to fight for their professional and tertiary qualification status to improve their wages, conditions and career structures, to enhance their skills and roles and, more recently, to protect hard-won gains over control of some aspects of the work process, in particular nurse–patient ratios (Bartram et al 2007a, McCoppin & Gardner 1994). International evidence shows that nurses join unions not only to improve their pay and conditions but also to protect and advance the profession and their own professional status (Bartram et al 2007a, Breda 1997). As any health minister knows, an industrial dispute with nurses very quickly becomes front-page news and a potential major embarrassment for the government of the day.

Together, nurses and medical practitioners represent the largest groups of professionals in the health sector, although allied health professionals and scientists and non-professional employees are of increasing importance in the hospital environment with influence beyond their numbers. Should medical scientists or radiographers decide to take industrial action, for instance, they can quickly bring surgery in a hospital to a halt and severely disrupt the production process (Bremner & Kelly 2000, Stanton 2006). Experience over the past decade demonstrates that these professional groups will take industrial action if they feel their interests are threatened. Rigoli & Dessault (2003) describe how in a range of countries including Costa Rica, Zambia, the Philippines and Israel, trade unions have strongly opposed health sector reform that threatened labour contracts, conditions of service and the roles of health professionals. The effect of this opposition limited governments in reorganising their public sectors.

Healthcare professionals are very mobile both domestically and internationally. They often migrate to areas where their services will be better compensated both by country migration and by emigration. As the Australian Productivity Commission (2005) notes, a major challenge for the sector is the international labour shortage in many key professional areas including nursing, medical specialists and allied health professionals. Solutions to this problem include encouraging migration from overseas, increasing university places for health professionals and substituting one group of workers with another. However, the solution for one country may have a detrimental effect on others, as developing countries struggle to provide good-quality medical care to their own citizens. Countries such as Ghana, Kenya, South Africa and Zimbabwe have been forced to seek other human resource solutions to counter the emigration of their highly educated and medically trained personnel (Kabene et al 2006). In developing countries such as Nicaragua and Bangladesh health professionals are drawn to the cities where they can find better opportunities for themselves and their families

(Kabene et al 2006). This trend is mirrored in Australia where there are acute rural and regional shortages of healthcare staff (Duckett 2005).

Not surprisingly, labour substitution has become increasingly popular with governments as a possible solution to the labour shortage problem. In Australia and the UK, patient care attendants now substitute their labour for some of the more routine work of nurses, allowing nurses to take on some of the work of medical practitioners in a process of 'skills escalation', and in the US there is extensive use made of nurses and other health professionals as physicians' assistants (Duckett 2005). However, in Australia the 'demarcation' of professional work is problematic as the issue of skill mix and labour utilisation at the organisational level is highly contested terrain. At the industry level professional associations have largely resisted changes to their work practices as other professions move on to their turf. Medical practitioners resist the development of nurse practitioner roles, and nurses in some states resist the use of patient care attendants.

Finally, the healthcare sector is highly feminised. In Australia, women account for almost 80% of health sector employees. They predominate in nursing and allied health professions and increasingly in general practice, although the higher income medical specialists remain largely male (Duckett 2005). Diallo et al (2003) note that female-dominated occupations such as nursing and midwifery are often not given their proper market value in line with their skill levels as the work is seen as 'women's work' and therefore of lesser value. Also increased participation by women in medicine is often accompanied by different work patterns and evidence shows that women work fewer hours than men and that part-time work is increasing. For example, in Australia in 2001 more than half of nurses worked part time (AIHW 2004) and the level and utilisation of casualisation in the sector has increased (Cregan et al 2003). Allan (1998) argues that casualisation is a managerial tool used to manage workflow. However, Lumley et al (2004) found that nursing shortages allowed nurses to choose to work casually and they did this to take control of their own work schedules, improve their balance of work and family life, and to have less responsibility and hence a more stress-free existence. This was not good news for hospitals that struggle to cover unpopular shifts and to provide acceptable standards of nursing care. In the longer term it might not be good for women either, as evidence shows that female nurses who take time out of the permanent workforce to bring up children fall behind their peers in relation to career development and salary levels (Pudney & Shields 2000).

From the evidence it is clear that workforce flexibility in the healthcare workplace is a major issue to be resolved, yet there is no agreement on what workforce flexibility means in practice, who benefits and how it is to be achieved. In 2004 the Council of Australian Governments commissioned research to examine issues that impact on the ability of the healthcare workforce to ensure 'the continued delivery of quality healthcare over the next 10 years' (Productivity Commission 2005:iv). The research undertaken by the Productivity Commission argued that a major objective was to develop 'a more sustainable and responsive workforce while maintaining a commitment to high-quality and safe health outcomes'. The commission sought views and submissions from a wide range of stakeholders and concluded that while all Australian governments agreed that successful healthcare delivery depended on 'the commitment, care and professionalism of the Australian healthcare workforce', a range of challenges faced the sector in reaching this objective. Included were workforce shortages of health professionals particularly in rural and remote areas; an increasing demand for health workforce services; the sheer numbers of institutions, agencies and organisations involved in healthcare delivery; and the difficulties of measuring productivity in such a complex industry. Recommendations to address these challenges ranged from changes in professional training and accreditation to changes to items covered in the Medical Benefits Schedule and better evaluation of service delivery.

In practice, however, healthcare decision making takes place within a complex political arena and many of the commission's recommendations missed the mark. Healthcare occurs largely in an organisational context and the delivery of healthcare services therefore 'relies fundamentally upon the human capacity and capabilities of healthcare organisations to train, develop, deploy, manage and engage their workforce effectively' (Hyde et al 2006:2). This takes place within a highly political and often emotive industrial context and a complex web of powerful key stakeholders whose activities can impact directly on the organisation's ability to manage its staff effectively. These stakeholders include not only the already-identified professional associations and trade unions but also both federal and state governments that provide funding and policy direction and sometimes direct management and control, as well as vocal consumer organisations and lobby groups. The healthcare workforce is a major focus of change, but attempts to do so often fail because the power of stakeholders is underestimated or ignored. The goals, interests and philosophies of these stakeholders conflict as they struggle over limited resources. While the demand for healthcare services grows, the industry faces increasing resource pressures and the community expects efficient, effective, accountable and quality services.

> **Pause for reflection**
>
> Understanding the role of key stakeholders in healthcare is essential, particularly in the employment relations arena where the professional groups and trade unions come into their own. Who are the key stakeholders in healthcare and what are their main interests?

Employment relations in healthcare

Healthcare systems in both developed and developing countries have undergone significant reforms as governments search for more efficient and effective service delivery. As Rigoli & Dussault (2003:3) argue, while these reforms were intended to 'improve the efficiency, equity of access, and quality of public services in general', in practice much of the focus has been in reducing operating costs and cutting budget deficits. In the search for greater efficiencies, governments introduced a range of policies including decentralising services from central to local level, creating internal purchaser–provider markets, competitive tendering and contracting out of services, introducing performance contracts, pay decentralisation and performance-based pay, downsizing services and re-engineering processes. Yet until recently the impact that such policies had on the work of clinicians was largely ignored.

Understanding the role of government policy in shaping organisational strategy is crucial in the healthcare sector, especially in the employment relations arena, and in particular the way staff are remunerated and rewarded. An emerging issue over the past 25 years has been the level of centralisation of industrial relations and the relationship between pay and performance. In their comparison of the industrial relations systems of the UK, the US and Canada in the early 1980s, Adams et al (1982) concluded that the largely centralised National Health Service (NHS) in the UK was becoming more flexible at a local level and the largely decentralised systems of North America were becoming more centralised. They argued that 'although collective bargaining in the health sectors started off by being decentralised in North America and centralised in

Britain, both were moving towards a similar state of fairly centralised bargaining with accommodation of local needs' (Adams et al 1982:186). The reason for this streamlining tendency is often the centralised nature of funding. The initiatives of the UK Government in the 1990s to encourage local pay and conditions bargaining to link pay to performance in the NHS failed due partly to the political sensitivity of public services, and also because governments fund public health services and allowed hospitals limited flexibility to fund wage increases. In practice, time and energy were absorbed in negotiations over fairly small amounts of money as managers sought short-term reduction in their overall pay bill by imposing changes in work organisation and labour utilisation (Bach & Winchester 1994, Thornley 1998).

The Australian experience tells a similar story. In Australia the federal government has largely driven both workplace and health sector reform, although it is state governments that have responsibility for hospital services that employ the largest numbers of staff and account for the greatest expenditure (Willis et al 2005). State governments provide policy direction to their healthcare institutions and are the main sources of funding. They set wage policies for their publicly funded services and strive to contain those policies within certain limits (Stanton 2006). Hence, state governments' decisions about wage policy, funding priorities and employment relations have a direct impact on organisational policy and on hospital employees.

Most Australian state governments pursued similar strategies to improve the productivity and efficiency of their health systems throughout the 1990s. These strategies included budget cutbacks and financial restraint, introducing new forms of funding mostly based on output, such as casemix funding, and outsourcing and privatising services such as catering, cleaning, pathology and radiology (Willis et al 2005). At the same time, both state and federal governments pursued the decentralisation of industrial relations through a move away from centralised award-based industrial arrangements to introducing bargaining at the enterprise level (Stanton 2006). In comparing the introduction and experience of enterprise bargaining in the health sector in New South Wales, Victoria and South Australia, Bray et al (2005) found that despite the different political, legal and historical differences there were similarities. A change of government from Labor to Liberal Coalition in each state led to a period of decentralisation within a rhetoric of increased efficiency and productivity that shifted control of wages and conditions away from state-wide awards based on occupation to local employers. But in reality, although the agreements in each state were signed at the local level, they had been centrally bargained with the active intervention of state governments. The return of the Labor Party to government in each state marked a return to a more open process of centrally agreed but locally implemented enterprise agreements.

Bray et al (2005) suggest that there are three key reasons for centralised bargaining in the healthcare sector: state governments fund healthcare and there are significant cost considerations; trade unions and professional associations have used their industrial strength to keep the bargaining processes centralised; and the fact that the healthcare industry is politically sensitive means governments carry out large-scale reform at their peril. Stanton et al (2004) also found that employer groups favoured some aspects of centralisation, especially of wages, as local employers had few extra resources with which to bargain, and local wage bargaining in a centrally funded system became meaningless. Nonetheless, employers wanted more control over local concerns such as labour utilisation and human resource management initiatives.

It can be argued that any efficiency and productivity gains made during this period were due to the implementation of budget cuts, outsourcing, managerialism and output-based funding rather than bargaining. Indeed, according to some employers the trade unions used the enterprise bargaining process to 'claw back' some of the gains that employers had won through these other means. In other words, enterprise bargaining, despite the rhetoric, did not lead to efficiency and productivity gains (Stanton 2006).

> **Pause for reflection**
>
> Should governments try to influence change through industrial relations reform in healthcare? How does this impact on health professionals in the workplace and on patient care?

A more efficient and productive health workforce?

The major questions that emerge from this story so far are: What are the actual outcomes from all of this rhetoric and activity? Is the healthcare workforce more efficient and productive? What does this mean for staff at the workplace?

At one level it is possible to argue that there is evidence that the health sector is now more efficient and productive. For example, evidence from Australia shows that by 1996, fewer staff in Australian hospitals were treating significantly more people at a much higher rate of patient turnover and a declining rate of stay (AIHW 1998). In other words, we are getting more from less. However, even the Australian Productivity Commission warns against such simplistic measures of productivity in the healthcare sector arguing that much better data is needed before such claims can be made (Productivity Commission 2006).

Also, debates about efficiency and productivity are generally silent on the outcomes for staff. Harrison & Pollitt (1994) argue that changes in health and industrial relations policy in the UK weakened the 'market relations' of health professionals, i.e. their pay and conditions, and at the same time changes in 'managerial relations' in the workplace led to an increasing control of the day-to-day work of health professionals and a challenge to their professional autonomy. In Australia, evidence suggests that working conditions have undergone dramatic changes due to a range of factors of which enterprise bargaining was just one. A range of empirical studies link technological changes, rationalisation, budget cuts, outsourcing, privatisation and the introduction of output-based funding to job loss, work intensification and staffing shortages, complaints of greater stress levels and ill health and a decline in staff motivation and morale (Willis et al 2005).

Evidence also shows that health professionals have faced greater managerial control and scrutiny with increased levels of monitoring (White & Bray 2005, Willis & Weekes 2005) and anecdotal evidence suggests that many government departments have developed a tendency to 'micromanage' their healthcare agencies under the auspice of improved accountability. Similar stories in the UK have led health professionals to turn to their professions and unions for collective support and resistance (Harrison & Pollitt 1994). The same phenomenon has happened in Australia (Bartram et al 2007b), for example, the growth of the Australian Nursing Federation is due not only to the federation representing its members' interests by arguing for better wages and conditions, but also through gaining control over workload via nurse–patient ratios and other initiatives. The federation has also appealed to consumers by presenting itself as the defender of the quality of health service delivery.

What this story makes clear is that the strategies of workplace and health sector reform that focus on efficiency and productivity have contributed little to developing a sustainable and responsive workforce. Even if the industry is now more efficient and productive at one level, there has clearly been a downside. The evidence suggests that the international labour shortage problem has been exacerbated and workforce planning and recruitment and retention of all healthcare staff has become a major issue for governments and organisations. In Australia, there is little evidence to demonstrate any major gains in workforce flexibility through these processes, and responsiveness or engagement of professionals and clinicians in positive change. In fact, it has often been the opposite, as professionals turn to their industrial organisations and professions to enable them to dig in and defend the status quo, and in turn the professions appeal to the general community for support against uncaring governments only focused on the bottom line.

> **Pause for reflection**
>
> In terms of workforce flexibility there is little evidence that progress has been made through industrial processes; any changes that have been made have often been in spite of enterprise bargaining. What new approaches to managing the health sector workforce need to be explored in view of the increasing cost pressures in the sector?

A sustainable and responsive health workforce

The evidence so far suggests that the complex nature of the healthcare industry requires sophisticated and cooperative responses from key stakeholders. Focusing on industrial relations and managerialist solutions to complex problems exacerbates the tensions within the industry and between the key players leading to discord and division. So, is there another way to achieve a sustainable and responsive health workforce?

Internationally, increasing attention has been given to a more systematic approach to HRM as a vehicle to improve organisational performance (Becker & Huselid 2006, Bowen & Ostroff 2004). The link between good people management practice and improved organisational outcomes has been demonstrated in a range of industries. While there is no agreement on exactly what configuration of HRM practices contribute to improved performance, evidence suggests that a range of high performance practices can be identified. These include selective recruitment, appropriate reward and recognition, career and developmental opportunities, teamwork, and employee participation and involvement in decision making (Buchan 2004, Macky & Boxall 2007). Evidence suggests that such practices engage employees and lead to high workforce commitment and hence high performance.

While the measurement of performance in the healthcare industry is contentious (Buchan 2004, Harris et al 2007), studies in the healthcare sector in the US and in the UK have linked such positive people management practices to improved patient mortality in acute hospitals (Aitkin et al 2000, West et al 2002). Such evidence has led the UK government to explore more inclusive approaches to improving efficiency and effectiveness in the healthcare workforce and more attention has been given in exploring the potential of HRM to engage the workforce in change processes. The NHS's 'HR in the NHS Plan' (DoH 2002) aims to do this to 'achieve more people, working differently'. Its key objectives include making the NHS a model employer, ensuring that the NHS provides a model career path through offering a skills escalator, improving staff morale and building people management skills. A range of initiatives have been introduced including establishing the Leadership Centre and the NHS Institute for Innovation and Improvement, as well as developing performance standards for HRM and pay modernisation. All of these initiatives demonstrate that governments do have a role in putting people management centre stage and creating the conditions for organisational development in this key area.

In Australia, on the other hand, there has not been the same degree of focus on the promotion of improved people management practices as a solution to complex workforce problems. Stanton et al (2004) examined the institutional context of people management practices in the Victorian healthcare sector by interviewing trade union and government officials and employers, and found a lack of understanding of the potential of HRM in this people-rich, knowledge-based service industry. HRM was seen as an administrative function with no measurable links to improved care delivery and organisational performance. Importantly, they found a general lack of interest or ability to explore the value of HRM despite evidence of labour shortages and high labour turnover in the sector. Government interviewees saw HR as the responsibility of the hospitals and employers worried that putting more resources into people management would be seen by the community as taking resources away from patient care. Employers also saw no benefit in encouraging government to follow the UK approach and drive HR in their industry, fearing that this would lead to increased micromanagement by government departments and unrealistic performance contracts.

Yet despite this negativity, evidence demonstrates that HR can play a crucial role in organisational performance in healthcare and more managers and practitioners are becoming aware of this potential. Organisational research points to four critical success factors in HR-led reform that create the conditions for successfully managing clinicians and improved outcomes. These are:

- leadership and commitment from the senior management team
- building managerial skill at every level
- engaging employees and giving employees a 'voice' in decision making
- understanding and valuing performance.

Leadership and commitment

Bowen & Ostroff (2004) argue that strong HR systems have three key characteristics:

- distinctiveness – this includes the features of the HR system that capture the attention and interest of staff in organisational goals
- consistency of message – this includes establishing unambiguous cause and effect relationships between desired employee behaviour and associated employee and organisational performance outcomes
- consensus between decision makers or 'within group agreement' and fairness of HRM practices.

In any organisation it is the senior management team that plays the key role in defining the strength of the HR system. They do this by agreeing on desirable patterns of behaviour and outcomes and in transmitting clear and visible messages throughout the organisation. Studying the cultural characteristics in high- and low-performing hospitals, Mannion et al (2005) found a strong relationship between hospital leadership and hospital performance. Those organisations that demonstrated clear accountability and information systems, developed HR policies and engaged in proactive external relationships tended to be high performers. Similarly in a study of three rural hospitals Young et al (2007) found that the role of the CEO in building a senior management team that valued the role of HR and embedded HR processes throughout the managerial hierarchy was crucial in engaging managers and employees and creating a high-performing workplace.

Governments can also have a role in creating effective organisational leadership. The introduction of a leadership development program within the NHS aimed to raise the profile of HR by developing HR professionals as full members of the team charged with building capacity and delivering change. The program aimed to embed a consistently high level of managerial skill across the NHS, combine academic knowledge with practical insight and develop an understanding of the needs and development of the NHS. An evaluation of the leadership development program in the UK found that it both raised the profile of HR in the NHS and had a positive focus on both individual and organisational development (Boaden 2006).

Building managerial skill at every level

All the evidence shows that good HR policies and practices, while essential, are only one component of high performance. It is also necessary to have managers who can understand and interpret these practices fairly and consistently and can build commitment within their teams. Hence building people management skills at all levels of management can have direct benefits for organisations if done well. This is particularly true in the healthcare sector where so much of the work takes place in multidisciplinary teams and clinicians have a certain amount of autonomy and independence. It is often the individual manager who makes the difference between a high-performing and a low-performing team.

Research shows that managers are often prepared to take a prominent role in HR functions such as selecting and developing staff and to share responsibility in areas such as equal opportunity, occupational health and safety, employee assistance and welfare, however they are not so keen on the time-consuming job of maintaining records (McConville & Holden 1999, Young et al 2007). Managers in the healthcare sector often experience high workloads, lack awareness of the source of HR policy and of strategic goals, and are not always aware of what is available to them in terms of advisory services from HR. Managers also experience pressure from both ends – from their employees and their superiors – and they are often held accountable for the outcomes of decisions that were made without their input, and for the activities and attitudes of their staff. McConville & Holden (1999) found that even though managers were willing to take responsibility for HRM, they often lacked financial, human and strategic resources to do so. Clearly the commitment of the leadership team to the engagement, training and support of managers at every level is central in developing good people management processes (Young et al 2007).

Employee participation in decision making

Closely linked to managerial skill is the concept of employee participation in decision making; the themes of collaboration, involvement and employee voice consistently emerge as key issues in the discourse on workplace change within the health sector. Participation can be defined as anything from an employee suggestion scheme to employee consultation committees and is usually seen as an important component of employee engagement and consequent high performance (O'Donoghue et al 2005). In healthcare, clinical governance can also be seen as a form of employee participation and Iedema et al's (2005) exploration of clinical governance as a mechanism of change indicates that a collaborative approach to leadership, teamwork, patient focus, changing culture and self-management is preferable to one based on monitoring, inspection and control. There is no doubt that employee participation is a key element in building commitment.

The literature on employee participation in decision making stresses the importance of management support, adequate resources and the perception of benefit if it is to work well (O'Donoghue et al 2005). However, even though many health sector managers, while in theory, might see employee participation as 'a good thing', in practice it can be seen to be time consuming and resource intensive, and the reality does not always match the rhetoric. Government can provide resources and training to support employers to engage with employees in a spirit of collaboration to improve the provision of healthcare services for both staff and consumers. In practice, however, government directions often require organisations to make quick reactive responses to change that are not conducive to building a climate of trust and collaboration necessary for real employee involvement in decision making.

Understanding and valuing high performance

Finally, an important but contentious area is the understanding, measurement and evaluation of HRM outcomes and the links to organisational performance. Performance management is often seen in a negative light as it appears to suggest monitoring and control and sometimes even punishment. Yet the evidence shows that organisations that collect, monitor, evaluate and feed back their performance data are able to identify and reward areas of good practice and fix up areas that need attention. The first issue here is that organisations actually do need to collect and utilise the data. Bartram et al (2007a) found that Victorian hospitals primarily monitored financial and volume indicators with little evidence of effective systems in place to benchmark or integrate performance management of employees. They also found a lack of consistency in measuring HRM outcomes such as labour turnover, sickness and absenteeism making it difficult to benchmark some items across the sector. However, they also discovered that a number of organisations did measure their HR outcomes and in a number of these organisations there were positive associations between espoused HRM practices and HRM outcomes (Bartram et al 2007a). In other words, organisations that claimed to have good people management practices and collected and analysed the indicators that proved this, such as lower rates of turnover, low staff vacancy levels, and low rates of sickness, absenteeism, accidents, industrial disputes and grievances, were able to demonstrate the relevance of HR and its contribution to their overall organisational outcomes.

The second issue here is ownership of the data and senior managers taking the lead rather than government forcing measurement on them. For example in the UK a focus on performance rating for HRM in the NHS, while intended to increase public awareness of quality of healthcare provision and improve standards of performance, was perceived by HR managers as a burden rather than a measure of good organisational performance. Givan (2005) found that meaningful comparison of performance depends on the availability of accurate data collected in a fair and transparent way and in the NHS the HR directors had no confidence in the quality of the data used to create the ratings and only trusted the results when they had been consulted directly rather than through a top-down collection of performance data. Managers felt that government was not responsive to their concerns and there was a general lack of consultation. HR managers wanted to have some ownership of the process at the organisational level. As with clinicians, these findings suggest that managers prefer to be included in decision making rather than having standards imposed upon them and then monitored for compliance. However, collecting such data is crucial if organisations are to know whether their people management practices are working well.

The third issue is valuing the data and recognising the contribution that good people management practices can make to organisational outcomes. The performance management system in the NHS has since been superseded by the 'Annual Health Check' comprising standards that include HR indicators. These standards measure hospital performance on a range of issues including 'the extent to which they support and recognise their staff contribution via personal development plans, appropriate recruitment, mandatory training and further professional development' (Harris et al 2007:453). However, the thrust of the new approach is to encourage local autonomy and flexibility, recognising the value of tailoring HR practices to suit local circumstances. All the evidence suggests that for this approach to be successful, leadership and commitment at every level is essential, and leaders need the skills and abilities to engage with their staff in order to encourage attitudes and patterns of behaviour that lead to excellent patient care.

Box 3.1 Leadership in practice – a tale of three case studies

Between 2004 and 2007 researchers in the Faculty of Law and Management and School of Public Health at Melbourne's La Trobe University explored HRM systems in three case study hospitals in Victoria. Two of the hospitals were identified as high performing and one low performing. The criteria used were financial targets, throughput, quality and industrial relations reputation. The study aimed to identify links between HRM and organisational performance in healthcare and focused on each organisation's HRM system's link to organisational strategy, the understanding, interpretation and operationalisation of HRM across the management hierarchy, and the measurement of HRM and linkage to organisational effectiveness. The study found that the clear differentiator between the high-performing and the low-performing hospitals was the leadership provided by the CEO. In particular, in each case study site the CEO's understanding and commitment to HR was crucial in terms of overall effectiveness. It was the CEO who gave HR legitimacy, provided leadership in making things happen, committed resources and provided the links between organisational strategy and HR strategy. In the two high-performing organisations, the researchers found clear evidence of CEO commitment and leadership in linking HR systems and organisational effectiveness. In the low performer, they found lack of support and understanding of the value of HR by the CEO.

The researchers also found that within-group agreement at the executive level and between-group agreement throughout the organisational hierarchy was also crucial. Again the role of the CEO in providing the leadership and gaining commitment for good people management practices throughout the organisation was essential. In the low-performing case study hospital there was a lack of within-group agreement at the senior executive level and there were confused and inconsistent messages across hierarchical layers, resulting in between-group inconsistencies on HR issues, perceptions of lack of fairness and trust, and confusion among lower level managers about desirable organisational behaviour and outcomes. This confusion led to managers spending valuable time reacting to staff grievances and industrial relations problems. In the high-performing organisations, the HRM system was seen as legitimate with strong senior management support and was highly visible, understandable and relevant to operational managers. Hence, there was more agreement on desirable behaviour and less time spent reacting to problems.

The researchers also found that the role of managers at all levels of the organisational hierarchy in operationalising HRM was crucial. The further away managers were from the strategy makers the more challenging it was to keep them informed, engaged and empowered, particularly in large and complex organisations. One of the high-performing hospitals put emphasis on resourcing lower level managers in time, knowledge and information in order to effectively and consistently translate strategy into practice. The executive team in this organisation recognised that information flows between and across hierarchical levels is imperative to ensure that silos, blockages and information overload do not occur. Such blockages impact on validity, consensus and consistency, and the larger and more complex the organisation the more difficult this is to achieve. Overall the message from these case studies was clear: good people management practices that improve organisational effectiveness can only be enacted with strong leadership and support from the top.

> **Box 3.2** Implications for practice – The human side of managing clinical processes
>
> It is clear that managers and clinicians have a key role in improving health service outcomes and creating change by building, managing and contributing to effective and collaborative teams.
>
> If you are a manager, what are the major skills and abilities you need to lead your team successfully?
>
> If you are a clinician, how can you play a constructive role in making your team a high-performing team?

Conclusion

This chapter has identified some of the key challenges facing the Australian healthcare sector if it is to develop a flexible and responsive workforce that provides high-quality healthcare services. These challenges concern engaging with the size, cost, strength and disparate nature of the workforce; the powerful stakeholder presence of government; and the political nature of the industry. In this context, there are difficulties in trying to re-direct management practice in organisations that are inextricably linked to a wider complex web of regulations, relationships and restrictions. These structural constraints impinge directly on management practice. While the evidence shows that the institutional framework can drive change, it is not always in the right direction and the impact on the organisation is varied, particularly where key stakeholders resist change.

The way of the future must surely be to engage stakeholders, specifically clinicians and managers at every level. While not always so easy at the macro level, there are clearly possibilities to do this strategically at the local level through positive HRM systems that illuminate, reward and encourage behaviour that leads to high-quality and responsive patient care. Organisational research points to the fact that action at the local level is more likely to succeed. However, to carry out policies that focus on long-term strategic development and staff engagement requires not only managerial commitment but also time, ability and resources that enable senior managers to focus on the future rather than just reacting to present circumstance. In reality, healthcare executives spend much of their time reacting to the vagaries of government policy and the responses of key stakeholders than in strategic organisational management. A key challenge for government is to create a set of conditions that encourage and nurture new initiatives that allow healthcare organisations to become truly high performing.

References

Adams G, Beatty D, Gunderson M 1982 Structural Issues of Centralised Bargaining in Health Services: Canada, USA and UK. In: Sethi A, Dimock S (eds) Industrial Relations and Health Services. Croome Helm Ltd, London

Aitken L H, Havens D S, Sloane D M 2000 The magnet nursing services recognition program: A comparison of two groups of magnet hospitals. The American Journal of Nursing 100(3):26–36

Allan C 1998 Stabilising the Non-Standard Workforce: Managing Labour Utilisation in Private Hospitals. Labour and Industry 8(3):61–76

Australian Institute of Health and Welfare 1998 Australia's Health 1998. Australian Institute of Health and Welfare, Canberra

Australian Institute of Health and Welfare 2004 Australia's Health 2004. Australian Institute of Health and Welfare, Canberra

Bach S 2001 HR and new approaches to public sector management: improving HRM capacity. Workshop on Global Health Workforce Strategy. World Health Organisation

Bach S Winchester D 1994 Opting Out of Pay Devolution? The Prospects for Local Pay Bargaining in UK Public Services. British Journal of Industrial Relations 32(2):264–82

Bartram T, Stanton P, Leggat S et al 2007a Lost in translation: exploring the link between HRM and performance in healthcare. Human Resource Management Journal 17:21–41

Bartram T, Stanton P, Harbridge R 2007b Protecting the Individual, the Profession and the Quality of Health Services: union growth in nursing. In: Buttigeig D, Cockfield S, Cooney R, Jerrard M, Rainne A (eds) Trade Unions in the Community: Values, Issues, Shared interests and Alliances. Heidelberg Press, Melbourne

Becker B, Huselid M 2006 Strategic Human Resource Management: Where do we go from Here? Journal of Management 32(6):898–925

Boaden R 2006 Leadership development: does it make a difference? Leadership and Organisation Development Journal 27(1):5–27

Bowen D, Ostroff C 2004 Understanding HRM-Firm Performance Linkages: The Role of the 'Strength' of the HRM system. Academy of Management Review 29(2):203–221

Bray M, Stanton P, Willis E et al 2005 The Structure of Bargaining in Public Hospitals in Three Australian States. In: Stanton P, Willis E, Young S (eds) 2005 Workplace Reform in the Healthcare Industry: the Australian Experience. Palgrave Macmillan, Basingstoke

Breda K 1997 Professional Nurses in Unions: Working together pays off. Journal of Professional Nursing (3) March/April: 99–109

Bremner J, Kelly R 2000 The Medical Scientists Association Of Victoria. Unions 2000: Retrospect and Prospect Conference. Monash University, Melbourne

Buchan J 2004 What difference does ('good') HRM make? Human Resources for Health 2 (6) http://www.human-resources-health.com/content/2/1/6

Cregan R, Duffield C, Forrester K 2003 Casualisation of the nursing workforce in Australia: driving forces and implications. Australian Health Review 26(1):201–208

Department of Health 2002 HR in the NHS – More Staff Working Differently. National Health Service, London

Diallo K, Zurn P, Gupta N et al 2003 Monitoring and evaluation of human resources for health: an international perspective. Human Resources for Health 1(3) http://www.human-resources-health.com/content/1/13

Duckett S 2005 The Australian Healthcare Workforce. In: Stanton P, Willis E, Young S Workplace Reform in the Healthcare Industry: the Australian Experience. Palgrave Macmillan, Basingstoke

Freidson E 1970 Profession of Medicine. Harper and Row. New York

Givan R K 2005 Seeing stars: human resource performance indicators in the National Health Service. Personnel Review 34(6):634–647

Gunderson M 1982 Health Sector Labour Market: Canada, USA and UK. In: Sethi A S, Dimock S (eds) 1982 Industrial Relations and Health Services. Croome Helm Ltd, London

Harris C, Cortvriend P, Hyde P 2007 Human resource management and performance in healthcare organizations. Journal of Health Organization and Management 21(4/5):448–459

Harrison S, Pollitt C 1994 Controlling Health Professionals. Open University Press, Buckingham

Hunter D 1996 The Changing Roles of Healthcare Personnel in Health and Healthcare Management. Social Science & Medicine 43(5):799–808

Hyde P, Boaden R, Cortvriend P et al 2006 Improving Health through Human Resource Management: mapping the territory. Research Report, CIPD, London

Iedema R, Braithwaite J, Jorm C et al 2005 Clinical Governance: Complexities and Promises. In: Stanton P, Willis E, Young S (eds) 2005 Workplace Reform in the Healthcare Industry: the Australian Experience. Palgrave Macmillan, Basingstoke

Kabene S, Orchard C, Howard J et al 2006 The importance of human resource management in healthcare: a global context. Human Resources for Health 4(20) http://www.human-resources-health.com/content/4/1/20

Lumley C, Stanton P, Bartram T 2004 Casualisation: friend or foe. New Zealand Journal of Employment Relations 29(2):33–48

Macky K, Boxall P 2007 The Relationship Between 'High Performance Work Practices' and Employee Attitudes: an investigation of additive and interaction effects. International Journal of Human Resource Management 18(4):537–567

Mannion R, Davies H T O, Marshall M N 2005 Cultural characteristics of 'high' and 'low' performing hospitals. Journal of Health Organisation and Management 19(6):431–439

McConville T, Holden L 1999 The filling in the sandwich: HRM and middle managers in the health sector. Personnel Review 28(5/6):406–424

McCoppin B, Gardner H 1994 Tradition and Reality: Nursing and Politics in Australia. Churchill Livingstone, Melbourne

O'Donoghue P, Stanton P, Bartram T 2005 Employee Participation in Victorian Health Services: The Rhetoric and the Reality. Employment Relations Record 4(1):67–80

Perkins R, Petrie K, Alley P et al 1997 Health Service Reform: The Perceptions of Medical Specialists in Australia (New South Wales), the United Kingdom and New Zealand. Medical Journal of Australia 167(18th August):201–204

Productivity Commission 2005 Australia's Health Workforce. Research Report Canberra

Pudney S, Shields M 2000 Gender and Racial Discrimination in Pay and Promotion for Nurses. Oxford Bulletin of Economics and Statistics. 62, Special Issue: 801–826

Rigoli F, Dussault G 2003 The interface between health sector reform and human resources in health. Human Resources for Health 1(9) http://www.human-resources-health.com/content/1/1/9

Stanton P 2006 Industrial Relations in the Public Hospital Sector. In Bray M, Waring P Evolving Industrial Relations. McGraw Hill, North Ryde

Stanton P, Bartram T, Harbridge R 2004 HRM practices in the public health sector: Lessons from Victoria, Australia. Journal of European Industrial Training 28(2/3/4):310–328

Thornley C 1998 Contesting Local Pay: the decentralisation of collective bargaining in the NHS. British Journal of Industrial Relations 36(3):413–434

West M, Borril, C, Dawson J et al 2002 The link between the management of employees and patient mortality in acute hospitals. International Journal of Human Resource Management 13(8):1299–1310

White, N, Bray M 2005 The Processes of Workplace Change for Nurses in NSW Public Hospitals. In: Stanton P, Willis E, Young S (eds) Workplace Reform in the Healthcare Industry: the Australian Experience. Palgrave Macmillan, Basingstoke

Willis E, Young S, Stanton P 2005 Health Sector Reform and Industrial Reform in Australia. In: Stanton P, Willis E, Young S (eds) Workplace Reform in the Healthcare Industry: the Australian Experience. Palgrave Macmillan, Basingstoke

Willis E, Weekes K 2005 Work Intensification for Personal Care Attendants and Medical Scientists In: Stanton P, Willis E, Young S (eds) Workplace Reform in the Healthcare Industry: the Australian Experience. Palgrave Macmillan, Basingstoke

Wilson L, Goldschmidt P 1995 Quality Management in Healthcare. McGraw Hill, Sydney

Young S, Stanton P, Leggat S et al 2007 The HR Department and Line Managers: roles, responsibilities and resources. Current management thinking: drawing from the Social Sciences and Humanities to address contemporary challenges. EURAM Conference Paris May 2007

PART 2

The operational environment

Managing clinical processes is based on having methods in place to do so. Transforming health services involves moving from a craft-based approach to healthcare delivery, to a production system grounded in systematising and standardising components of care around core services based on common clinical case types. Particular tools and processes are therefore important in organising and managing healthcare as a production system, recognising that managing healthcare is a multifaceted endeavour, including technical, social and organisational factors. If performance is a collective and collaborative process, methods are needed to coordinate purposeful activity among all those involved in it. What type of new skills will be required to manage this new system? What incentives will motivate people to engage in the type and extent of change envisaged?

In this respect, the relationship between evidence and practice is a key one in health, and relates not only to evidence on which clinical outcomes can be judged in relation to treatment, but also evidence on which organisational outcomes can be judged based on managing clinical processes. Here the question is: What types of tools and techniques are appropriate and effective in finding evidence of what works and applying the evidence? Relatedly, the question also becomes: How can the disparate, complex and diverse activities in health be organised among multidisciplinary clinicians and managers to ensure application of evidence and good patient outcomes? The contested issue of rules also arises in health, constituted as it is by clinical caregivers with a high degree of clinical autonomy expressed as freedom of decision making. Healthcare is a social process and rules are important to manage behaviour, expectations and outcomes. What rules are appropriate? Who should make them? Who should abide by them? When can they be broken?

Teams are being positioned as the vehicle that produces and delivers healthcare, constituted by multidisciplinary clinicians with a range of different knowledge and expertise about health and healthcare. While teams are not a new concept, their current manifestation in healthcare is, as the place of individual professions in the healthcare environment changes and a more democratic approach to decision making emerges. This new direction in healthcare is important not only for effectiveness, but also for recognising that healthcare is co-produced and placing patients and families at the centre of care. Even though strongly promoted, teams are also problematic in terms of their dispersed accountability and different levels of skill and remuneration, as well as the interpersonal aspects of team functioning. What types of attributes are associated with high-performing teams and how can they be fostered in an environment strongly characterised by clinical autonomy?

In the following chapters we discuss different ways in which health care is 'produced' and organised, the continuity of care, the organisation of care, the place of multidisciplinary team care in healthcare production and the importance of consumer participation in healthcare decision making.

Chapter 4

Producing health

Tanya Claridge & Gary Cook

Introduction

Healthcare economies worldwide are subject to the pressure of rapid advancements and adoption of new technologies and treatments. This is just one of myriad pressures on the health system, that include changing demographics and organisational cultures, increasing demands on system performance and concerns about the quality, safety and sustainability of the care received by patients. As a result the traditional 'push' or 'individual practitioner'-led delivery of healthcare has become outmoded over the past two decades, overtaken by a significant shift to healthcare being delivered as a 'pull' or 'population based', co-produced healthcare system.

This chapter discusses the characteristics and use of clinical pathways as commonly used tools in healthcare delivery to organise and manage, sometimes previously tacit, clinical processes into a more seamless and patient-oriented production system. Care is organised around clinical case types, for example patients with chronic obstructive airways disease; thus the 'pull' rather than the 'push' philosophy embodied within clinical pathways means that the production system is defined by the evidence-based needs and the expectations of the patient population instead of the 'push' from the healthcare system. Clinical pathways contribute to the production system by integrating low-tech patient-related activities with healthcare technology, information technology and social and management practices. Well-designed clinical pathways have the potential to reduce or eliminate wasted time, money and energy in healthcare, contributing to systems that produce safe, efficient, effective, and continuously improving and responsive healthcare.

From push to pull – moving from individual practitioner-based care to a co-produced service

Healthcare as a system

An evolution has occurred in the understanding of and emphasis given to the provision of healthcare. This evolutionary change shifts healthcare from an individually orientated pattern (with rudimentary batching and queuing of patients with different treatment needs grouped in 'individual silos') of delivery (see Figure 4.1), to one of a multidisciplinary systems-orientated pattern of patients grouped by similar conditions, treatments or healthcare needs (Figure 4.2). This evolution relates to the conceptualisation of healthcare as an industry comprised of complex systems and subsystems of healthcare organisation and delivery that incorporate dynamic and goal-orientated processes. In the first model, each different service manages a variation as if it were unique to each process and each (differently shaped) patient with little generalisation to similar patients or processes. In the second, variations are managed for populations of patients that stabilises the process, integrates the change and applies it to all subsequent patients treated for that particular case type (same shape).

Figure 4.1 Individual practitioner-orientated healthcare delivery

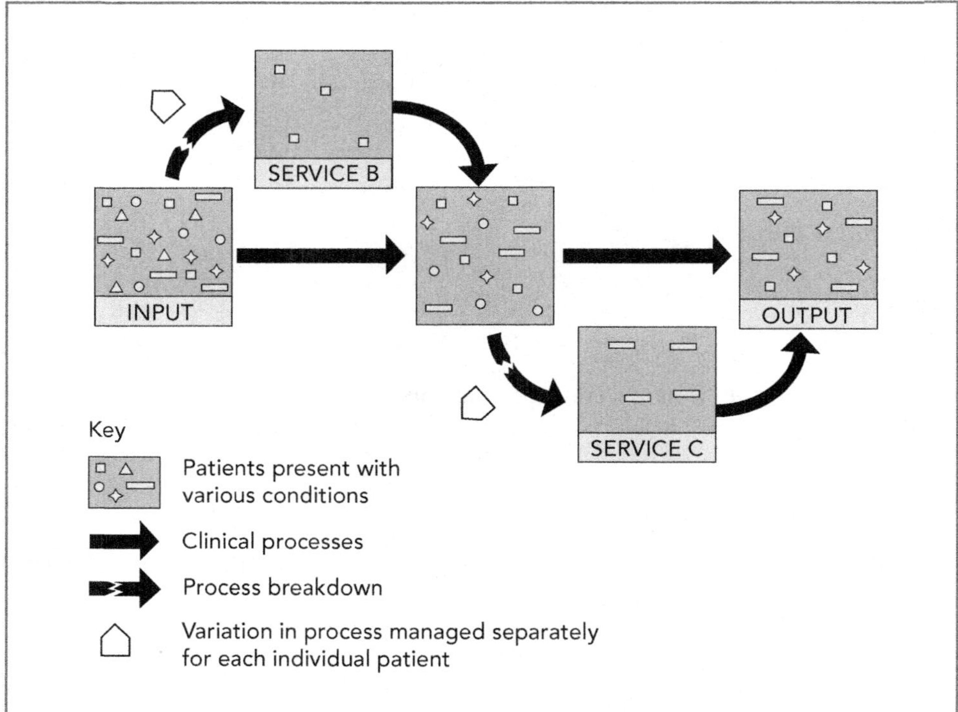

In this context, healthcare delivery should be viewed as transdisciplinary and integrative. This conceptualisation of healthcare is underpinned by the assumption that reducing or removing a process from the whole system reduces the system's overall effectiveness. This view stresses the interdependence between groups of individuals, structures and processes that enable the organisation to function and hence to result in a 'co-produced' service. Primacy is given to these interrelationships, and not, as with more traditional models of healthcare delivery (that centre on the effectiveness of individual practitioners, structures and departments), to the separate elements of the system.

All systems are determined by their inputs, outputs, processes, feedback and control mechanisms and environmental factors. This chapter explores how and why management of clinical processes within a healthcare system is needed to 'produce health', in terms both of improving process flow and of managing process variation.

Figure 4.2 Population-based systems-orientated healthcare delivery

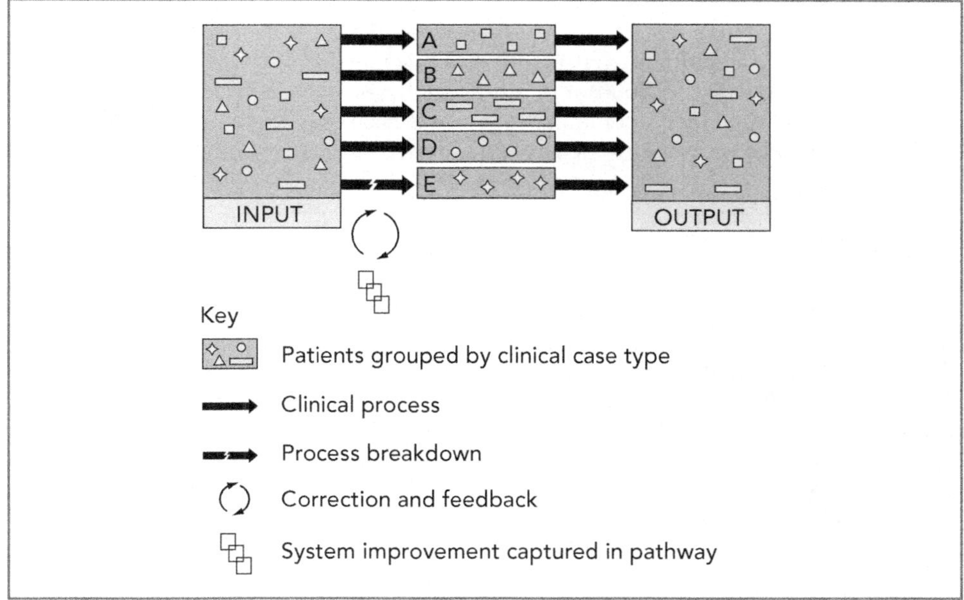

Why manage clinical processes?

The development of organisational capability to deliver sustainable, accountable, patient-focused and quality-assured, safe healthcare is the aim of healthcare systems and organisations worldwide (Nicholls et al 2000, WHO 2000). However the context of healthcare delivery is complex and healthcare systems are subject to myriad pressures. These pressures include:

- changing patterns of supply and demand (Frankel et al 2000)
- the cost of innovation
- changing organisational structures
- patient and public expectations
- the diverse and complex nature of healthcare delivery.

At its simplest, clinical process management enables healthcare organisations to respond to these pressures by putting procedures in place to ensure individual practitioners/teams or services execute critical activities required to concurrently measure, improve or sustain the productivity, quality (Lilford et al 2007) and safety of care and guarantee a level of control to best manage and evaluate the system. Process management in any system can involve managing the 'flow', managing any variance in the process or both.

Managing process flow – lean thinking

The flow of work through healthcare systems is complex and costly, although the actual work involved is often routine. By delineating, standardising, synchronising and managing every step in the process of healthcare delivery, both in patient-focused systems and in wider networks of care (Keen et al 2006), the work can flow in line with actual demand. This is the premise of 'lean thinking'. Lean thinking is not currently widely associated with healthcare organisations though the encouraging results produced in a variety of sectors all round the world have generated interest in the healthcare community (Institute of Health Care Improvement 2005). While the ideology was developed in Japanese manufacturing (Eisert 2006) it is just as applicable in healthcare, where waste (of time, money and supplies) is common, as it provides an opportunity to increase productivity, reduce waiting times, lower costs and improve services by improving processes.

Managing process variance – critical pathways

Critical Path Method (CPM) or Critical Path Analysis was developed in the 1950s for managing maintenance projects (DuPont Corporation and Remington Rand Corporation) and formalised within social science in the 1960s (Lucas 2001). It is now commonly used with many forms of projects that involve concurrent interdependent activities in diverse sectors including construction, research and engineering. CPM is essentially an algorithmic method for scheduling project activities. It produces, in diagrammatic form, the longest path of planned activities to the end of a project, the process of development determining both 'critical activities' and those that have 'total float' (i.e. can be delayed without making the project longer). Thus project managers can either prioritise actions to ensure the project is completed effectively, 'fast track' (by performing more activities concurrently) or direct resources (e.g. staff or equipment) to the critical path from activities that have 'total float'. This is known as 'crashing the critical path'.

Critical pathways are administrative models with close links to CPM, utilised in industry (Industrial Engineering 1992, Kallo 1996) as tools to improve the efficacy of production by streamlining work processes (Every et al 2000). Any variance on a production line in industry will have an effect on its efficacy. Using critical pathways to define and time processes enables the identification of problematic areas, the measurement of any variation and hence allows improvements to be made.

Identifying clinical processes

In order for clinical processes to be managed within the production systems of a health organisation they have to be identified. This is usually done by identifying the processes that support different 'core services'. A core service of a healthcare organisation could be as generic as a patient appointment with a doctor. However if considered in the context of population-based healthcare, a core service of a healthcare organisation would be the provision of care for patients based on clinical case types. This approach to identifying 'core population-based services' of health organisations is just as relevant to primary care services as it is to secondary and tertiary care. Examples of some core services offered by healthcare organisations can be found in Table 4.1.

Pause for reflection

Healthcare economies are subject to multiple pressures including rapid technological advances, changing demographics and concerns about the quality and safety of the care received by patients. In response to these pressures there has been a shift from individual practitioner-led healthcare delivery to the co-production of care using a population-based systems approach that incorporates dynamic and goal-orientated processes. Process management techniques allow the management of flow, management of variance or management of both thus increasing standardisation and predictability within the system. Why is this important in managing healthcare?

Table 4.1 Some core population-based services of healthcare systems

Core product	Example
Assessment	of the psychosocial wellbeing of women in the early postnatal period (Yelland et al 2007)
Education	of caregivers of patients with dementia (Kazui et al 2004)
Surgery	Total joint replacement (Ho & Huo 2007, Saufl et al 2007) Oesophagectomy (Low et al 2007)
Prevention	of primary bacteraemia (Juan-Torres & Harbarth 2007)
Diagnosis and treatment	of septic arthiritis (Merino Muñoz et al 2007)
Support and signposting	of pregnant teenagers (Logsdon & Koniak-Griffin 2005)
Multidisciplinary identification and treatment	of distress in palliative care (Vitek et al 2007)
Public health	Preventive dental care (Tay et al 2006)
Management	of the technology-dependant child in the community (see example later in chapter)

Managing clinical processes – protocol-based care

Developing and implementing rules is one of the most common ways to manage behaviour in complex organisations (Hopwood 1974) to promote the uptake of clinical management practices. Promoting both quality and safety is one area of organisational behaviour in which rules feature heavily. For instance, Reason's (1995) model of organisational safety indicates that rules, in the form of procedures, protocols and guidelines, are one of the principal defences necessary to ensure a safe organisation. In recent years there has been a proliferation of formal or semi-formal rules in healthcare worldwide, often in the form of policies, protocols, guidelines or clinical pathways in order to standardise and manage clinical processes both to improve the quality and measurability of healthcare systems and to try to ensure the safety of patients receiving care.

One of the key features of organised society is the development of a system of social rules and behavioural norms. The principal functions of such systems are to reflect societal and cultural values, and to safeguard things of value. Rules come in many different forms, including conventions, laws and social norms. Some are based on fundamental moral principles (it is wrong to commit murder), while others serve as a form of social control, proscribing antisocial behaviour (it is wrong to drop litter). Many rules exist purely in order to ensure that social affairs run smoothly. For example, driving on the right-hand side of the road is not intrinsically safer than driving on the left, but in many countries there is a rule (in this case, with the force of law) that all drivers will keep to the right. This rule has been imposed as a way of introducing standardisation and increasing predictability in a complex system.

Semi-formal and formal rules in various guises have been used for a number of years in all sectors of healthcare to regulate safety-critical ancillary processes (for instance storage of controlled and prescription drugs (Yee 1998) and hand washing (McCarthy et al 1999)). They have also been used with reference to clinical processes, for instance, guidelines on clinical technique and history taking are often presented in handbooks on clerking patients (Swash & Hutchinson 2001) and within the nursing process (Roper et al 1983).

However, in recent years healthcare policy worldwide has begun to focus on the use of rules embodied in clinical pathways as a way of managing both quality and safety.

The implementation of evidence-based medicine (EBM), the doctrine that professional clinical practice should be based on sound research evidence (Sackett et al 2000), is one area in which rules governing clinical processes have been used as a vehicle for improving quality. Previously, even when clinical effectiveness was supported by apparently rigorous evidence, this proved insufficient to produce related changes in practice. For example, Schuster et al (1998) postulated that 30–40% of patients do not get treatment of proven effectiveness and 20–25% patients get care that is not needed or is potentially harmful. In response to the slow pace of progress towards evidence-based practice (EBP), policy interest increased in the use of rules to promote it (Grol 2001). For instance, the UK National Health Service (NHS) Plan (Department of Health 2000:86) specified that 'by 2004 the majority of NHS staff will be working under agreed protocols' and that there will be 'a major drive to ensure that protocol-based care takes hold throughout the NHS'.

In terms of patient safety, there is also a move internationally towards using rules to regulate clinical processes and the behaviour of healthcare professionals (Kohn et al 2000). In 2002 the World Alliance for Patient Safety was formed and passed a resolution urging the World Health Organization to take the lead in developing global norms and standards. The assumption is that, as in other high-risk industries, patient safety can be improved by increasing standardisation and predictability in the system.

The drive for quality improvements, coupled with increased awareness of patient safety issues in recent years, has seen a proliferation of formal (active) or semi-formal (passive) rules, developed in order to standardise and manage the behaviour of healthcare professionals. The most common type of rule in healthcare is a protocol, which is essentially a set of instructions that can be formatted in a variety of different ways and used in many different clinical contexts.

Passive protocols (Coiera 2003) such as guidelines are semi-formal. They do not direct patient management, but provide guidance and add to the information resources available. Passive protocols are accessed or used at the discretion of the healthcare professional. In contrast, active or formal protocols (clinical pathways) are prescriptive, actively managing clinical processes. Active protocols are fundamentally different from passive protocols, in that they are central to the way the patient is managed, rather than an optional accessory. The way protocols are formatted also varies. Active protocols can be computer based and include alerts when there is deviation from the protocol (e.g. GP prescribing software). However, the majority of active protocols are paper based, allowing their effect on actual practice to be evaluated through audit of adherence and outcomes. Protocols in any format are seen by their exponents as 'tools that ensure service development is driven by evidence of clinical or cost effectiveness, for improving the safety of and consistency of care, and for coordinating health services' (Dillon & Hargadon 2003). In other words, protocols are tools that manage clinical processes within healthcare systems that should lead to improvements in the quality of care and in patient safety.

Managing clinical processes – clinical pathways

Clinical pathways (underpinned by an ideology similar to critical pathways described above) have been used worldwide (Hindle & Yazbeck 2005) for over a decade to systemise and support a process-centred vision of healthcare delivery. Clinical pathways have been variously known as anticipated recovery paths (ARPs), CareMaps®, multidisciplinary pathways of care (MPC), care protocols, integrated care management, pathways of care, care packages, collaborative care pathways, critical care pathways, care profiles and integrated care pathways. They are mass customisation disease- or symptom-specific case management plans that display goals for patients based on their clinical presentation and provide the sequence and timings of key elements of care based on EBM necessary to achieve these goals with optimal efficiency (Pearson et al 1995). They are generally conceptualised as vehicles for implementing collaboratively developed (multidisciplinary) care programs focused on population-based and patient-centred care. In theory fragmentation and duplication of care and treatment are therefore reduced, and coordination and communication are improved (De Bleser et al 2006, National Electronic Library for Health 2006).

Clinical pathways provide the opportunity to manage both clinical process flow and variance using lean thinking and critical pathway ideologies. They are developed by mapping and modelling clinical and non-clinical processes related to specific clinical case types or client groups. Opportunities for multidisciplinarity and skill mixing are identified based on roles, competencies and responsibilities rather than on individual disciplines alone. Both priorities and sequencing of actions are identified and processes and outcomes are incorporated (adapted from Venture Training 2005). The documentation – either paper or electronic – that supports the clinical pathway is designed to capture variations between the clinical processes planned and those experienced by the patient. The presence and implications of any variance can be analysed and assessed. Changes can then be made to the clinical process if necessary.

Clinical pathways and outcomes

Programs to develop and introduce clinical pathways aim to improve a range of clinical and financial parameters through decreased length of stay, preventing readmissions and reducing resource use (Vanounou et al 2007). There are few papers describing rigorous financial testing of clinical pathways. Those that are available tend to use algorithms to estimate savings based on the above objective process, throughput and outcome measures. Vanounou et al (2007) described a new model to evaluate the clinical and economic impact of clinical pathways. They used deviation-based cost modelling to determine the contribution of clinical pathway implementation itself to cost savings beyond usual secular trends in measuring improvements in care. The core product of the system involved in their study, a pancreaticoduodenectomy, was delivered using clinical processes that shortened length of stay, reduced resource use and decreased costs compared with before the clinical pathway was introduced. However, in a review of several case studies Lee & Anderson (2007) found that only one out of five clinical pathways implemented showed an association with a statistical significance in decreasing the length of stay. In another study an acute inpatient clinical pathway for psychosis and depression was trialled for a 12-month period and discontinued after it failed to demonstrate any improvement in terms of either clinical or financial parameters (Emmerson et al 2006). The authors suggested that the complexity, individuality and variability of mental disorders meant that clinical pathways were not beneficial in mental health settings.

It is difficult to establish whether or not all clinical pathways will have a direct impact on patient and/or financial outcomes. It may therefore be more important to explore the impact clinical pathways can have on clinical processes themselves. This involves ceasing dependence on inspecting clinical outcomes to achieve quality and eliminating the need for inspection on a mass basis by building quality into the process in the first place and monitoring the processes themselves (adapted from Deming 2000, Lilford et al 2007).

It is a natural assumption to make that a clinical pathway designed to delineate a pre-determined, evidence-based clinical process will have an effect on that process. It may also be reasonable to assume if the anticipated process is delivered to the expected standard then the desired outcomes will also be achieved. However, there are few tools available to assess how a clinical pathway influences clinical processes in the production of core healthcare services (Vanhaecht et al 2007). This may be due to a general lack of clarity about the concept of clinical pathways, but also related to the preoccupation of healthcare organisations with achieving financially motivated targets, for instance length of stay and readmissions. Vanhaecht et al (2007) have developed a care process self-evaluation tool designed to assess the organisation of the clinical processes embedded in an acute clinical pathway. The tool allows an assessment of the impact of a clinical pathway on clinical processes in terms of multiple domains including the coordination of care, cooperation with primary care and monitoring of the clinical process.

Clinical pathways are thus a potentially effective instrument in ensuring high-quality, effective and safe clinical processes because, in theory, they decrease process variability and improve process flow. This is because they are tools that can be used both at a macro level to delineate system design and integration and at a micro level to influence and regulate the behaviour of healthcare professionals at the patient care interface. The role of clinical pathways in ensuring effective clinical processes at these different levels of a system is discussed in more detail below.

Influencing system design – supporting patient focus and coordination of care

Developing a clinical pathway requires mapping the current state of the process critical to the delivery of the 'core service' under scrutiny (Hunter & Segrott 2007). This is often where 'lean thinking' can facilitate changes in the process to place the patient at the centre and to better coordinate care, removing unnecessary steps, even before the clinical pathway has been produced. Consider the case study in Box 4.1, and the diagrammatic representation in Figure 4.3.

Box 4.1 Case study – Product: provision of specialist equipment for technology-dependent children in the UK

In the UK, care and support for technology-dependent school-age children living at home and their carers is delivered by both multiple provider services operating within primary care trusts (e.g. health visiting, nutrition and dietetics, school nursing, equipment and adaptations) and external agencies (e.g. secondary care, tertiary care, social care and hospices). One of the core services required for this patient population is the needs assessment and provision of specialist equipment (for instance enteral feeding, airway management and continence supplies). Complaints from relatives of technology-dependent children and anecdotal information from healthcare professionals highlighted both the complexity and lack of accountability within the system. Mapping of the clinical and non-clinical processes for this core service revealed that time and resources were wasted on non-clinical processes and there was a lack of clarity about roles and responsibilities of practitioners within the system. Box 4.4 contains a diagrammatic representation of this original individual practitioner-led 'push' system. The time taken for new equipment to be ordered could take up to a month, causing potential delays to patient discharge from secondary care and distress and frustration to both the family of the patients and the healthcare professionals involved.

Figure 4.3 Clinical and non-clinical processes operating in order to provide specialist equipment to a technology-dependent child living at home in primary care in the UK

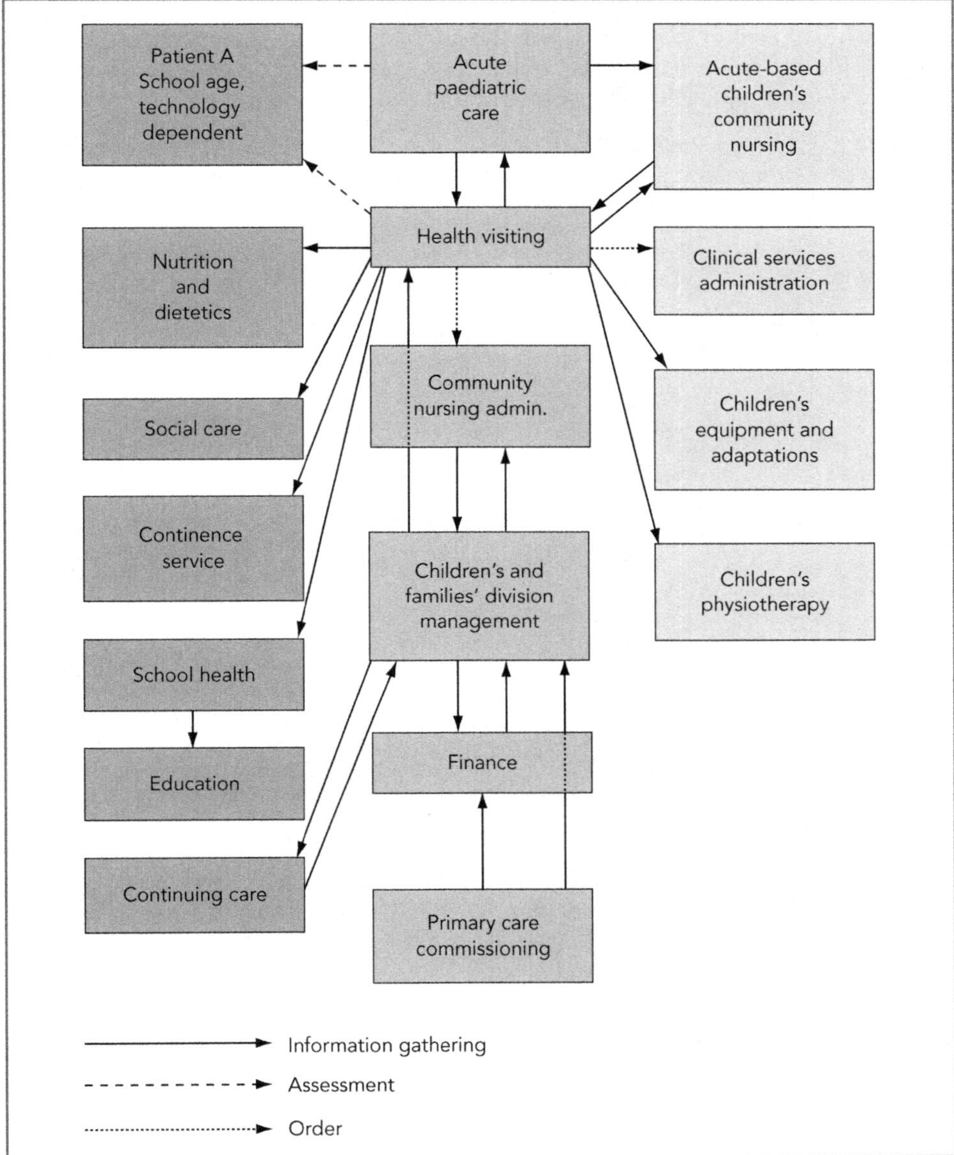

In the diagram above, it is clear that the clinical processes involved are complicated and dependent on a health visitor to assess (registered general nurse with an additional specialist community practitioner/public health qualification) even though the visitor has no day-to-day contact with the child (in the UK health visitors manage the child health surveillance and safeguarding of preschool children). The health visitor, with little or no expertise in the care of a technology-dependent child, has to consult with numerous other professionals and administrators. The health visitor also has no control over the equipment budget from which the cost of the order has to be met. Any order has to be agreed with senior managers and the finance department. Primary care trusts in the UK are divided into departments with a commissioning function and multiple discrete provider units (shaded boxes). There are few established communication systems and there is no clarity as to which provider unit should be commissioned to fund and provide the equipment for the child. Now consider the same process organised using a pathway approach in Figure 4.4.

Figure 4.4 Potential clinical and non-clinical processes supported by the development of a multi-agency clinical pathway needed to order specialist equipment for technology-dependent school-age child in primary care

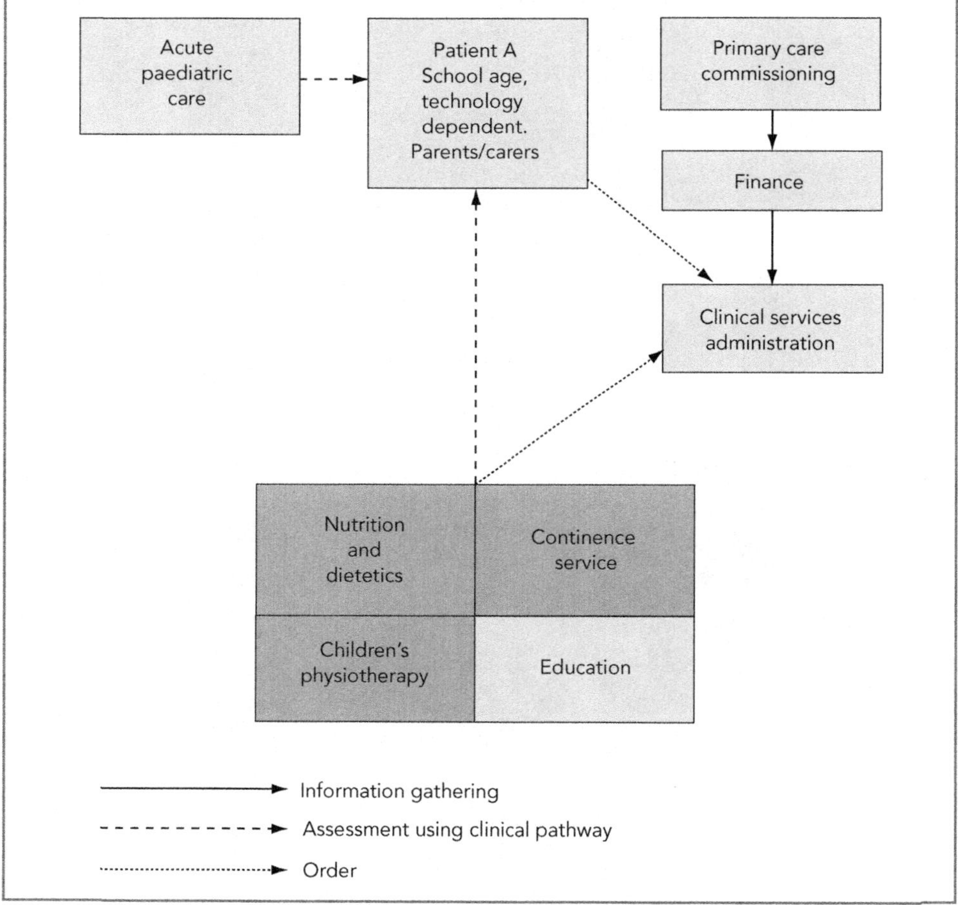

Figure 4.4 shows a visual representation of how the clinical and non-clinical processes could be refined by removing unnecessary steps and defining the 'critical path' essential to produce the core service. Delineating and structuring the clinical processes within a clinical pathway can facilitate the delegation of decision making about the provision of equipment to both healthcare professionals involved with the family and the family itself.

This case study provides examples of how managing clinical processes supported by a clinical pathway can rationalise systems of healthcare delivery, facilitate the involvement of patients/carers in decision making despite the population-based approach (Edwards & Elwyn 2001) and promote multidisciplinarity to ensure any service is co-produced.

Influencing system design – promoting multidisciplinarity

From the early 1980s it has been recognised that the complexity and demands of many tasks and decisions in healthcare are often too great for any individual to conceptualise and manage (Kahneman et al 1982). For this reason multidisciplinary teamworking is central to the performance of healthcare systems. Because of their ability to process large amounts of information, teams of healthcare professionals comprising members with different areas of expertise, skills and knowledge are now ubiquitous in medical contexts. However teams of healthcare professionals tend to be hierarchical with distributed expertise as well as distinguishing characteristics (Phillips 2001). Distributed expertise refers to the fact that team members differ in the type of information and expertise they contribute to the clinical process. Status differences can exist among the team members and decision responsibility may be distributed unequally among them.

The co-production of healthcare services from healthcare systems (i.e. those produced through transdisciplinary integrative clinical processes) is a goal that is therefore not easy to achieve in a healthcare context. There are numerous barriers to the changes needed to ensure optimum teamworking, ranging from clashes of personalities to occupational structures. Further, the way in which health professions are organised as vertical hierarchies is one of the barriers to effective teamworking (Mackay 1993). Professional boundaries can become barriers to innovation (Walby et al 1994) and they can also become a refuge when collaboration is difficult to achieve (Greenwell 1995).

Meta-analysis of participative decision making has shown that participation is generally related to greater satisfaction, motivation and task performance (Wagner & Gooding 1987) although some studies in the US have shown a fairly strong negative relationship (Phillips 2001). Phillips suggested that the mixed findings regarding the effectiveness of collaborative decision making may be due to the lack of attention paid to team performance in general. Effective collaboration between professional staff has long been recognised as essential to maximising possible health gain (Greenwell 1995) and is therefore axiomatic in enhancing the effectiveness of healthcare systems.

Mapping clinical processes illustrates the interactive and dynamic nature of healthcare systems. It is clear that to improve multidisciplinary collaboration, communication systems must play a central part in co-producing core services. These communication systems are diverse and include multiple, disparate non-electronic technologies (charts, telephones, patient records) and electronic technologies (electronic prescriptions, pathology reporting systems). Accurate and effective communication within and between services and professional teams involved in a clinical process is essential to achieving both efficiency and effectiveness.

Communimetric tools (Lyons 2006) are specifically designed to communicate the clinical process between healthcare professionals of different clinical backgrounds and allow the use of technology to support improved care. Introducing the electronic patient records is an international preoccupation that aims to facilitate this process of communication. However, a conceptual and representational view of the processes needs to be developed in order to fully understand existing clinical processes (Berg 1999) before such tools can be integrated into the clinical processes related to producing core health services. Healthcare systems are inherently complex and developing clinical pathways can contribute to this conceptual view by providing a multidisciplinary-representational model of low-tech patient-related activities integrated with healthcare technology, information technology, social conventions and management practices.

Influencing system design – clinical process monitoring

The analysis of valid criteria within clinical processes (derived from information contained within clinical pathways) can provide a sensitive, useful and cost-effective method of monitoring the quality of the system of healthcare delivery. Lilford et al (2007) identify four advantages that process measures have over outcome measures. These are:

1. the reduction of casemix bias by using the opportunity for clinical process error as the denominator (which is heightened with sicker patients) rather than number of patients being treated (Lilford et al 2007)
2. the focus on improving steps within clinical processes rather than labelling systems as failures; for instance, Read & Levy (2006) describe clinically important, positive impacts on clinical processes related to the assessment and care of patients who had suffered a stroke as a result of the implementation of a clinical pathway irrespective of whether those impacts affected outcomes such as mortality or length of stay
3. the multidisciplinarity of clinical processes and clinical pathways that result in applying multidisciplinary solutions to any problems, in turn resulting in wider action within the system; for example, Wolff et al (2004) used the assessment of compliance with key process measures, determined as best practice in stroke care to conclude that significant improvements in the quality of patient care could be made by incorporating multidisciplinary reminders and checklists about relevant clinical processes in a clinical pathway
4. clinical process monitoring that can contribute to the root cause analysis of delayed adverse events.

The findings of ongoing clinical process monitoring should also be able to contribute directly to, and provide structure for, risk management and other clinical governance activities within healthcare systems, enabling organisations to be 'scanning the horizon' for potential risks and deal with them in a proactive way (Kirk et al 2007).

Pause for reflection

Managing population-based clinical processes and developing clinical pathways are central to the planning, development and monitoring of healthcare, but also to delivering safe, effective care at the patient care interface.

While the actual mapping of clinical processes and the development of related clinical pathways may promote multidisciplinary working by creating an inclusive collaborative environment for developing healthcare systems and an opportunity to monitor the quality of care received by patients, unless the clinical pathways are used as they are designed the multidisciplinary working and the integrity of the clinical processes they support will not be sustained.

Why is it not sufficient to consider the co-production of health through healthcare systems (underpinned by clinical processes and supported by clinical pathways) purely in terms of the systems and system artefacts? Why is it essential to explore the potential impact of clinical pathways at a micro level (at the patient care interface)?

Managing clinical processes and provider behaviour

Most clinical care occurs within the context of the patient–provider interface and any effects of clinical process management are mediated through this interface. Provider behaviour is therefore one of the most proximal determinants of whether the clinical processes delineated in the clinical pathway are translated into practice. In order to develop a better theoretical understanding of professional behaviour it is essential to explore determinants of provider behaviour to better identify both modifiable and non-modifiable factors (Claridge 2006).

The presence of clinical pathways to manage clinical processes and to promote quality and safety in healthcare is not enough to ensure the quality and safety of care provided. Clinical pathways are essentially rules designed to influence and control behaviour. In order to have an effect the rules have to be followed. It is crucial that they are both understood and accepted by those expected to use them. It is also important to know whether the widespread non-compliance with guidelines that has been noted (Grol et al 1998) is the result of genuine error or of deliberate decisions on the part of the individual. This distinction between mistaken non-compliance (error) and deliberate non-compliance (violation) has been shown to be crucial in other contexts (Parker et al 1995) as they require different remediation.

Classifications of the determinants of rule-related behaviour have been developed and studied in a variety of settings, including driver behaviour (Parker et al 1995), in organisational terms (Reason et al 1998), in healthcare (Parker & Lawton 2003) and in communication (Shimanoff 1980) and are often closely related to theoretical considerations and investigation of human error. While a number of taxonomies of rule-related behaviour have been developed in diverse settings, striking similarities are evident. All include some element of deviation (Reason 2000, Senders & Moray 1991), although rule-related behaviour is generally seen as being controllable (Parker et al 1995, Shimanoff 1980) in that the agent is responsible for the behaviour and can either perform the behaviour or not. It is also often seen as criticisable (Parker et al 1995, Reason 2000, Shimanoff 1980). Evidence that supports the criticisability of the behaviour can be found in judgments of appropriateness, negative sanctions and repairs of deviations (Shimanoff 1980). Rule-related behaviour is therefore contextual, part of a behavioural pattern and connected with particular situations. Reason et al (1995) outline a way of classifying rule-related behaviour that focuses on ways in which people behave in relation to procedures, and on the outcome of such behaviour in terms of achievement of goals based on research into driving errors, driver violations and accident involvement (Parker et al 1995).

Unintentional non-compliant behaviour (error)

Human error has been defined as 'the failure of planned actions to achieve their desired outcome without the intervention of chance or unforeseeable agency' (Parker et al 1995:1036). Errors in healthcare have been described as 'the failure of a planned action to be completed as intended; or the use of a wrong plan to achieve an aim' (Kohn et al 2000:1). These definitions of human error allow a separation of two distinct types of error, namely:

- Slips or lapses that occur when the plan is adequate but the associated actions do not go as intended, i.e. they are skill based, and are thus failures of execution. Slips can be seen as relating to observable actions and can be correlated to attention failures. Lapses are internal events and relate to failures of memory (Reason 2000). An example of these errors could be connecting oxygen tubing to IV tubing or forgetting essential details of a patient's treatment at shift handover.

- Failures of intention (mistakes) that occur when the actions may go entirely as planned but the plan is inadequate to achieve its intended outcome, a rule is applied incorrectly or the actions do not achieve the intended outcome due to knowledge deficits.

Mistakes can be subdivided into rule-based mistakes and knowledge-based mistakes (Reason 2000). The implications here are that the failure occurs at a higher level in terms of the mental processes involved in an action, that is, the development, implementation and evaluation. Rule-based mistakes can occur when a person has some sort of pre-packaged solution to an issue, for instance in terms of training or guidelines. This gives rise to the error occurring in various forms such as the misapplication of a good rule (in the wrong circumstance), the application of a bad rule or the non-application of a good rule (Reason 1990). On the other hand, knowledge-based mistakes occur in novel situations where the solution has to be developed on the spot.

Reason (2000) reduced error-producing conditions to eight broad categories:

1. high workload
2. inadequate knowledge
3. ability or experience
4. poor interface design
5. inadequate supervision or instruction
6. stressful environment
7. mental state
8. change (major factor in absentminded slips of action) (Reason & Mycielska 1982).

Intentional non-compliant behaviour (violations)

Clinical pathways introduce procedures to regulate behaviour. Procedures introduced for this reason can give rise to a type of behaviour that is very difficult to deal with in terms of managing risk in healthcare systems or any other organisation, that is, the intentional deviation from procedures or procedural violation (Free 1994, Reason 2000, Lawton & Parker 1998).

Violations fall into four main groups:

1. *Routine violations* – cutting corners whenever such opportunities present themselves. If staff are not 'punished' by the system (perhaps by a safety incident or peer disapproval) they become incorporated into the normal way of working. If rules are increased or made more restrictive in response to routine violations, a heightened opportunity for routine violations and their reward or reinforcement is created.
2. *Optimising violations* – occur for personal gain or to alleviate boredom.
3. *Situational violations* – occur when the rule cannot be carried out in the circumstances when it is expected to be used.
4. *Exceptional violations* – occur in exceptional circumstances, where time pressure or even emotion may prevent people from following even the most basic rules.

Violations are characterised as being a social phenomenon and as having a broad organisational context. Though the precise conditions in which they are promoted are not especially well understood, they are, however, generally associated with resistance to change and motivational problems (e.g. low morale, the failure to reward compliance or to sanction non-compliance) occurring in a regulated social context (Reason 2000).

Why is the distinction between error and violation important?

Until recently, in healthcare, the relevance of this distinction had not been explored in a systematic way (Claridge 2006). In a recent study Claridge (2006) encountered difficulty in establishing quantitatively a clear, consistent distinction between errors and violations. The concept of, and therefore the recognition of, a violation appeared to be relatively novel to healthcare professionals and their managers. Violations can only occur when known rules are in place to manage behaviour. In healthcare, there is a general preoccupation with error reduction, usually by increasing the layers of organisational defences (which include procedures, checking and electronic support) (Reason 2000), error reporting systems (for instance the National Reporting and Learning System (NPSA 2005)), where violations and errors are not distinguished or distinguishable, and identifying system factors contributing to adverse events (e.g. root cause analysis (NPSA 2005)). Claridge (2006) suggests that the management of rule violations in healthcare is a challenge that those involved with clinical process and risk management have not yet acknowledged. Violations are dangerous as they can bypass organisational defences, yet their impact on the performance of clinical processes and ultimately the safety of patients has not been assessed.

Research and development in high-risk industries (e.g. nuclear and petrochemical industries) provides useful information about factors that encourage violations (Battman & Klumb 1993, Hudson et al 1998, Williams 1997) and preferred actions to decrease violations (Hale et al 2003, Leplat 1998, Perin 1993). It is essential to apply this existing knowledge to the consideration of rule-related behaviour in clinical process management. This application should contribute directly to developing and implementing clinical process management in healthcare systems worldwide.

Conclusion

Clinical pathways can be used to organise and manage clinical processes related to specific 'core services' to structure a system of healthcare delivery that spans organisational and geographical boundaries. The patient trajectory through the system is pre-defined, risks are pre-assessed and monitored and waste is minimised. Clinical pathways seek to embed quality and safety assurance at the point of care delivery (micro context), while providing evidence for service planning, budgeting and subcontracting (macro context). Acquired information through variance analysis can be used to identify causes of medical error, areas of high cost both in terms of the organisation and for the patient and also potentially to shape improvement or restructuring of clinical processes to manage costs and improve both quality and safety. Such improvements in resource use and reductions in poor outcomes and harm enhance the overall contribution of healthcare systems to the wider health of the community.

Crucially, clinical pathways need to be used by healthcare professionals at the patient care interface to be effective in the ways described above. The rule-related behaviour of healthcare professionals should be a central consideration when developing clinical pathways; clinical process management invariably involves change, sometimes at the expense of short-term goals or aspects of the process that professionals feel comfortable with. Change is one of the significant factors in an environment that make violations more likely. Clinical process management also imposes a structure on the delivery of healthcare. Claridge (2006) found that this structuralisation caused the most dissatisfaction among healthcare professionals with clinical pathways, compared with the evidence on which they were based and their appearance. This dissatisfaction could lead to intentional non-compliance with the clinical pathway at the patient care interface.

In healthcare organisations worldwide structures such as clinical governance, risk management and financial assurance and quality control are remote finite entities (Degeling 2006) and clinical process management is often indistinguishable from a collective of service development and improvement initiatives. In order for the status and function of clinical process management to be clear to healthcare professionals, these structures need to be embedded within clinical processes rather than distinct entities. For instance, a safety management system can be embedded within a healthcare system, expressed within clinical process management and clinical pathways. Therefore clinical processes that cut across disciplines or professional groups and that operate within and between different care settings and producing core services to diverse patient populations require a responsive integrated management infrastructure (Degeling 2006) (including governance/finance/risk) that supports all functions and features of the healthcare system, its component clinical processes and supporting clinical pathways.

References

Battman W, Klumb P 1993 Behavioural economics and compliance with safety regulations. Safety Science 16(1):35–46

Berg M 1999 Patient care information systems and health care work: a sociotechnical approach. International Journal of Health Informatics (55):87–101

Claridge T 2006 Human factors, human error and health care professionals: The attitudes of health care professionals towards integrated care pathways. Doctoral Thesis

Coiera E 2003 Guide to Health Informatics. Hodder Arnold, London

De Bleser L, Depreitere R, De Waele K et al 2006 Defining pathways. J Nurs Manag 14(7):553–63

Degeling P 2006 Realising the developmental potential of Clinical Governance. Clin Chem Lab Med 44(6):688–91

Deming E 2000 Out of the Crisis. MIT Press, USA

Department of Health 2000 NHS Plan: A plan for investment. A plan for reform. London: Stationery Office, London, www.nhs.uk/nhsplan

Dillon A, Hargadon J 2003 What is protocol based care? NHS Modernisation Agency. National Institute for Clinical Excellence. Online. Available: http://www.modern.nhs.uk/protocolbasedcare 3 Jan 05

Edwards A, Elwyn G 2001 Developing professional ability to involve patients in their care: pull or push? Quality in Health Care 10:129–130

Eisert S 2006 Applying Lean Toyota Production System Methods to Improving Health Care Systems Paper presented at the annual meeting of the Economics of Population Health: Inaugural Conference of the American Society of Health Economists, Madison. 2006-10-05 from http://www.allacademic.com/meta/p91599_index.html

Emmerson B, Frost A, Fawcett L et al 2006 Do clinical pathways really improve clinical performance in mental health settings? Australasia Psychiatry 14(4):395–8

Every N R, Hochman J, Becker R et al 2000 Critical pathways: a review. Committee on Acute Cardiac Care, Council on Clinical Cardiology, American Heart Association. Circulation 101:461–5

Frankel S, Ebrahim S, Davey Smith G 2000 Education and debate. The limits to demand for health care Commentary: An open debate is not an admission of failure. BMJ 321:40–45

Free R 1994 The role of procedural violations in railway accidents. PhD thesis. University of Manchester

Greenwell J 1995 Patients and Professionals. In: Soothill K, Mackay L, Webb C Interprofessional Relations in Healthcare. Edward Arnold, London

Grol R 2001 Successes and failures in the implementation of evidence-based guidelines for clinical practice. Medical Care 39(8):1146–54

Grol R, Dalhuijsen J, Thomas S, in 't Veld C, Rutten H, Mokkink H 1998 Attributes of clinical guidelines that influence use of guidelines in general practice: observational study. British Medical Journal 317:858–861

Hale A R, Heijer T, Koornneef F 2003 Management of safety rules: the case of railways. Safety Science Monitor III

Hindle D, Yazbeck A M 2005 Clinical pathways in 17 European Union countries: a purposive survey. Aust Health Review 29(1):94–104

Ho D M, Huo M H 2007 Are critical pathways and implant standardization programs effective in reducing costs in total knee replacement operations? Journal of American College of Surgeons 205(1):97–100

Hopwood A G 1974 Accounting systems and managerial behaviour. Saxon House. Hampshire

Hudson P T W, Verschuur W L G, Lawton R L et al 1998 Bending the Rules II: Why Do People Break Rules or Fail to Follow Procedures, and What Can You Do About It? Report to Shell SIEP, the Hague

Hunter B, Segrott J 2007 Re-mapping client journeys and professional identities: A review of the literature on clinical pathways. International Journal of Medical Inform 76(2–3):151–6

Industrial Engineering 1992 Critical Path Software Smooths Road for Automotive Supplier. Industrial Engineering 24:28–9

Institute of Health Care Improvement 2005 Going Lean in Health care. Institute of Health Care Improvement, Cambridge

Juan-Torres A, Harbarth S 2007 Prevention of primary bacteraemia. International Journal for Antimicrobial Agents Aug 22; [Epub ahead of print]

Kallo G 1996 The reliability of critical path method (CPM) techniques in the analysis and evaluation of delay claims. Cost Engineering 38:35–37

Kahnemann D, Slovic P, Tversky A (eds) 1982 Judgement Under Uncertainty: Heuristics and Biases. Cambridge University Press, Cambridge

Kazui H, Hashimoto M, Nakano Y et al 2004 Effectiveness of a clinical pathway for the diagnosis and treatment of dementia and for the education of families. International Journal of Geriatric Psychiatry 19(9):892–7

Keen J, Moore J, West R 2006 Pathways, networks and choice in health care. International Journal of Health Care Quality Assurance 19(4):316–327

Kirk S, Parker D, Claridge T et al 2007 Patient safety culture in primary care: developing a theoretical framework for practical use. Journal of Quality and Safety in Health Care 16:313–320

Kohn L, Corrigan J, Donaldson M (eds) 2000 To Err Is Human: Building a Safer Health System. Committee on Quality of Health Care in America, Institute of Medicine National Academy Press, Washington

Lawton R L, Parker D 1998 Procedures and the professional: The case of the British NHS. Risk Decision and Policy 3:199–211

Lee K H, Anderson Y M 2007 The association between clinical pathways and hospital length of stay: a case study. Journal of Medical Systems 31(1):79–83

Leplat J 1998 About implementation of safety rules. Safety Science 29(3):189–204

Lilford R, Brown C, Nicholl J 2007 Use of process measures to monitor the quality of clinical practice. British Medical Journal 335:648–650

Logsdon M C, Koniak-Griffin D 2005 Social support in postpartum adolescents: guidelines for nursing assessments and interventions. Journal of Obstetric Gynecological and Neonatal Nursing 34(6):761–8

Low D E, Kunz S, Schembre D et al 2007 Esophagectomy – It's Not Just About Mortality Anymore: Standardized Perioperative Clinical Pathways Improve Outcomes in Patients with Esophageal Cancer. Journal of Gastrointestinal Surgery. Aug 31; [Epub ahead of print]

Lucas G 2001 Critical Approaches to Fieldwork: Contemporary and Historical Archaeological

Lyons J 2006 The Complexity of Communication in an Environment with Multiple Disciplines and Professionals: Communimetrics and Decision Support Care. In: Huyse F J, Stiefel F C Integrated care for the complex medically ill. Medical Clinics of North America July

McCarthy G M, Koval J J, MacDonald J K 1999 Compliance with recommended infection control procedures among Canadian dentists: results of a national survey. American Journal of Infection Control 5:377–84

Mackay A 1993 Team up for excellence. Oxford Press, New York

Merino Muñoz R, Martín Vega A, García Caballero J et al 2007 [Evaluation of a clinical pathway for septic arthritis] [Article in Spanish] Annals of Pediatrics (Barc) 67(1):22–9

National Electronic Library for Health 2006. Online. Available: http://libraries.nelh.nhs.uk/ Pathways/ 5 May 2006

National Patient Safety Agency (NPSA) 2004. Online. Available: www.npsa.nhs.uk 12 May 2006

Nicholls S, Cullen R, O'Neill S, Halligan A 2000 Clinical Governance its origins and its foundations. Clinical Performance and Quality Health Care 8(3):172–8

Parker D, Lawton R L 2003 Psychological contribution to the understanding of adverse events in health care. Quality and Safety in Health Care 12(6):453–7

Parker D, Reason J, Manstead A et al 1995 Driving errors, driving violations and accident involvement. Ergonomics 38:1036–1048

Pearson S D, Goulart-Fisher D, Lee T H 1995 Critical pathways as a strategy for improving care: problems and potential. Annals of Internal Medicine 123:941–948

Perin C 1993 The dynamics of safety: the intersections of technical, cultural and social regulative systems in the operations of high hazard technologies. Paper to the 11th NeTWork Workshop: the use of rules to achieve safety. Bad Homburg, 6–8 May

Phillips J M 2001 The role of decision influence and team performance in member self-efficacy, withdrawal, satisfaction with the leader and willingness to return. Organizational Behaviour and Human Decision Processes 84(1):122–147

Read S J, Levy J 2006 Effects of care pathways on stroke care practices at regional hospitals. International Medical Journal 36(10):638–42

Reason J, Mycielska K 1982 Absent-Minded? The Psychology of Mental Lapses and Everyday Errors. Prentice-Hall, Englewood Cliffs, New Jersey

Reason J T 1990 Human Error. Cambridge University Press. Cambridge

Reason J T, Parker D, Lawton R, et al 1995 Organisational controls and the varieties of rule-related behaviour. In: Loomes G (ed) Risk and Human Behaviour. Economic and Social Research Council, York

Reason J 1995 A systems approach to organisational error. Ergonomics 38:1708–21

Reason J T, Parker D, Lawton R 1998 Organisational controls and safety: the varieties of rule-related behaviour. Journal of Occupational and Organisational Psychology 71:289–304

Reason J 2000 Human error: models and management. British Medical Journal 320:768–770

Roper N, Logan W, Tierney A (eds) 1983 Using a Model for Nursing. Churchill Livingstone, Edinburgh

Sackett D, Straus S, Richardson W et al 2000 Evidence Based Medicine: How to teach and practice EBM. Churchill Livingstone, Edinburgh

Saufl N, Owens A, Kelly I et al 2007 A multidisciplinary approach to total joint replacement. International Journal of Nursing Studies May 22 [Epub ahead of print]

Schuster M A, McGlynn E A, Brook R H 1998 How good is health care in the United States? Milbank Quarterly 76:517–63

Senders J W, Moray N P 1991 Human error: Cause, prediction and reduction. Erlbaum, Hillsdale, NJ

Shimanoff S 1980 Communication rules. Sage, Beverly Hills

Swash M (ed) Hutchinson R 2001 Hutchinson's Clinical Methods, 21st Edition. WB Saunders, London

Tay H L, Raja Latifah R J, Razak I A 2006 Clinical pathways in primary dental care in Malaysia: clinicians' knowledge, perceptions and barriers faced. Asia Pacific Journal of Public Health 18(2):33–41

Vanhaecht K, De Witte K, Depreitere R et al 2007 Development and validation of a care process self-evaluation tool. Health Services Management Research 20(3):189–202

Vanounou T, Pratt W, Fischer J E et al 2007 Deviation-based cost modeling: a novel model to evaluate the clinical and economic impact of clinical pathways. Journal of American College of Surgeons 204(4):570–9

Venture Training 2005. Online. Available: http://www.venturetc.com/ 23 May 2007

Vitek L, Rosenzweig M Q, Stollings S 2007 Distress in patients with cancer: definition, assessment, and suggested interventions. Clinical Journal Oncology Nursing 11(3):413–8

Wagner J A, Gooding R Z 1987 Effects of societal trends on participatory research. Administrative Science Quarterly 33:241–62

Walby S, Greenwell J, Mackay L et al 1994 Medicine and nursing: professions in a changing health service. Sage, London

Williams J C 1997 assessing the likelihood of violation behaviour – a preliminary investigation. Paper to the Institution of Nuclear Engineers Conference COPSA 9th October

Wolff A M, Taylor S A, McCabe J F 2004 Using checklists and reminders in clinical pathways to improve hospital inpatient care. Medical Journal of Australia 181(8):428–31

WHO World Health Report 2000. World Health Organization, Geneva, Switzerland

Yee S K 1998 What you need to know: guidelines to medical practitioners for proper maintenance of drugs and dispensing records (including controlled drugs). Singapore Medical Journal 39(11):520–2

Yelland J, McLachlan H, Forster D et al 2007 How is maternal psychosocial health assessed and promoted in the early postnatal period? Findings from a review of hospital postnatal care in Victoria, Australia. Midwifery 23(3):287–97

Putting the patient in the middle: managing chronic illness across organisational boundaries

Hannele Kerosuo

Introduction

Public sector organisations, including healthcare organisations, operate within multiple sets of co-existing organisational, professional and practice boundaries. Boundaries in healthcare are created mainly through medical specialisation and bureaucratic forms of organisation that can fragment healthcare services and their delivery. Yet the changing nature of healthcare (predominantly the ageing of the population), changing methods for allocating funding and expectations that health services integrate, challenge boundary continuance.

Boundaries hamper patient care especially for patients suffering from multiple and chronic illnesses because their care is characterised by a multiplicity of intertwining health problems and needs that themselves are increasing in complexity and in turn cause difficulties for effective service provision (Davis et al 2000, Plsek & Greenhalgh 2001, Wagner & Groves 2002, Wilson & Holt 2001). Further complexity is added as medical and drug technology and treatment advances not only for acute conditions but also for chronic diseases (Wagner & Groves 2002). Patients with chronic disease are generally simultaneously in the care of several specialists who are often geographically separated in numerous clinics providing different levels of care. In any one episode, this can lead to no one taking overall responsibility for coordinating the patient's care, and hence patients are left 'in the middle', 'in no-man's land of care' where care needs are not necessarily attended to as they should be (Kerosuo 2006:2).

Managing the boundaries in chronic illness is an urgent task. As advanced medical technology, pharmacology and treatment help people live longer, they require care for longer periods of time. How, then, can we improve the organisation of healthcare that requires clinicians with different clinical and professional orientations to collaborate, particularly where care relationships are characterised by individual clinicians delivering episodic care to individual patients? This chapter considers the impact of organisational, professional and practice boundaries on patient care, specifically the care of patients with multiple and chronic illnesses. Ameliorating the effect of boundaries means re-interpreting the outcomes of care, the role of the patient and the responsibility of treating clinicians that in turn mean creating new ways to conceptualise and deliver care within the context of organisation and organisations.

As with many of the health systems represented in this book, the Finnish healthcare system is segmented into primary, secondary and tertiary care sectors provided by different levels of government: primary and general hospital care by local municipal authorities; secondary and tertiary care by hospital districts and regions. Healthcare is further segmented by clinical specialties that have created their own clinical communities and their own specialty-specific care practices. Thus, patient referrals within and between clinical specialties and patient pathways within and between the different levels of care presage changes not only in the patterns of care, but also in clinical practice, clinician collaboration and organisational integration. In this chapter, we consider the organisation of patient care having regard to:

- patient trajectories of care
- the boundaries within care trajectories
- the use of collaborative tools to span the boundaries.

Patients' care trajectories as a developmental challenge within the intervention

We use the concept of a patient care trajectory to understand how illness is managed. The concept allows us to construct a comprehensive view of care for chronic illness within the context of inter-organisational care, that is, care that is carried out by a multiplicity of independent, specialist 'organisations', including for instance that provided by multispecialties and multidisciplines where comorbidities exist in the patient's presentation. The concept encompasses the temporal progress of events in caring for a person with a chronic illness. Strauss et al (1984:8) caution that a patient's care trajectory describes 'not just the physical course of illness but all the work that patients, staff and kin do to deal with the illness, and all the social/psychological consequences that encircle the illness course (its intrusiveness on relationships, temperament and so forth)'. The multiple illnesses that accompany patient comorbidities can involve different levels of care and different types of work that bring complexity to the division of labour and raise confusion about the coordination of care (Strauss et al 1984). Trajectories help us 'see' the care as one connected episode, and alert us to the problems, disturbances, tensions, gaps and innovation efforts that can occur in daily practice as they act as drivers of development and changers in intervention (Engeström 1987:174).

These trajectories of care can be constructed from observation, interviews and video clips that describe the actual care setting as well as from parts of patients' health documentation. We focus on data from a number of case histories to develop our approach to care trajectories. The data are drawn from an ethnographic study of organisational activity – actions and interactions in routine and developmental practice carried out in two phases in the specialties of internal medicine that included cardiology, endocrinology, pulmonary diseases, rheumatology and nephrology. Phase one involved mapping the problems and discussing them in intervention sessions organised by the researchers in inter-organisational care for 16 patients and their providers from two healthcare centres, five secondary care hospitals and three university hospital clinics in Finland. Phase two involved creating and testing new collaborative tools as solutions for inter-organisational care fragmentation and involved 10 patients and a pilot group of 13

Table 5.1 Patient 'Hugo'

Patient	Patient 6: Male aged 54
Observation	Field diary and videos of care settings
Interviews	The patient (15.3.200X) Internist, secondary care clinic (29.3.200X) Cardiologist, university hospital (4.4.200X) General practitioner, primary care (5.4.200X) Nurse, primary care (5.4.200X) Nurse, secondary care clinic (6.4.200X) Clinician, university hospital (11.4.200X) Pulmonary specialist, university hospital (14.4.200X)
Patien's health documents	Health centre (14 pages) Secondary care hospital (9 pages) University hospital (32 pages)
Laboratory session	Held 19.4.200X
Follow-up interviews	The patient (16.8.200X, 28.3.200X)

doctors and three nurses (Engeström et al 2003, Kerosuo 2006). We present the data of a patient case as an example of a trajectory developed through the research is presented in Table 5.1.

The care trajectory for Hugo depicted above illustrates the inter-organisational care for the multiple chronic illnesses that Hugo suffers, namely hypertension, high cholesterol, diabetes, degenerative arthritis and eye trouble (cataract). He is overweight and not able to move well because of arthritis. Hugo's illness and care trajectory can be described figuratively, as in Figure 5.1.

In Hugo's case, Figure 5.1 shows there were five care trajectories contained in one primary care clinic, one secondary care clinic and three university hospital clinics. The care of hypertension, high cholesterol and diabetes occurred together. Transitions from one provider to another are depicted with arrows. The broken arrows depict disruptions between the providers representing the different levels of care.

The problems emerging in Hugo's care relate to communication disjunctions between the different providers. The first disjunction in communication occurred when clinicians at the health centre clinic transferred Hugo's care for diabetes to the secondary care hospital. They expected the secondary care clinic to take care of the hypertension, elevated cholesterol and tests for blood consistency. The patient also expected that. However, the tests for blood consistency were not done at this clinic, and the patient did not know that it was important to have the tests for blood consistency done at least once a month.

The second and third disruption in the flow of information related to communication between the university hospital and the primary health centre clinic. The care document concerning the angiography for heart disease from the university hospital clinic to the primary health centre clinic did not reach the other end. Therefore, the primary health centre clinician lacked the information from cardiology about the follow-up for heart failure to be conducted at the primary health centre. The patient thought that the cardiology clinic did the follow-ups; he was wondering why it was taking so long for the cardiology clinic to give him an appointment, especially because he was afraid that he was going to have another infarct before receiving treatment.

The patient's experience was that his overall care was not conducted as it should be. He was expecting to be operated on for his heart and his knees. He was having the

Figure 5.1 Patient 'Hugo's' illness and care trajectory

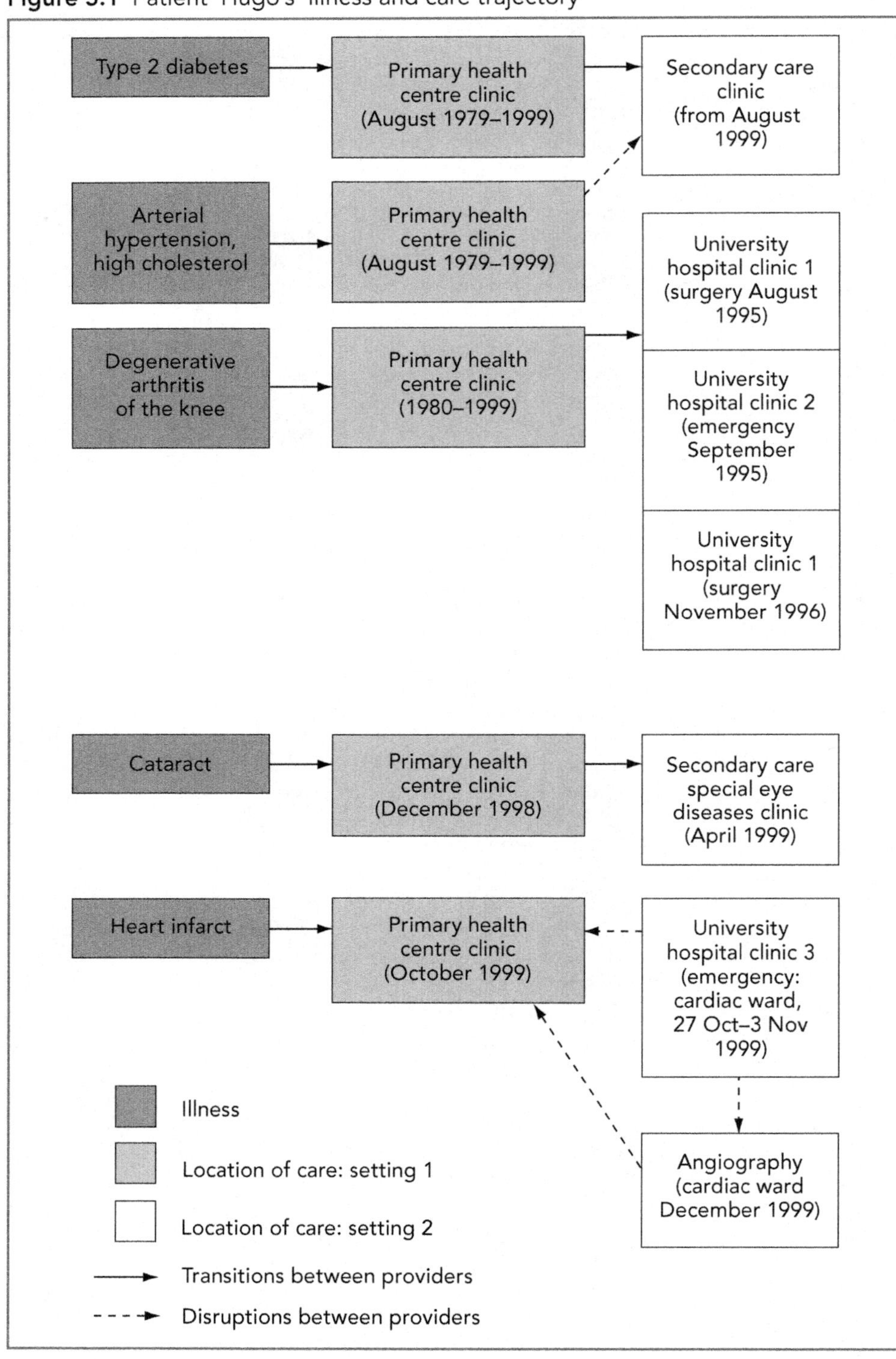

same laboratory tests run in two different places and the providers kept changing his care. The professionals were quite surprised by the disjunctions in the patient's overall care but thought they were not the only ones to blame for the disjunctions – the patient himself was also passive in his care. A possible 'solution' was for the providers to negotiate to eliminate the disjunctions in Hugo's case. The patient himself was present during the first negotiation arranged by the researchers but not the second negotiation, conducted by the primary health centre providers and a specialist from the university hospital clinic.

The general opinion was that Hugo's overall pattern of care was not run properly. The cardiology specialist commented that there were too many providers involved at the second negotiation: seven specialists treated the patient during the last episode at the cardiology clinic (in 1999), and two primary health centre clinicians and two secondary care clinicians treated the patient in primary and secondary care. The providers could not negotiate a solution to secure the overall care. One barrier related to the providers' opinion that the patient had become non-compliant when in fact he did not know how the healthcare system worked. Beginning to solve the pattern of Hugo's care involves drawing a map of the overall view of care, as in Figure 5.2. The locations of care are marked in boxes; one box represents one location of care. The connections between locations are depicted with double-headed arrows representing the long-term care relationships and single-headed arrows representing a single visit.

Hugo's case shows that many boundaries crosscut the care of patients with multiple and chronic illnesses. Two types of organisational boundaries emerge: one is the organisational division between the levels of primary, secondary and tertiary healthcare, the other, clinical boundaries inside each level of organisation. The consequences of these boundaries for Hugo's care were disruptions and gaps in the flow of information and the lack of an agent with an overall responsibility for care provision. How, then, do patients experience the effects of boundary divisions?

Pause for reflection

Who should have overall responsibility for patient care, when it involves multi-specialties and multi-professionals, as well as the patient and their family members?

The effects of boundaries

Boundaries between levels of care emerge as disruptions, gaps and overlaps (Kerosuo 2007). In one instance, data relating to the experience of an elderly woman show that primary and tertiary professionals treated her ailments without each other's knowledge. These data are drawn from the ethnographic research described earlier in the chapter. The patient suffered from asthma, circulatory disorders, infection of the urinary tract and osteoporosis. She had mainly been treated at the pulmonary clinic at the university hospital and at the health centre clinic. She was uncertain about the treatment for urinary tract infection since the care she received from the primary and tertiary clinicians varied. Not surprisingly, she felt that she was not treated properly. Her account of her care follows.

Patient: If I go to [the pulmonary clinic] specialised care there is a different doctor every time who prescribes a different medicine. Then I visit the doctor [at the health centre clinic] and she says that you cannot take that medicine [for your urinary tract infection] now. And I am confused because I do not know whom to believe and what to believe and

Figure 5.2 A map of Hugo's care provision in 1999–2000

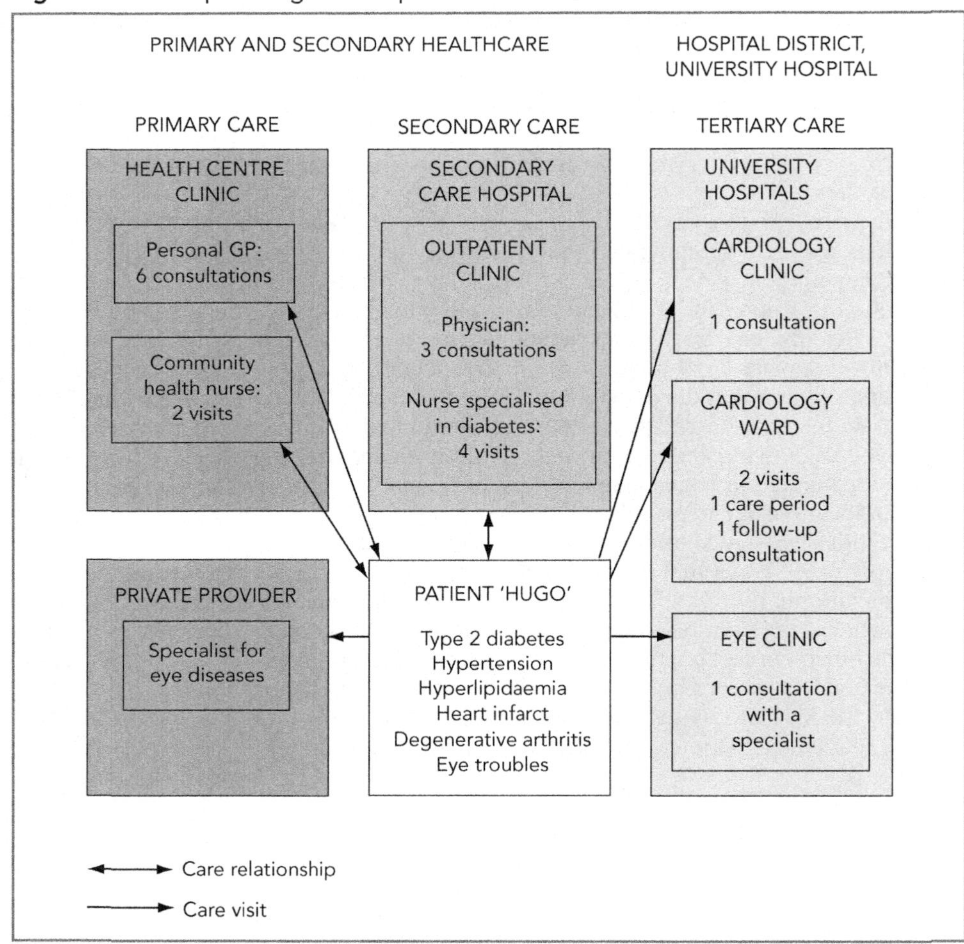

what is wrong with me … They have not fixed [my condition], no one has fixed it; no one has cared for me.

(10 December 2001)

The unconnected nature of inter-organisational practice emerges as it becomes evident that professionals believe that 'others' are taking the responsibility for care. A further patient with coronary artery disease, diabetes, COPD, swelling and pulmonary symptoms had been a patient at the health centre clinic for seven years and also visited the university hospital in emergency situations. The disruption and gaps between the levels of care affecting the patient emerged in meetings between the university hospital physician, the health centre physician and the home care nurse as the professionals became aware that nobody was looking after the patient's diabetes and lipids. The health centre physician thought that the university hospital was in charge of care and vice versa.

A further example shows that not only is clinical care uncoordinated, so too is the organisation of tests. In the next instance, a relative reports on her mother-in-law's experiences. Her mother-in-law, an elderly woman with memory problems who needed the help of her relatives, required treatment for a fracture of the thigh, pleura in the lungs and convulsions, for which she received care at three hospitals in short intervals. The discoordination of care concerned laboratory tests – the same laboratory tests were run in the health centre clinic, the health centre hospital and the university hospital on successive days.

> *Patient's relative:* She is not able to walk very well, and therefore I tried to ask whether the tests taken over there [at the health centre clinic] are enough. [The tests] were taken the day before. Or was it after? But in any case they said that they take their own tests over there [at the health centre clinic], and we take our tests here.

> *Patient's physician:* This is unfortunately true. Our laboratories do not communicate with each other; they have different computer systems.

> (15 February 2001)

Disruptions in the flow of information between levels of care are an example of problems in healthcare that are difficult to solve. Some relevant information, for instance medication or changes in care, may not be transferred between providers. The primary care physician often lacks relevant information from other locations of care. In one case, for instance, a primary care physician provided care for a patient with severe heart failure. She did not, however, know about the heart failure because she had not received any information about it from the university hospital where the patient was treated. The patient for his part thought that the information was shared because he had signed a form giving permission for this to occur.

In other cases, patients sometimes act as postmen, carrying documents between clinicians in the different levels of care. Some patients collected their own personal files that they used when they felt that information was not flowing properly. One patient, worried about the professionals' lack of acquaintance with the information concerning his illnesses, actually took charge of delivering information to the health centre hospital. Because he was uncertain that the hospital had all the relevant information about his renal treatments, he asked his wife to bring all his medical documents from home. He then asked the physician at the ward, and later the senior physician, to read through the documents in order to prescribe the proper medication for his current ailments.

> *Patient:* [The senior physician] said that he would get acquainted with [my medical documents]. I said no, I will give them to you now and you will see what is in there, and we will then see what the diagnosis from these [symptoms] is … The senior physician sat down and read and said that it is quite clear now. Here we have plain orders what we should take, what medication we should use. And the physician at the ward agreed. And that was the end of the [ailments].

> (3 May 2000)

Boundaries between specialties

Occupational groups and professions establish communities to sustain their interests, privileges, specialised training and their occupational identity (Freidson 1970). These communities are internally divided by further sub-specialties and stratification (Freidson 1988). Besides the division between generalist and specialist medical practice, the profession of medicine has evolved into diversified specialties and subspecialties. This specialisation manifests as numerous clinics that provide specialised services, for example at the university hospital. Ideally, the collaboration between specialties is perceived as seamless, and specialists commonly refer to the exchange of information through the shared documentation in the hospital clinics. In practice, however, collaboration between the specialties is difficult, as the following discussion between an endocrinologist and patient illustrates.

> *Endocrinologist:* This pattern between primary and secondary care, although it limps, it is still easier than ... the internal exchange of information at the university hospital ... Although, it is perhaps difficult for a layman to understand ... Why does one not [have all the information available regarding a patient] when it is [in] the same building? ... We are unbelievably far away [from each other], sometimes it feels like a light year away.
>
> *Patient:* It is because some are on the eleventh floor, and the others are on the ground floor.
>
> *Endocrinologist:* Yes, and those are, in practice, very ... specialised divisions ...

> (20 June 2001)

For a patient, the overlaps in healthcare services sometimes seem odd. One patient, who suffers from diabetes and associated diseases including ailments with his lower limbs, and treated by a surgical specialist and endocrinologist in parallel, reports an incident about the use of surgical stockings as an example of inter-specialty collaboration difficulties.

> *Patient:* I could tell ... how I felt from my point of view. Over there at the outpatient clinic for treating legs [poly-neuropathy] they had the opinion that I needed a surgical stocking for the blood circulation in the leg ... I had reservations about it ... but then I went to a store [that] specialised in health products and ordered the stocking. But then I had a visit with the surgical outpatient clinic the next day, and I went there. And I happen[ed] to mention this stocking. Then the surgeon said ... cancel it immediately. So, this is how I got contradictory information. You see, a patient gets a little lost when he does not know. There are two [opinions]; these are specialists – educated specialists in medicine – who take opposite views.

> (20 June 2001)

Here, the differences between the specialty content and actual clinical practice created boundaries, often associated with the temporality of contact between the different specialists. Cardiac patients, for instance, are often treated for a short period at a hospital cardiology department, while in the rheumatology clinic, specialists have long-term relationships with their patients. Because of this difference, the opportunities that these specialties have to collaborate are specific. The cardiologists have limited opportunities for inter-organisational collaboration concerning individual patients, while rheumatologists can collaborate on a longer term basis.

Further, as demands for cost-effective care increase, there is a flow-on effect on the practices of clinical specialties. Through cost shifting, different specialties transfer costly treatments to other specialties to minimise their own costs. If an orthopaedist finds out that a patient treated in rheumatology needs an instrumental aid in his or her care, they do not order that aid due to the costs but refer the requirement for the aid to the rheumatology clinic. Clearly, while this may advantage the budgets of individual clinical departments, it does not help individual patients. Changing the focus of care, then, from the interests of the provider to those of the patient will require a range of solutions, including changes in attitudes clinicians have to the way they treat patients, the centrality of patients' interests when plans of care are being made and treatment is being delivered, and importantly, in the ways that clinicians relate to each other, to achieve the goals of care for patients whose care they share.

> **Pause for reflection**
>
> Who should take responsibility to eliminate the disruptions to care that can arise from administrative arrangements, such as budgets and performance outcomes?

Spanning boundaries – creating new tools for collaboration

Providers who represent single specialties tend to focus on single ailments or symptoms and risk losing sight of the overall picture of care (Kerosuo 2003). By encountering providers who represent other levels of care, an experience of collective learning is automatically created. While prevailing boundaries are challenged and defended, simply by encountering others, new rules are created for information exchange and new divisions of care responsibility between providers are negotiated. In the case of Hugo, when challenged, providers agreed to organise a negotiation session to improve problematic aspects of care. Patients also become learners as 'Mark' reflected on his experiences.

Patient: Suddenly I realised … that I would have to go around like an orphan [to receive care]. I think that it was the attitude of the senior specialist that was really important there. That he considered and was prepared to take overall responsibility for my care in the clinic.

(5 March 2001)

For Mark, it became clear that his overall care was organised by a system of care providers and that it was in danger of becoming disrupted. He learnt that the division of care responsibility could be negotiated with the providers across organisational boundaries. Providers also learn as they come together to create and test new collaborative tools. A package consisting of a care calendar, a care map and a care agreement become the core tools through which clinicians can reorient and re-order their patient care processes across their organisational and professional boundaries. Central to the re-ordering is the coming together of the different clinicians from their different levels of care to discuss specific patients, not just as clinicians, but as members of a team that also includes the patient and representatives from the diverse healthcare organisations that provide care to the patient.

Learning is an elemental part of creating and implementing new tools. As Béguin & Rabardel note (2000:175) 'an artifact only becomes an instrument through the subject's activity'. The new care calendar, care map and care agreement are templates to be modified as the context and situation dictates. Taking the case of Hugo from Figure 5.1, and in listing the history of Hugo's diseases, his descriptions of his symptoms and illnesses and his diagnosed illnesses and their treatments reported in the patient's health documents, the care calendar acts as a template within which to contain and sequence complex, dislocated, *shared* information. The care map template depicts prevalent care relationships, the information exchange between the providers and the division of care responsibility. The care agreement epitomises the joint negotiations between patient and provider, including knowledge about the patient's illnesses and symptoms and their concerns about those illnesses. Through the care agreement, patients are no longer passive receivers of expertise, but become experts themselves in their own care, or perhaps, rather, are given the opportunity to contribute the expertise that they have always had (Engeström et al 2003).

Professionals enrich the tools as they use them (Kerosuo & Engeström 2003). Through use, clinicians communicate between each other and thereby create new meaning as they engage in new sense-making activities. An example is the doctor who began sketching an illness model of a client at the community health centre as an amoeba – the several 'legs' of the amoeba marked the various illnesses of the patient in the model. Yet another clinician brought new insights to the care calendar as depicted in Figure 5.3, by using it not only as a means of describing the patient's care provision to others, but also as a tool for managing the patient's present care. We use this clinician's example to illustrate the use of a care calendar to reconfigure a patient's care trajectory.

Developing new collaborative tools is complex (Kerosuo & Engeström 2003). It requires a long process of experimentation and their use is often resisted. But in taking

Figure 5.3 Johan's care calendar

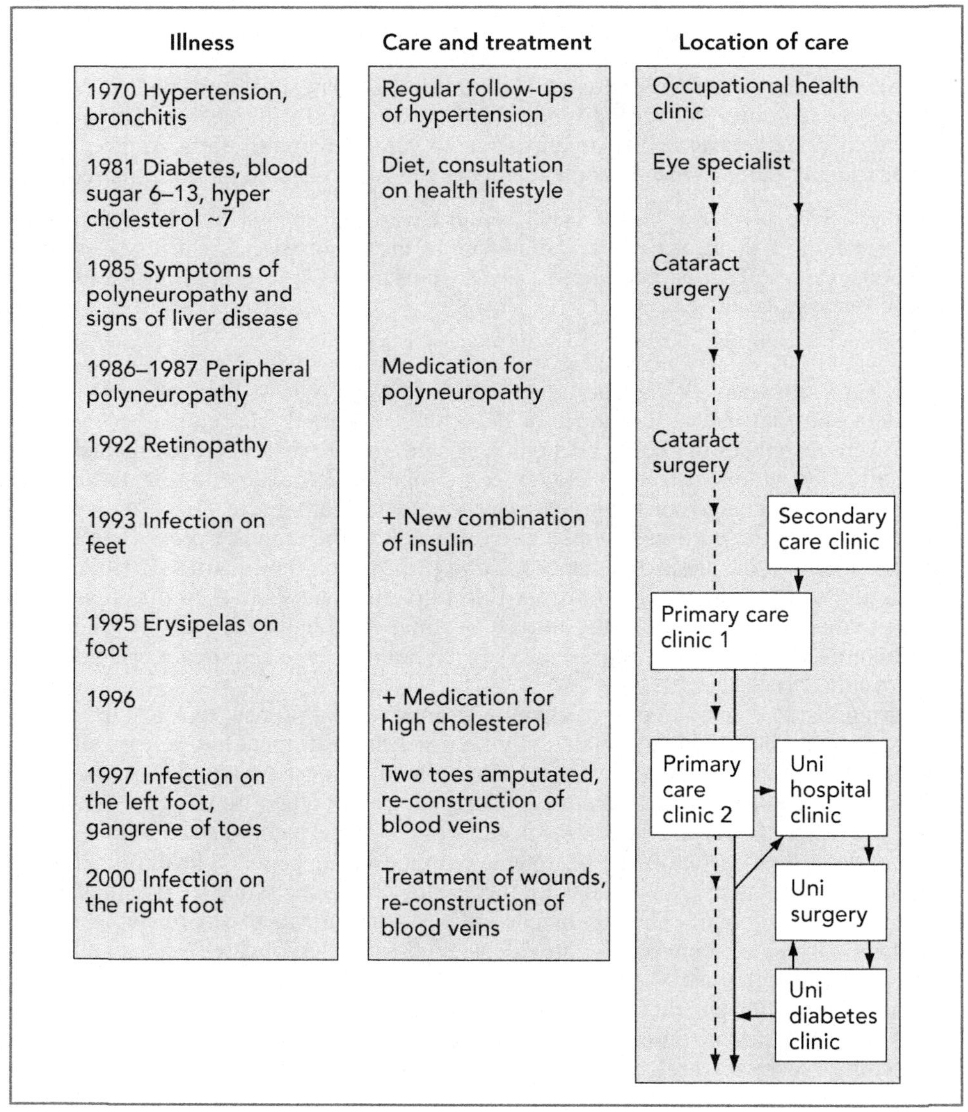

Nicklas's case (see Figure 5.4), we show how a turning point is created. As one specialist began using the care agreement template as a part of her regular clinical work to ensure Nicklas's overall care, she and Nicklas completed the form together during his regular visit to specialised care. Then, using the form, she telephoned the primary care clinician after the visit and told the clinician about the care provided at the specialised clinic. Using the form, she ensured that the clinician was aware of the care expected to be carried out in the primary care clinic. Finally, she posted the care agreement form to the primary care clinician.

Figure 5.4 The care agreement form for patient 'Nicklas'

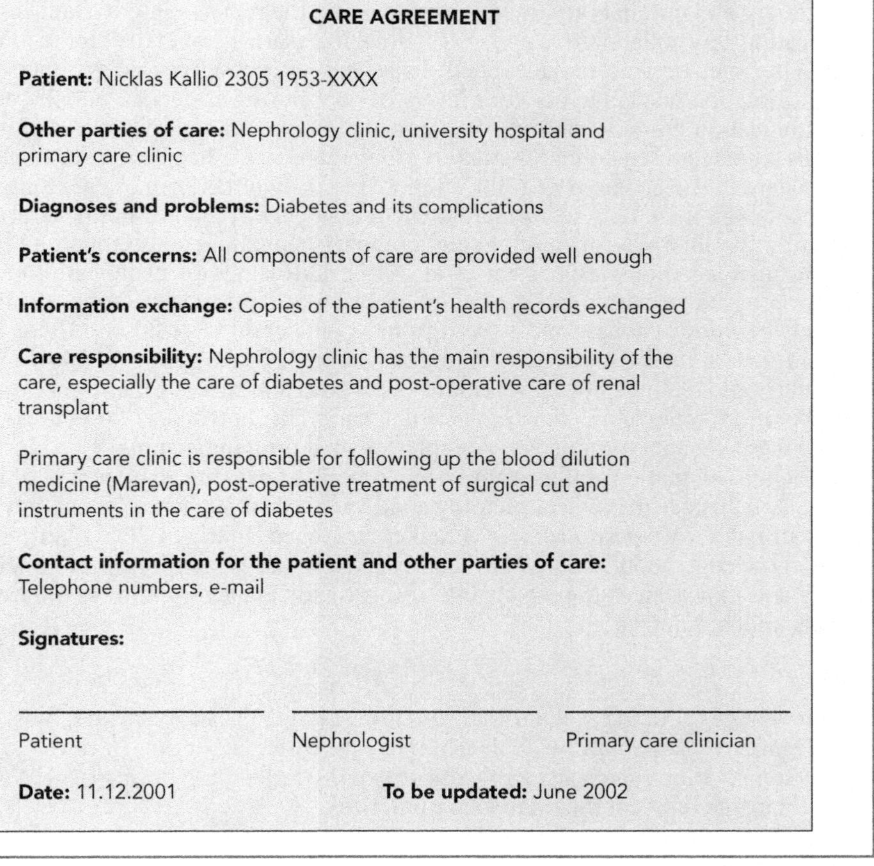

CARE AGREEMENT

Patient: Nicklas Kallio 2305 1953-XXXX

Other parties of care: Nephrology clinic, university hospital and primary care clinic

Diagnoses and problems: Diabetes and its complications

Patient's concerns: All components of care are provided well enough

Information exchange: Copies of the patient's health records exchanged

Care responsibility: Nephrology clinic has the main responsibility of the care, especially the care of diabetes and post-operative care of renal transplant

Primary care clinic is responsible for following up the blood dilution medicine (Marevan), post-operative treatment of surgical cut and instruments in the care of diabetes

Contact information for the patient and other parties of care:
Telephone numbers, e-mail

Signatures:

___________________ ___________________ ___________________

Patient   Nephrologist   Primary care clinician

Date: 11.12.2001   **To be updated:** June 2002

These new tools not only enabled organisational boundaries to be crossed, they encouraged, necessitated even, new forms of practice. By compiling information comprehensively and sequentially in one location, clinicians see new patterns that allow them to reflect on and alter their own practices. Disruptions, disjunctions and problems, once hidden within the logic and fragmentation of single, episodic disease-specific management, are illuminated and resolved as the multiplicities of complex comorbid conditions are exposed, information exchanged, care agreed and division of responsibilities negotiated. This care negotiation emerged as a new clinical practice with defined phases: choosing a patient; using the care calendar and care map to compile and view overall care; ensuring appropriate functioning of care provision; attending to care gaps; agreeing care; and updating the care agreement (Kerosuo & Engeström 2003).

Conclusion

Organisational, professional and practice boundaries cannot be crossed easily. Organisationally based sets of cultural rules and resources bind the behaviour of healthcare providers into separated units of actions. Creating critical pathways of care has improved the inter-organisational care for single diseases but our findings demonstrate that the overall care for patients with multiple and chronic disease is crosscut by boundaries affecting the overall process of care. Patients experience boundaries as bringing uncertainty and unreliability to their care and turn the patients into bystanders.

Creating new collaborative tools is essential to ensure the overall chronic illness care within the inter-organisational context. The electronic patient record system is improving information exchange between levels of care but its effects on collaboration and communication are still missing. Implementation and spread of clinical innovations such as the one presented in this study is problematic in the healthcare sector generally. For instance, Buchanan et al (2007) report the difficulties of implementing clinical innovations in the UK. According to their findings, the spread of innovations is influenced by the interplay of multiple and complex contextual, substantial, and process factors in innovations (Buchanan et al 2007). Diffusions of healthcare innovations do not proceed smoothly but are inhibited by inter- and intra-professional boundaries between professionals and expert groups (Fitzgerald et al 2002). These kinds of discontinuities can be mended by 'bridging actions' (Engeström et al 2007). Managerial decisions creating new organisational structures and spaces for inter-organisational collaboration, establishing new projects that enrich the outcomes of previous ones and launching personnel training are examples of such bridging actions.

Patient participation is important. While reports of patients' experiences of illnesses have a long history in medical sociology, only a few deal directly with patients' experiences of healthcare *organisations* (Frankel & Treger Hourigan 2004). Since patients have knowledge about the overall health services that professionals often lack, their views and experiences are a valuable resource for managing chronic illness across organisational boundaries.

Box 5.1 Implications for practice – Managing across organisational boundaries

Interweaving the fragmented care for chronic patients can be secured by creating new collaborative tools and related practices.

Tool creation represents a process of expansive learning during which participants reinvent their daily care practices.

Healthcare management needs to be alert to creating opportunities for expansive learning.

References

Béguin P, Rabardel P 2000 Designing for Instrument-Mediated Activity. Scandinavian Journal of Information Systems 12:173–190
Buchanan D A, Fitzgerald L, Ketley D 2007 The Sustainability and Spread of Organisational Change. Routledge, London and New York
Davis R M, Wagner E G, Groves T 2000 Advances in managing chronic illness. British Medical Journal 320:525–526

Engeström Y 1987 Learning by Expanding: An Activity-theoretical Approach to Developmental Research. Orienta-konsultit, Helsinki

Engeström Y, Engeström R, Kerosuo H 2003 Discursive construction of collaborative care. Applied Linguistics 24:286–315

Engeström Y, Kerosuo H, Kajamaa A 2007 Beyond discontinuity: Expansive organisational learning remembered. Management and Learning 38:319–336

Fitzgerald L, Ferlie E, Wood M et al 2002 Interlocking interactions: the diffusion of innovations in healthcare. Human Relations 55(12):1429–49

Frankel R M, Treger Hourigan N 2004 Thirty-five voices in search of an author: What focus groups reveal about patients' experiences of managed care settings. Communication & Medicine 1:44–58

Freidson E 1970 Professional Dominance: The Social Structure of Medical Care. Atherton Press, New York

Freidson E 1988 Profession of Medicine. A Study of the Sociology of Applied Knowledge. University of Chicago Press, Chicago

Kerosuo H 2003 Boundaries in health care discussions: an activity theoretical approach to the analysis of boundaries. In: Paulsen N, Hernes T (eds) 2003 Managing Boundaries in Organisations: Multiple Perspectives. Palgrave Macmillan, Basingstoke

Kerosuo H 2006 Boundaries in Action: An Activity-theoretical Study of Boundaries in Health Care for Patients with Multiple and Chronic Illnesses. Helsinki University Press, Helsinki- http://ethesis.helsinki.fi/julkaisut/kay/kasva/vk/kerosuo/boundari.pdf

Kerosuo H 2007 Renegotiating disjunctions in interorganisationally provided care. In: Iedema R (ed) The Discourse of Hospital Communication: Tracing Complexities in Contemporary Health Care Organisation. Palgrave Macmillan, Basingstoke, Hampshire, UK and New York

Kerosuo H, Engeström Y 2003 Boundary crossing and learning in creation of new work practice. Journal of Workplace Learning 15:345–351

Lindberg K, Czarniawska B 2006 Knotting the action net, or organising between organisations. Scandinavian Journal of Management 22:292–306

Plsek P E, Greenhalgh T 2001 The challenge of complexity in health care. British Medical Journal 323:625–628

Strauss A L, Fagerhaugh S, Suczek B et al 1984 Social Organisation of Medical Work. Transaction Publishers, New Brunswick and London

Wagner E H, Groves T 2002 Care for chronic diseases: The efficacy of coordinated and patient centreed care is established, but now is the time to test its effectiveness. British Medical Journal 325:913–14

Wilson T, Holt T 2001 Complexity and clinical science. British Medical Journal 323:685–688

The collectivity of healthcare: multidisciplinary team care

Eileen Willis, Judith Dwyer & Sandra Dunn

Introduction

This chapter examines the concept of multidisciplinary team care (MTC), drawing on broader organisational literature but focusing on team care in health organisations. We argue that MTC represents a new direction in healthcare and is of interest not only because of its importance in approaches to improving the effectiveness of care, but also because teams are critical to the goal of placing patients and their families at the centre of healthcare. We review available evidence about the barriers and facilitators for effective MTC. We then draw out strategies for developing and supporting healthcare teams at several levels – within the team; in the organisation; and at the level of the health system and health policy.

Threaded through this discussion are excerpts from a case study of the care of a single child with brain cancer ('Teamwork for Keown') presenting the perspectives and insights of four members of this family's healthcare team in ways that we hope illustrate the major themes in current thinking about teamwork in healthcare. We use both a narrative and thematic approach drawing on the experiences of: a paediatric oncologist; a paediatric palliative care nurse practitioner; a physiotherapist with experience in paediatrics, oncology, adult rehabilitation and domiciliary care teams; and Sandra, mother of five children and professor of nursing. Professor Sandra Dunn is an author of this paper in both capacities, and her family has consented to this use of Keown's story.

In 1998 Keown, Sandra and James's youngest child, was diagnosed with medulloblastoma, cancer of the brain. He died in 2003 at the age of 10. Interviews and thematic analysis were conducted by the first two authors following ethics approval and focused on the participant's experiences and beliefs about client/family-centred multidisciplinary care. The framing of these interviews was based on a review of the literature and a reading of the narrative account presented by Sandra, although the focus of the interviews was not on Keown exclusively, but rather on teamwork more generally. We use the case study to remind the reader that in the last analysis the organisation of clinical treatment is about dealing with human need and suffering. The first narrative of the case study is below.

Box 6.1 Case study – Teamwork for Keown

Sandra: On 15 August 1998, aged five years and four months, Keown James Dunn, my youngest son, was diagnosed with a medulloblastoma, cancer of the brain. In the coming years my husband and I learned more than we ever wanted to know about the paediatric oncology experience – from the parent's side of the looking glass.

Keown had had maybe a year of occasional morning headaches, sometimes vomiting – not enough to get much attention in the chaos of getting seven people off to school and work. Then one morning came the call from school – 'Keown has a bad headache. He's crying and the light hurts his eyes.' The nurses in the ER stood with me and my husband, listened to our questions, told us what was said when our ears were too full of fear to hear the doctors' discussion. Then the CAT scan, the first set of films, the radiologist arriving to inject contrast. For me, it truly started then. Then surgery. There were no real choices. With that presentation, there weren't options; there wasn't time.

Post-op … waiting. Did they get it all? Will he wake up? And if he does, will he still be our son? As Keown lay in paeds ICU, the neurosurgeon came to see us, telling us what had happened, reassuring us that the surgery had gone well. The nurses answered and re-answered our questions, the same questions over and over, reassuring, moving with purpose and skill.

After surgery came the looking for answers: How do we help our son? We didn't even know the questions, let alone the answers.

Teamwork in organisations

The concept of the team is an old one, originally referring to harnessed animals pulling loads together and now used extensively for groups of people playing sport or working together. It implies interdependence, common goals and effort, and its positive meaning is related to the idea that the whole is more than the sum of its parts. A team can be defined as two or more individuals performing a range of interdependent tasks with a clear division of labour (Baker et al 2006). More technically, it is defined as

> [A] collection of individuals who are interdependent in their tasks, who share responsibility for outcomes, who see themselves and are seen by others as an intact social entity embedded in one or more larger social systems and who manage their relationships across organisational borders.

> (Cohen & Bailey 1997:241)

Teams can be lasting structures – such as the staff of a dialysis unit or a community health centre – or short-term groups that form to meet the needs of an individual family or situation such as those responding to a local outbreak of infection in a child care centre, or a project team introducing a new system or service.

Over the past several decades attention to teamwork has been a strong component of contemporary management theory with a number of experts suggesting that it contributes to increases in efficiency, productivity, problem solving and workplace creativity (Morris 1996). Management literature in the 1980s and 1990s on the flexible firm and flexible specialisation suggested that teamwork produced flatter structures and a breakdown of the rigid division of labour, bringing the production process closer to the customer and their needs (Mathews 1989, 1991, 1992a, 1992b, Robbins & Barnwell 2002). As Sutcliffe and Callus (1994:67) note the aim is to enhance the links between the market and the organisation in an arena where technological change increasingly requires more flexible work practices. Two questions arise from this work: first, it is not clear from the literature what exactly it is about teamwork that brings the production process closer to the customer; and second, whether the rationale for team-based work outlined by Mathews (1991, 1992a) and others as suitable for industry is directly transferable or desirable for healthcare settings. Teamwork is after all a means to an end, not a goal in itself, and like all methods, has limits to its application. Further, there are real costs to effective teamwork, and attention must be paid to ensuring that costs are contained and proportional to the benefits (West et al 2002).

Teamwork is the totality of methods of collaboration in pursuit of shared purposes used by members of a team. Given this definition much is made of the importance of multidisciplinary teamwork in healthcare (e.g. Moorin 2005), which is seen as both vitally important and difficult to achieve. It is important because the different professions or disciplines (including specialties within professions) bring different skills and perspectives. These skills and perspectives need to be integrated to ensure that goals and decision making are based on the best available understanding and that commitment to the decisions is shared by team members. However, teamwork is difficult to achieve not only because it requires time and attention to the way people work together, but also because the training of health professionals tends to emphasise individual accountability and skill (and a preference for working with one's own profession), as do systems for remuneration and reward (Leggat 2007).

What is multidisciplinary team care?

In authentic multidisciplinary care, team members rely on cross-disciplinary input in planning their own clinical care, in the development of a collaborative individual treatment plan for a patient (National Breast Cancer Centre 2003:2), and in emergence of new activities arising from this collaboration. There is a clear understanding of the array of professional expertise, but a willingness to be flexible, to share skills and in some cases to tolerate role substitution, collective ownership of the care plan and a capacity to reflect on these processes. Bronstein (2003:114) extends this to suggest that team members have to see the collaboration as positive and believe that the goals could only be achieved through collaboration with each other. Perhaps more than in other industries, multidisciplinary teamwork in healthcare is achieved through a combination of structural units (such as the oncology unit) and 'virtual teams' – the health professionals who work together across organisational units to plan and deliver the care for an individual or a group of patients (such as pharmacists, radiologists, pathologists and others working with the oncology unit).

The significant characteristic of MTC is that the various professionals come together to pool their expertise in all relevant aspects of the patient's care, and together plan a program of care tailored to each patient (Herrman et al 2002; Liberman et al 2001). Why this approach should emerge at this point in history is partly explained by

> **Box 6.2** Case study – The patient, his family and the healthcare team
>
> Keown's carers defined multidisciplinary teams as a small core group of professionals, as well as others who may at times form part of the group, but are often on the outer rings. In the acute phase (post surgery), the core team was the oncology unit, along with the pharmacist, radiologist, play therapist and pathologist. They did not regard the patient or his family as core members of the team, but recognised the family's role in decision making about treatment options.
>
> In the palliative phase, the team is 'a virtual team' drawn from those available in the patient's community – every health professional who can contribute and is willing to work with the team philosophy. In this phase, the family was seen as the centre of the team – the palliative care nurse practitioner saw her role as 'creating a nest for that family' while they coped with the reality of their child dying. Perhaps because of their inability to change the course of Keown's illness, the professionals worried that they may have let Keown's family down in the palliative phase, but Sandra felt that her whole family had been supported and cared for.
>
> In the professionals' view the inclusion of patients and their families into the team has emerged at the current time because of the need for the treating team to share the same goals as the patient. They note that sometimes clinicians have goals directed towards a 'cure at any cost', while clients may wish to pursue quality-of-life approaches. In such situations decision making requires bringing the client into the team as an equal member, entitled not just to consent to treatment, but to be able to say what treatment is provided and of course to know their treatment options. Keown participated in decisions to do with his own quality of life and brain function. He knew he *had bad cells and good cells* and that the radiotherapy would attack the bad cells and also damage good ones. At age nine, with the hindsight of seeing other children, he said to his parents, 'I don't want to do that, I don't want to be like X (who had a brain injury from treatment); I know I can die from this, but if all the good cells are going to die, I don't want to do that.'

developments in healthcare and in society. Cancer care has been a focus of attention to MTC because it requires a set of complex decisions to be made over diagnosis, treatment options, and efficacy for specific individuals. Chronic illness more generally requires the interventions of an array of health professionals over an extended period. Further, sick individuals are not only clinically specific, they are also patients with rights, and are increasingly well informed.

Some commentators and researchers have used definitions with lower thresholds for multidisciplinarity – any care involving more than one discipline (Britton et al 2006, Karjalainen et al 2007). However, an important criterion in our definition is that the group of health professionals bring their *shared expertise* to the diagnostic, treatment, rehabilitation and/or care processes. Treatment and care may come from any member of the team at various stages in the patient's illness. As a consequence senior medical professionals may not always take the lead. Leadership may come from the patient's GP, their specialist nurse, or dietician (Wilson et al 2005).

Further ambiguity in defining MTC occurs in the Australian context, where team members may work across significant geographical distances. Recognising this, the National Multidisciplinary Care Demonstration Project (NMCDP) in breast cancer developed a set of five essential principles in defining multidisciplinary care (National Breast Cancer Centre 2003:5). These are:

1. a team approach involving core disciplines integral to the provision of good care, with input from other specialities as required (the 'core' disciplines are surgery, radiology, medical and radiation oncology, pathology and supportive care)
2. communication occurs among team members regarding treatment planning
3. access to the full therapeutic range for all women, regardless of geographical remoteness or size of institution
4. care is provided in accordance with nationally agreed standards
5. involvement of the woman in decisions about her care.

The limitation of confining the team to medical specialists has been highlighted in the care of patients with cancer, who usually require input from several clinical disciplines in the acute phase, but also in rehabilitation and palliative phases of care (National Cancer Control Initiative 2003).

In the Australian context multidisciplinary care teams can be found in intensive care units (ICUs), cancer and palliative care, in geriatric and rehabilitation services (Karjalainen et al 2007), in crisis mental health teams (Joy et al 2006), in the organisation of care for people with chronic conditions, in aged care and in many other areas. In the UK multidisciplinary teamwork has been endorsed as the major way to organise care for cancer patients (Fleissig et al 2006:935), and in Canada as the major approach to re-structuring the healthcare system in the light of increasing expectations, rising costs and the ageing population (Canadian Health Services Research Foundation (CHSRF) 2006). Multidisciplinary care teams appear to operate best in situations where patients require long-term healthcare interventions across a variety of areas requiring input from a range of professionals, or where care is provided in small and cohesive units such as ICUs or community mental health teams. MTC is also found where diagnosis and treatment are characterised by ambiguity or lack of certainty.

Clinical effectiveness of multidisciplinary team care – the evidence

Evidence on the value of MTC in relevant aspects of healthcare is growing. In a major review of the evidence for MTC in the treatment of cancer, Moorin (2005) reported on 14 studies that provided evidence of reduced mortality and increased quality of life for patients receiving multidisciplinary care. However, some of those studies simply demonstrated the value of the learning curve (that is, better outcomes for those surgeons experienced with and specialising in, for example, breast cancer) and the use of multiple therapies and/or the existence of defined relationships with other disciplines (which may relate to a multidisciplinary team approach) rather than MTC directly (Sainsbury et al 1995). Five of the studies limited the definition of MTC to medical specialists, and one examined the effect of introducing a specialist breast nurse with a role in support and coordination for patients (National Breast Cancer Centre 2003). Several studies examined patient satisfaction and other indicators (such as reduced time to treatment) (Gabel et al 1997) and higher levels of physical functioning (Frost et al 1999).

Proponents of MTC argue that multidisciplinary teams provide benefits for patients ranging from ensuring equal access to specialist services for patients with similar diagnosis, smoother referral between services as communication between treating team members is enhanced, less duplication and delay of diagnostic tests, speedier implementation of treatment plans that conform to internationally accepted standards, less variation in patient survival rates, and increases in the recruitment of patients into clinical trials (Burns & Lloyd 2004, Fleissig et al 2006, Moorin 2005). These and other authors conclude that the benefits are the result of consensus decision making within the team, and a wider awareness of the treatment options available, and in the case of cancer care, possible differences in the staging of treatment (Howard et al 2001). What is clear is that a MTC approach results in increased patient satisfaction arising from enhanced support and a clearer sense of the organisation of care (Fleissig et al 2006, Moorin 2005).

Box 6.3 Case study – The purpose of MTC for Keown

Sandra began her interview by telling us how terrible the healthcare system is for patients – it is like a machine, set up to serve itself, she said. There is a cost to families in attending, waiting, and undergoing routine tests, and time for ordinary activities is lost. Hospitals appear not to have the capacity to schedule appointments to suit daily life, so that clients have to make daily, but significant adjustments. Sandra found she had to struggle to make the treating team aware of her child's practical needs, and R[*] and M[*] both saw negotiating between patients and 'the system' as one of their primary roles. For Sandra in her role as mother this meant ensuring Keown got to kindergarten to play with his friends irrespective of appointments for radiotherapy, for R it meant rescheduling appointments to reduce the client's discomfort, costs, and disruption. For M it meant supplying letters of referral when Sandra and her family went on holiday and during the palliative stage in case they might need to call an ambulance or take Keown to the emergency department. In effect the clinical team worked to soften the system, so the family felt cocooned and able to get through the rigours of painful treatment, and then what was going to be a bad outcome. These observations are consistent with the research evidence that patients report speedier services, treatment schedules that reduce waiting times and less impact on their daily lives.

---

[*]clinical members of the multidisciplinary team

The review by Joy et al (2006), and a similar one by Karjalainen et al (2007) (focused on rehabilitation for neck and shoulder pain among working-age adults), found no differences in clinical outcomes, including deaths, or discernible differences in mental and social wellbeing, and no differences in hospital admissions or repeat admissions pointing to little by way of cost savings. Similarly the studies cited by Moorin (2005:43–44) on cost savings are not conclusive, although Moorin notes that one of the key findings of the Australian National Cancer Demonstration Projects was that costs associated with multidisciplinary team meetings reduce as they become better established. The exception to this is a study done by Ettner et al (2006) who were able to demonstrate that it was cheaper to care for the patients in an intervention (multidisciplinary) group than patients who received 'usual' care.

MTC and psychological wellbeing

While the jury is out on the clinical and cost effectiveness of MTC, the evidence on the value for the psychological wellbeing of clients is overwhelmingly positive. In the studies by Joy et al (2006) and Karjalainen et al (2007), not only did participants report improved wellbeing, their families also reported less disruption to their lives and higher levels of satisfaction with the care provided. In the Joy et al study, this was despite the

Box 6.4 Case study – Evidence and decision-making

Sandra: For a child with a medulloblastoma, maybe, on a good day, there might be a 15% chance of survival without any treatment. But these stats are old, and might well be confounded by misdiagnosis or other error. There are no good recent stats on survival without treatment – the study design problems are obvious. So, we are left with old, probably unreliable evidence of a 15% survival rate without treatment.

With each step in treatment there are benefits, but there are also enormous risks. For a child with a medulloblastoma, following neurosurgery alone there may be approximately 45% survival depending on the site, extent and type of tumour. Setting aside those risks associated with any surgery, neurosurgery for cancer risks permanent brain damage (motor control, memory, sensory, cognitive) and hormonal system damage (growth, hunger, diuresis, sexual maturity, etc).

Add radiotherapy to the surgery and survival increases from 45% to around 55 or 60% – survival for two or three more children out of every 20. However, with that improved survival comes more treatment-related risks and side effects: cognitive defects, sensory deficits, secondary cellular dysplasia or cancers, radiation burns, nausea and vomiting. Keown said, 'Throwing up, Mum. Don't forget throwing up.'

Chemotherapy. Add 48 weeks of triple therapy and survival increases to maybe 65 or 70% – another two or three kids out of every 20 who get to survive. Additional side effects and risks include death from ordinary childhood illnesses (chicken pox, viruses), renal damage, major hearing loss, sterility, cardiac damage, vomiting and hair loss. The cumulative effects of treatment – a 70% chance of survival and certainty of complications.

Keown is sick, he is tired, he looks funny. He can't go to school much of the time. He can't play with his friends. If we go out anywhere, we take along a throw-up bag and a pee bottle because he's also got diabetes insipidus. 'Will this kill the bad cells, Mummy?' 'I don't know, my love.'

We are not doing something merely for the sake of action. Every decision carries with it enormous risks and we must balance the benefits with those risks. And the risks are to my son, and my family, and I love them very much. What does this evidence tell me about Keown? Not enough. How do I balance a 15% increase in survival with a 60 to 75% risk of him having a developmental delay?

So I followed the evidence, I followed the European Consortium on their trials. I called Dr X in the United States and asked him if he had any unpublished results for his low-dose radiation/long-term chemo regime. We could not choose survival at any price. So we went with low-dose radiotherapy and long-term chemo. We traded an unknown percentage of survival for a different, but still unknown, percentage of life – quantity for quality – the lady or the tiger – never knowing what was behind either door – the terror of getting it wrong. 'I wouldn't do it if it was my son' said one healthcare professional. 'If only it were your son', I thought.

Sandra is clear that the health professionals can't be expected to make the value judgments needed to choose the treatment that is best for any individual. That choice is the right and responsibility of the patient and his or her family. The paediatric oncologist and the nurse practitioner believed just as strongly that it's not fair to patients to present them with treatment options without a clear explanation not only of the costs and benefits but also of why this decision needs to be made now, and a clear recommendation. They saw it as an ethical responsibility – to give advice, and not to leave the family potentially with 'blood on their hands'. Two different, but reconcilable, perspectives.

fact that sick clients continued to live with their families during their illness episode. The National Demonstration Project in Breast Cancer (Moorin 2005:37) study found improvements in the women's mental health, and significantly, major improvements in decision making by the women. In our own interviews client decision making was a major issue for both the client and the clinicians. We report on the participant's views below.

> **Box 6.5** Case study – Teams and patient decision making
>
> There was a surprising consistency between the four participants in our case study on how patients might exercise their decision making within the team, and how health professionals might facilitate this. The physiotherapist, drawing on her work with clients in rehabilitation, saw it as a *duty of care* to ensure that they made realistic decisions and set reachable goals. To do this required taking time out to inform patients of all the treatment options and the available evidence and also allowing for mistakes where this could be accommodated – in her experience clients sat in on team meetings and took an active role.
>
> The oncologist similarly noted the need to take time to bring patients into the decision making as partners regardless of the additional time or effort required. He did not see this as ensuring they had the same scientific knowledge, but rather ensuring they understood the nature of the evidence and its limitations and were agreed on the way forward as a family unit, without family divisions or regret. For both the oncologist and the nurse practitioner, this required sharing their own knowledge about the patient's condition, providing the range of options, explaining their own recommendations and reasoning, but clearly outlining other options. As one noted, 'Few parents have the capacity to weigh the numbers on risks and benefits; they want their kid to "have a chance" – they are not able to reflect on statistics.'
>
> This approach brings the patient into the decision-making team, but consistent with the principles of MTC does not leave one member totally alone in their choices. Sandra noted that she never felt abandoned by the clinical team in making decisions, but at times she did defer to them; at other times she went against individual clinicians' recommendations.

The patient and family as 'partners' in care?

The management research on teams suggests that team structures allow the production process to be brought closer to the customer and their needs (see Box 6.5). The research on patient satisfaction and the care process suggests that one of the major benefits of MTC is that it can clarify and improve the relationship between patients and families and their care providers. The sense that the input of the various professionals is coordinated, and that the organisation is taking responsibility for that coordination, is important for managing client relationships in any professional business, and no less in healthcare.

Much of the rhetoric about patients and families as 'partners in care' has been just that – rhetoric driven by public relations goals and enthusiasm rather than a substantive change in the way the health system and its staff relate to and engage patients in their care. The case for such engagement has a particular logic when the patient is a sick child, and when the episode of care extends beyond the acute phase. Parents are in fact involved in looking after their children and managing their care both in hospital and in the community. Children's hospitals have recognised this reality for many years, and have changed some aspects of their care in response (such as the 'negotiated care' philosophy at the Children's Hospital at Westmead (Children's Hospital at Westmead 2005:29)). We suggest that greater recognition, and to some extent formalisation, of the active roles of patients in managing their disease, in achieving their personal goals for life with their disease, and in coordinating the care for sick family members, would improve the relationship between healthcare teams and patients, rather than simply complicate care. This is one of the benefits of MTC that could be better utilised, as we hope our case study of a particularly well-informed 'partner' family (Keown's story) illustrates.

What makes for effective multidisciplinary teams?

While research on the benefits of MTC continues, the model has been strongly embraced by health and medical authorities such as the Royal Australian College of Surgeons, the National Health and Medical Research Council and National Breast Cancer Centre (Moorin 2005). For example, the Australian Council on Safety and Quality in Healthcare states that: 'A culture of safety in healthcare will be reflected in a system that … supports multidisciplinary team approaches' (ACSQHC 2000:25). This raises the question of how MTC might be implemented more broadly.

Effective performance of multidisciplinary teamwork in complex healthcare settings depends on four major prerequisites: the structures within the healthcare system (policy and funding mechanisms) that would allow MTC to flourish; systems and procedures within health organisations that nurture teams; the process employed by the team itself; and the qualities of individual team members (Liberman et al 2001, Moorin 2005). We turn first to examine structural factors.

Structural and financial factors

We found little literature that explored the structural barriers to the development of MTC although a cursory examination of where the bulk of the research literature comes from might provide a clue. While the range of English-language clinical studies appeared to be spread proportionately across the US, UK, Canada, Australia and New Zealand, the majority of government-funded and -commissioned reports emanated from those countries with robust public health services providing free-to-the-consumer or subsidised healthcare. This is not to suggest that nations with universal health services are able to experiment with MTC without dealing with structural barriers, but it does point to the capacity to make national policy directives and to implement strategies to overcome the structural impediments of fee-for-service market-based health systems.

For example Moorin (2005) reports on a number of developments at the national level in Australia, New Zealand and the UK that facilitate the development of MTC. These developments include national policy and priority setting, funding of demonstration projects, and reimbursement to doctors and other health professionals for engaging in MTC. The British National Cancer Collaboration funded the formation of networks made up of private providers, trusts, health authorities, local authorities and the voluntary sector for the treatment of patients with cancer. One of the major outcomes of these network projects was a reduction in waiting times and an increase in patient satisfaction with the service for patients receiving treatment from multidisciplinary teams. This attractive outcome for government ensured that MTC became a standardised approach to cancer treatment in all cancer networks in the UK. Similar national policy directives in Australia have assisted in the development and routinisation of MTC. For example in 1996 cancer was identified as one of seven national health priorities. The National Health Priority Report published in 1997 noted the importance of MTC, as did the 2003 report (Moorin 2005:17).

On the other hand, in Australia, fee-for-service Medicare payments were found to encourage the sequential referral model that moved the patient from GP to a private specialist with little incentive for cross-referrals (because of risk of loss of income) and less incentive to engage in time-consuming MTC (Senate Community Affairs Reference Committee 2005:128). Remuneration methods for allied health professionals in the private sector are also generally not structured so as to enable participation in multidisciplinary team activities. There is little doubt that government funding for innovation assists MTC practices to become routinised in public hospitals and health services and it is not surprising that the major developments in MTC have occurred in the public sector. Access to MTC for rural and remote patients is a related problem.

The introduction of Enhanced Primary Care (EPC) items in the Medical Benefits Schedule (the list of fee-for-service payments that can be claimed from Medicare) is another important example of efforts to remove structural barriers to MTC. These items enable GPs, and their practice nurses, to engage with other service providers in planning and coordinating the care of older patients with chronic conditions. An item specifically for leading or participating in a multidisciplinary case conference to plan care for cancer patients has also been recently introduced, and other items support such activities for various specialties in caring for complex patients.

Lack of substantive research on the economic benefits of MTC is also a major impediment to implementation across the public and private sectors. The evaluation of the National Multidisciplinary Care Demonstration Project (NBCC 2003) found costs were higher for new initiatives, that the costs of personal time to attend meetings needed to be factored into the overall funding estimates, but that average costs per staff per meeting tends to reduce as the programs become established, especially if existing facilities and resources are used.

Organisational systems and process as enablers to MTC

Supportive policy and health structures are necessary but not sufficient requirements for effective multidisciplinary teamwork. Teamwork is also highly dependent on the systems in place within health units, and clearly articulated procedures and protocols outlining the roles, goals and functions of each team member or unit (Grumbach & Bodenheimer 2004, Liberman et al 2001). Baker et al (2006) refer to the high need for synchronisation of tasks across the hypercomplex system of hospitals as 'tight coupling'. The work of the various professional groups is highly interdependent and interlocked and the systems in place within hospitals need to support this.

Fleissig et al (2006) and Herrman et al (2002) report on difficulties with team processes. They found disaffection within multidisciplinary teams about leadership and decision making with significant gaps between team decisions and the treatment followed by clinicians, reluctance on behalf of clinicians to change their mind on management of the patient, and poor recording of decision making. This last factor points to the need for teams to have sufficient administrative support. The evidence points to a need to schedule meeting times on a regular basis, and this in turn is dependent on organisational factors supporting MTC, such as protecting meeting times from competing events and of course finding a regular time that everyone can attend. Where meetings require tele- or video-conferencing then technical support needs to be readily available. Invariably these requirements point to a need for adequate funding, a major issue for optimum MTC. An additional finding of the National Multidisciplinary Care Demonstration project was resistance by some clinicians to put the psychosocial issues of clients on the agenda (Moorin 2005).

> **Box 6.6** Implications for practice – Organisational requirements for Keown's team care
>
> According to the professionals we interviewed, effective teams:
>
> - are ideally geographically collocated with opportunity for regular contact time
> - quarantine time for regular meetings
> - need continuity in membership to achieve full capacity for care
> - are resourced for the costs of working as a team (including administrative support)
> - have some opportunities for relaxed time together, like 'first Friday drinks'
> - make benefits like staff development opportunities and conference attendance available to all professions.

Dynamics within the team

The dynamics of team meetings to a large extent depend on inter-professional respect for the role each discipline plays in the care of the client. The highly regulated division of labour represents one of the processes of teamwork (Mickan & Rodger 2000). It provides clear guidelines for role differentiation, leadership responsibilities and levels of accountability which in turn are reflective of a highly organised culture (Baker et al 2006, Herrman et al 2002, Mickan & Rodger 2000). Where health professionals operate according to and within the bounds of their professional expertise, roles are clear, conflict can be resolved and the possibility of adverse events is contained. The practicalities of this inter-professional collaboration are reflected upon by the oncologist we interviewed (see Box 6.7).

> **Box 6.7** Case study – Working with other disciplines: a medical perspective
>
> Reflecting on his early training the oncologist talked frankly about his first experience of a nurse telling him what he needed to do for a child (initiate IV therapy). He was taken aback at her frank assertiveness, but agreed with her assessment. The ability to communicate assertively is highlighted in the literature as something taught to airline pilots as a way of ensuring teamwork enhances safety (Baker et al 2006). The nurse, observing the child over an eight-hour shift, recognised the clinical signs, however putting in an IV line was the responsibility of junior doctors. In interview the oncologist noted that the difficulty here for the responsible clinician is to accept the observations of other professionals within the team, who pass these observations on for implementation. This does not mean taking the nurse's observations on faith or that there needs to be a move to role substitution. Medicolegal responsibilities mean that each professional is accountable for their role in treatment, and this in turn requires independent decision making as well as taking up advice when it is given.

However team members are often also required to modify their routines and methods to accommodate the priorities or logistics of others, and to adopt new technologies. Edmondson et al (2001) reported on the learning process of surgical teams that were introducing a new method of cardiac surgery. They found it was factors at the team (rather than hospital) level that made the difference for successful implementation; and that success was based on leader (surgeon) behaviour that encouraged team members to question and adapt established routines to the new technology, rather than treat it as a 'plug-in'. Members of teams also need to develop processes for effective communication and this is dependent on strong and informed leadership and opportunity for trial and error. A number of authors note that there appears to be an optimum size for effective team management. Four to 12 members is cited by Liberman et al (2001) as the ideal before communication begins to breakdown, although the National Multidisciplinary Care Demonstration Project reported up to 18 participants in care planning meetings (Moorin 2005).

Leadership as an enabler in teams

Leadership in MTC is a major issue in the literature, and no doubt in practice. A number of authors note that senior doctors expect to be team leaders (Herrman et al 2002, Lebrasseur et al 2002, Parker-Oliver et al 2005, Wilson et al 2005). It is often assumed that the professional with the longest educational preparation and highest status and salary automatically should lead the team. Herrman et al (2002) make a distinction between leadership of the team and clinical responsibility, autonomy and authority to perform a particular treatment or exercise in care. They suggest that leadership is earned within the team, while clinical responsibility arises out of education and accreditation, and the two qualities should not be confused (Bronstein 2003, Lebrasseur et al 2002, Parker-Oliver et al 2005).

Haward et al (2003) conclude that the most effective teams are those with shared leadership for clinical decision making and Liberman et al (2001) suggest that a case manager is the ideal project manager for the team. They note that leadership of multidisciplinary teams in large organisations like hospitals is presumed to be the responsibility of the senior medical clinicians and it is hard to imagine how other professional groups would have either the autonomy of day-to-day practice or the political clout. Despite this, they argue that what is needed in teams is a group of professionals with a set of competencies that range from acute through to rehabilitation care and that leadership may not necessarily be best performed by the doctors in all phases. The primacy of the doctor's skills, like those of the physiotherapist or social worker, vary according to where the patient or client is on the continuum of care. Interestingly, the Australian Cancer Network and National Breast Cancer Centre in its clinical guidelines (2003) notes that 'any member of the multidisciplinary team may, with the woman's approval, become the lead person for ongoing communication about her care' (Moorin 2005:30). The distinction between structural team leadership and (shared) clinical leadership in the care of individual patients and families is a useful one.

Individual qualities as enablers to MTC

At the individual level team members need a high level of professional and self-knowledge, and skills and attitudes that enable them to develop a shared understanding of the tasks to be performed by all involved. This includes a clear idea of each other's role, skills and knowledge and a capacity to anticipate the needs of other members of the team (Baker et al 2006, Mickan & Rodger 2000) in order to meet the individual needs of clients (Liberman et al 2001). Baker and colleagues also identify an ability to adjust to team decisions, along with a capacity to use the range of communication mediums in place whether this be case notes, emails, telemedicine or face-to-face interactions. They also cite mutual trust as a key quality for effective teamwork as does Bronstein (2003).

Box 6.8 Case study – Leadership in Keown's team

The four case study participants suggested that leadership in the team ebbed and flowed according to the task to be done. At times different members of the team took the lead, although this shift in leadership did not necessarily impact on team structure, since there needed to be a constant team manager. Among the physicians, one took the primary role as the point of coordination and communication with families. Leadership tensions were avoided by all members of the team having clear ideas about the roles and skills of each team member which in turn engendered respect. There were some individuals who found the team model difficult, and they sometimes left the team. Others needed support and coaching to relinquish 'solo operator' models of work, which had previously been expected and rewarded. An important factor in the success of the team was strong support and an expectation from management at all levels that MTC was the process of care.

Professional jealousies can be a major issue for effective teamwork and patients readily pick up these tensions. In the interviews R reflected upon the frustration felt by nurses at the power of doctors to make medical decisions, while J mused on the opportunities afforded to nurses to develop a deep and trusting relationship with the client who gave them insights into the patient not enjoyed by the doctor. These interprofessional tensions spill over into practice blurring the boundaries especially for young doctors in training who look to the consultant for leadership and decision making, while experienced nurses espouse a model of shared care arrived at through discussion at weekly team meetings.

Box 6.9 Implications for practice – Other barriers to teamwork

Additional barriers were identified by the case study participants. For them the rapid turnover of patients in the acute sector worked against MTC leading them to reinforce the idea that this approach to clinical work was best achieved in long-term care of chronic conditions – in the acute setting, at best, the team was the doctor and the nurse. Coupled with this they argued that work intensification meant more pressure on staff to get the work done and the patients through the system. Spending time on meetings was viewed as not cost effective. They also noted that the move to autonomous practice – especially in community health – worked against teamwork. In the community, teams may be multidisciplinary in composition, but often operate as autonomous practitioners, rarely meeting each other face to face.

Conclusion

This chapter has used a case study and narrative interwoven with the literature to explore the definition of multidisciplinary care, its effectiveness, barriers and facilitators. It has explored the implications of the client being seen as a member of this team, although like other team members their position is not constant. They may opt in or out depending on their capacity to engage in the processes and, importantly, on their capacity to grasp the implications of the knowledge underpinning clinical decision making. In the case study Keown's mother represents the extreme on the continuum of an informed family member. This continuum extends from other clients like her, trained health professionals with a capacity to do their own research on the evidence, to those with little knowledge of diagnosis or the various treatment modalities, or limited ability to assertively make their needs known. Some clients may make decisions to seek or refuse treatment that the team sees as dangerous. Knowledge of the diagnosis, treatments available and the implications mean clients and their families will be differently positioned within the team, and make demands on other team members in different ways. Clients with little knowledge will require more time for education and information; others will need time to deal with the complexity of decision making. Families and patients also differ from other members of the team in attachment to the outcomes. They are not health professionals seeking to provide value-neutral care for their client in a spirit of all that is positive in professional detachment. For families and clients their emotional attachment is, as it should be, self-centred.

The case study focuses on client-centred MTC in paediatric oncology. In the accounts provided by the four participants the MTC was most active during the outpatient treatment and palliative stages. We have already noted that MTC seems to be more prevalent where the patient or client has a chronic condition, where cure is not the major goal. At this point MTC can offer a wide range of care incorporating symptom management, family support, coordination of community services, and counselling. Of course there are other areas of healthcare that espouse client-centred MTC, including aged care and rehabilitation. In these areas, clients are often able to engage in the team process, understand the goals set for their care and report back to team members on the efficacy of interventions. These long-term relationships with adult clients are well suited to patient and family-centred MTC. What is needed to further client-centred MTC is rigorous research of a qualitative nature that investigates the impact of teamwork on diagnosis and treatment, and quantitative studies that evaluate the clinical and financial gains to be made by taking a team approach. A distillation of the 'take home messages' we garnered from our reading, discussion and writing of this chapter, and a final word on Keown, are provided in Boxes 6.10 and 6.11.

Box 6.10 Implications for practitioners – Multidisciplinary team care

The following principles are offered as a guide to health professionals in establishing MTC or extending its practice.

Structural: MTC depends on some enduring team structures along with the coming together of shorter term teams to meet the needs of particular patients or situations. Team structures need to be supported with good policy and systems. More innovation and experimentation is needed, as well as a stronger evidence base.

Financial: Remuneration in support of clinicians (particularly those funded on fee-for-service) engaging in teamwork is needed. The costs of setting up MTC are real, but so are the benefits (potentially including reduced utilisation of some interventions), and mature teams can develop efficient teamwork practices.

Systems: Managers and senior clinicians can enhance MTC through financial and human resource support for the smooth functioning of the team. Information systems can make teamwork easier.

Box 6.10 Implications for practitioners – Multidisciplinary team care – cont'd

Process: Effective MTC requires a commitment to regular meetings, and resources for implementing team decisions. Strong leadership is required for day-to-day management of enduring teams, but flexibility is needed to allow the most appropriate member to take leadership for particular patients or kinds of team tasks.

Respect: Teams need to operate from a basis of deep respect and understanding for each other's roles, and clear shared ideas of each member's roles and responsibilities. This has implications for formative and continuing education. There also needs to be a recognition that not all professionals are effective team players.

Individual professionals: Members of teams need to be confident in their own discipline boundaries, and comfortable to make suggestions in support of the client's care. This includes the ability to provide patients with treatment options and risks, and facilitate patient decision making, along with a capacity to be flexible in the face of decisions made by patients or other members of the team.

Patients and their families: The shared goal of meeting patient needs underlies the methods of MTC. Patients and families benefit from confidence that the care they receive is provided by a responsible team that they can rely on. They need to be factored into planning and decision making, and time is required to acquaint them of options, benefits and risks, and respect their choices about the extent of their engagement in decision making and caregiving.

Box 6.11 Case study – A final word on Keown

Sandra: Keown didn't live to see his 10th birthday. I received the call from our oncologist one morning. Doctor: 'Ah, hello. We have the report from the MRI. It's not looking good. The tumour has spread. It's all through the ventricles … I can't be sure, but there could be a bit in the base of the spinal cord …'

Keown lived his final 18 months of life with all his heart and all his soul. We visited Movie World. He rode his scooter – preferably very fast down hill and around corners – until he could no longer walk. He knew he was dying. 'I don't want to die, but when I do I want you to remember me as brave and strong and smart.'

And when we celebrated his life, at his final 'goodbye for now' party, his oncologist, his nurses, his GP, his palliative care nurse practitioner, his friends, his school mates, his family and his neighbours – we were all there, all part of the team, all there to send Keown on his way.

We can live with the decisions we made over those five and a bit years. Knowing what we know now, we wouldn't change them. Our brave, loving son was in the care of a team we trusted, and we were part of that team.

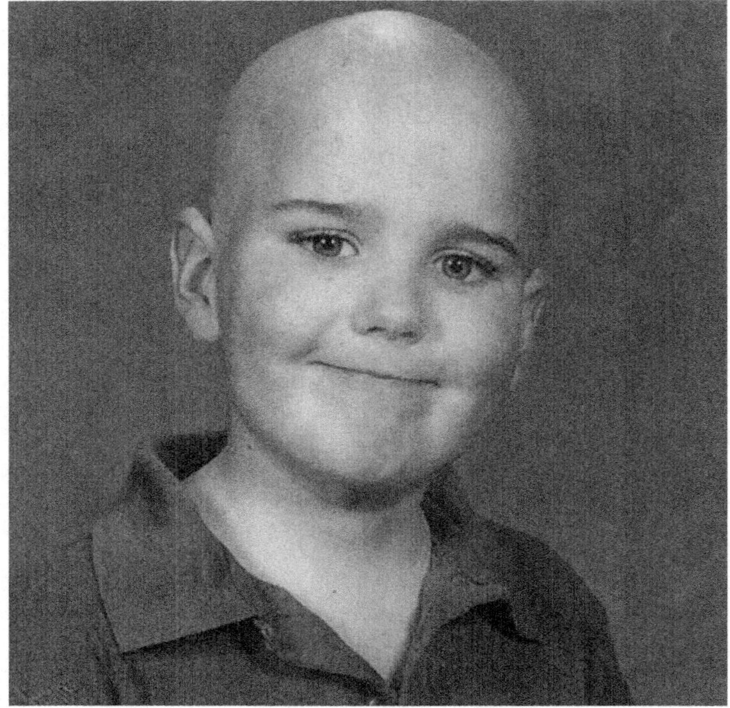

Keown: The youngest of Sandra and James's five children – brave, strong and smart forever.

Acknowledgement

We are grateful for the contributions of Ms Sara Fleming, Dr Michael Rice and Ms Michelle Todd whose experience and perspectives informed this chapter. Our thanks also to Anne Cahill Lambert for her assistance in developing the literature review for this article.

References

Australian Commission for Safety and Quality in Healthcare (ACSQHC) 2000 Safety and quality council action plan 2001. Australian Government, Canberra

Baker D, Day R, Salas E 2006 Teamwork as an essential component of high-reliability organizations, Health Services Research, Health Research and Educational Trust

Britton A M, Hogan-Doran J J, Siddiqi N 2006 Multidisciplinary Team Interventions for the management of delirium in hospitalized patients. (Protocol) Cochrane Database of Systematic Reviews, Issue 2. Art. No.: CD005995

Bronstein L 2003 A model for interdisciplinary collaboration, Social Work Research 48(3): 297–306

Burns T, Lloyd H 2004 Is a team approach based on staff meetings cost effective in the delivery of mental healthcare? Current Opinion in Psychiatry 17(4):311–314

Canadian Health Services Research Foundation (CHSRF) 2006 Teamwork in healthcare: promoting effective teamwork in healthcare in Canada: policy synthesis and recommendations. CHSR, Ottawa

Children's Hospital at Westmead 2005 A Handbook for families. CHM, Sydney.

Cohen S G, Bailey D R 1997 What makes teams work: Group effectiveness research from the shop floor to the executive suite. Journal of Management 23(4):238–290

Edmondson A C, Bohmer R M, Pisano G P 2001 Disrupted routines: team learning and new technology implementation in hospitals. Administrative Science Quarterly 46:685–716

Ettner S L, Kotlerman J, Afifi A et al 2006 An alternative approach to reducing the costs of patient care? A controlled trial of the multi-disciplinary doctor-nurse practitioner (MDNP) model. Medical Decision Making 26(1):9–17

Fleissig A, Jenkins V, Catt S et al 2006 Multidisciplinary teams in cancer care: are they effective in the UK? Lancet Oncology 11:935–943

Frost M, Arvizu R, Jayakumar S et al 1999 Multidisciplinary healthcare delivery model for women with breast cancer: patient satisfaction and physical and psychosocial adjustment. Oncology Nursing Forum 26(10):1673–80

Gabel M, Hilton N, Nathanson S 1997 Multidisciplinary breast cancer clinics: do they work? Cancer 79(12):2380–2384

Grumbach K, Bodenheimer T 2004 Can healthcare teams improve primary care practice? JAMA 291:1246–1251

Haward R, Amir Z, Borrill C et al 2003 Breast cancer teams: the impact of constitution, new cancer workload, and methods of operation on their effectiveness. British Journal of Cancer 89(1):15–22

Herrman H, Trauer T, Warnock J 2002 The roles and relationships of psychiatrists and other service providers in mental health services. Australian and New Zealand Journal of Psychiatry 36(1):75–80

Howard G, Thomson C, Stroner P et al 2001 Patterns of referral, management and survival of patients diagnosed with prostate cancer in Scotland during 1988 and 1993: results of a national retrospective population-based audit. British Journal of Urology 87(4):339–347

Joy C B, Adams C, Rice K 2006 Crisis intervention for people with severe mental illnesses. Cochrane Database of Systematic Reviews, Issue 4. Art. No.: CD001087

Karjalainen K, Malmivaara A, van Tulder M et al 2007 Multidisciplinary biopsychosocial rehabilitation for neck and shoulder pain among working age adults. Cochrane Database of Systematic Reviews, Issue 2. Art. No.: CD002194

Lebrasseur R, Whissell R, Ojha A 2002 Organisational Learning, Transformational Leadership and Implementation of Continuous Quality Improvement in Canadian Hospitals. Australian Journal of Management 27(2):141–162

Leggat S 2007 Effective healthcare teams require effective team members: defining teamwork competencies. BMC Health Services Research 7(17). doi:10.1186/1472–6963–7–17

Liberman R P, Hilty D M, Drake R et al 2001 Requirements for multidisciplinary teamwork in psychiatric rehabilitation. Psychiatric Service 52(10):1331–1342

Mathews J 1989 From Post-Industrialism to post-fordism. Meanjin 48(1):139–152

Mathews J 1991 Ford Australia plastics plant: Transition to teamwork through quality enhancement, UNSW Studies No 3. University of New South Wales, Sydney

Mathews J 1992a New production systems: a response to critics and a re-evaluation. Journal of Political Economy 30:91–128

Mathews J 1992b The Australian Taxation Office: Modernisation through People Structure and Technology, UNSW Studies No 6. University of New South Wales, Sydney

Mickan S, Rodger S 2000 Characteristics of effective teams: a literature review. Australian Health Review 23(3):201–208

Moorin R 2005 Inquiry into Service and Treatment Options for People with Cancer: briefing paper: Multidisciplinary Care, Centre for Health Services Research. School of Population Health, University of Western Australia, Perth

Morris R 1996 The Age of workplace reform in Australia. In: Mortimer D, Leece P, Morris R (eds) Workplace reform and enterprise bargaining. Harcourt Brace, Sydney

National Breast Cancer Centre (NBCC) 2003 Multidisciplinary Care in Australia: a National Demonstration Project in Breast Cancer, Summary Report, NBCC, Sydney. Online. Available: http://www.nbcc.org.au/resources/resource.php?code=MDS 3 Apr 2007

National Cancer Control Initiative 2003 Optimising Cancer Care in Australia: A consultative report prepared by the Clinical Oncological Society of Australia, Melbourne, The Cancer Council Australia and the National Cancer Control Initiative. Online. Available: http://www.ncci.org.au/pdf/OCCA/Optim_Cancer_Care.pdf 3 Apr 2007

Parker-Oliver D, Bronstein L, Kurzejeski L 2005 Examining variables related to successful collaboration on the hospice team. Health & Social Work 30(4):279–286

Robbins S, Barnwell, N 2002 Organisation Theory: Concepts and Cases. Pearson Education Australia, Frenchs Forest

Sainsbury R, Haward B, Rider L et al 1995 Influence of clinician workload and patterns of treatment on survival from breast cancer. The Lancet 34:1265–1270

Senate Community Affairs Reference Committee 2005 The cancer journey: Informing choice, Report on the inquiry into services and treatment options for persons with cancer. Commonwealth of Australia, Canberra

Sutcliffe P, Callus R 1994 Glossary of Australian Industrial Relations terms, ACIRRT & ACSM. University of Sydney, Sydney

West M, Borrill C, Dawson J et al 2002 The link between the management of employees and patient mortality in acute hospitals. International Journal of Human Resource Management 13(8):1299–1310

Wilson D, Moores D, Woodhead Lyones S et al 2005 Family Physicians' interest and involvement in interdisciplinary collaborative practice in Alberta. Canada Primary Healthcare Research and Development 6:224–231

Chapter 7

Co-producing care

Rick Iedema, Roslyn Sorensen, Christine Jorm & Donella Piper

Introduction

There is a shift in the role patients play in their healthcare. While the body of the patient has always been central to care, the place of patient cognition – the exercise of opinion and will – is a current focus. There has been a shift: from a passive view of patients as undiscriminating recipients of care defined by others ('patient centred' or not); to routine disclosure of information that affects them and their participation in decision making; through to encouraging discriminating consumers who are actively involved as care recipients with the power to choose the services they prefer; and finally to the notion of the patient/consumer as a co-producer of healthcare. Such recipients are not only involved in decision making about their care, but also actively assist and collaborate in designing the product that they consume. The emerging importance of co-produced healthcare is borne out by reference to the concept in numerous chapters in this book (see particularly Mooney, Chapter 13; but also Claridge & Cook, Chapter 4; Kerosuo, Chapter 5; Willis, Dwyer & Dunn, Chapter 6; and Jorm, Banks & Twohill, Chapter 12).

The place of patients/consumers of healthcare is moving from that of stakeholders with the limited power of 'being satisfied' or not with the care they receive to 'prosumers' of care. Coined by Alvin Toffler in 1979, the word 'prosumer' is gaining currency in many industrial and manufacturing circles. This term links the idea of consumer with that of producer. It encompasses the added consumer power of defining the product through consulting and negotiating with healthcare professionals. This suggests that the range of meanings inherent in patient-centred care is related to those who have the power to define the type of healthcare available, offered, accepted and delivered. That is, patients are becoming more involved, not just in accepting what is offered, but in determining the care they prefer and the manner in which it is provided. Further, the role of citizen in healthcare is becoming prominent, not only as the potential recipients of healthcare services, but also from the democratic basis that all citizens (not just service users) should have a say in how their services are designed and delivered.

This patient/consumer/prosumer prominence has far-reaching implications for the way the healthcare system, services and programs and clinical processes are planned, delivered and evaluated. As the conceptualisation of active patients who participate in their care moves from those who ask 'lay questions' to recognising that consumers themselves have expertise in managing their own diseases, illnesses or conditions, their relationships with health professionals must change concurrently. This is desirable, particularly since the evidence suggests that active participation is strongly associated with better patient outcomes. Thus the power dynamics between clinicians and patients will continue to become more complex and less privileging of the clinical professional as the final arbiter of what is appropriate care. This in turn has implications for what kinds of people will populate health, given we are talking about a new type of work involving new types of workers – professionals who besides enacting their expertise, are capable of acknowledging care limitations, exhibiting humility, accepting others' views, and embracing others' expertise.

Against this background, in this chapter we discuss:

- the changing place of patients in healthcare
- the experience of open disclosure
- the implications for practice of co-production.

The changing place of patients in healthcare

The place of patients and the public generally in healthcare is changing. Lay people are taking on more prominence, whether as individuals interested in managing their own chronic conditions; as members of active stakeholder groups who express growing legitimate interests in the quality, outcomes and experience of specific strands of healthcare; or as patients (or family members) becoming involved in the investigation of their (relative's) unexpected treatment outcomes. These interests and forms of participation need to be acknowledged and incorporated within an evolving concept of 'the healthcare product'. According to Irwin & Richardson (2006) patient-focused care includes four broad areas of intervention: communication with patients, partnerships, health promotion and physical care (i.e. medications and treatments). In their view, patient-focused or patient-centred care is constructive in achieving the 'three Cs' of care, namely communication, continuity and concordance. While this model seeks to counterbalance existing technology-based, disease-centred models (Irwin & Richardson 2006), it does not go so far as to envisage the potential for consumer involvement in the (re)design of healthcare services and treatment practices.

In effect, 'taking the consumer into account' constitutes a spectrum of engagement, ranging from clinicians and health services acting as experts in healthcare responding to patients' biological needs and preferences, to lay consumers with the power to pass judgment on the quality of care and hence the right to choose services and treatments, to 'prosumers' co-producing healthcare and practice improvements through collaboration with clinicians in (re)defining the product they desire to consume. The prosumer concept describes a rapidly evolving model of patient-centred care (Mansell et al 2005) whose intent is to increase the participation of patients in decisions within the medical–clinical encounter, and of the public in decisions about healthcare in general (see Mooney, Chapter 13). The word epitomises the rapidly developing view of the patient/consumer/prosumer[7] being a partner in producing healthcare processes and outcomes.

---

[7] These terms are used interchangeably throughout the chapter.

Consumer participation is being supported by a range of policy instruments, particularly at the medical-encounter level. Two policy instruments are prominent that reflect the changing place of the consumer, namely informed consent and open disclosure. Open disclosure is used as an example here and reference is made to informed consent.

First, informed consent is defined as a patient-driven decision-making model that applies, besides an evidence-based decision-making model, a public-participation model (Carey-Hazell 2005). Recognising the limited scope of existing informed consent policy, a recent report recommends extending informed consent from advice about and negotiation concerning medical risk (the epidemiological chance of surviving a treatment in conjunction with the patient's condition), to also covering clinical risk (Who will be operating on me today? Who will be supervising? What technological resources are there? Who is providing clinical and technical support?), and organisational risk (What are this department's or health facility's cross-infection risks, medication error rates, etc?) (Iedema et al 2007). This advice recognises a consumer's right to be informed and think about more than merely the scientific dimensions of care, particularly since medical treatment does not take place in a neutral clinical-organisational environment of predictable staffing and standard technologies.

Second, open disclosure guides hospital staff in openly communicating with patients and their nominated support person following an adverse event (Bauman et al 2003). In the case of open disclosure, guidelines and codes of conduct support the standard's implementation, although in Australia, the Australian Medical Association's code of conduct does not contain an express patient disclosure provision (Madden & Cockburn 2007). Statutory protection exists for those who express regret that an error has occurred,[8] but there is no corresponding statutory obligation to disclose personal or organisational responsibility (Madden & Cockburn 2007). In contrast, a legal obligation exists in Canada for doctors to fully disclose information, thereby enabling patients to participate in decisions about how the unexpected outcome is to be handled (Legare et al 2007).

What these policy initiatives have in common is that they drive the clinician–consumer relationship towards more 'democratic' or shared forms of decision making. Not surprisingly, in recent years shared decision making (SDM) has gained considerable importance (Simon et al 2007). In outlining the current position of SDM in Australian healthcare, McCaffery et al note that support exists in the form of guidelines and interventions (McCaffery et al 2007). They assert however that there is no clear overall policy framework, that resources and infrastructure are limited and that there is no clear implementation strategy for SDM. Despite this, SDM is increasingly embedded in specific initiatives involving the public such as open disclosure (Iedema et al submitted, Iedema et al 2007).

Work is also occurring internationally in relation to SDM. For example the Canadian government has established a Canadian Research Chair entitled the 'Implementation of Shared Decision Making in Primary Care' because of the steady increase of the number of diagnostic tools and treatment options available and the amount of information on healthcare services. Healthcare professionals were increasingly required to play a new role as 'decision brokers' and patients were being asked to participate actively in decision making on their health. Hence, decision-making processes were seen to be transforming. However the process of SDM is not widespread. Nor is the

---

[8] An 'expression of regret' is a 'partial apology' (such as 'I am sorry this happened to you'). This contrasts with a 'full apology' that acknowledges fault and which is admissible in court in all Australian states except New South Wales and the Australian Capital Territory (Vines 2005).

concept clearly understood (Charles et al 2003). The Canadian initiative is seeking to gain a better understanding of the needs of professionals delivering primary health-care and prompt them to promote SDM, develop the tools needed to apply this new professional technique, build the most effective strategies for introducing the tools, and assess their impact. The program aims to design effective intervention systems for implementing a SDM process in primary healthcare.

In the UK, Evans et al (2007) note two particular areas where implementation of SDM is proceeding, namely in the education curricula and in patient decision sup-port technologies (PDSTs), including around informed consent (Loh et al 2007). The medical education initiative appears to be limited, however, and PDSTs are described as unplanned and fragmented, although gaining momentum in some clinical domains (Evans et al 2007). Scholars associated with the UK's National Patient Safety Agency are exploring ways of involving consumers in patient safety and practice improve-ment. Some of these approaches are proactive and engage patients in infection control initiatives (Davis et al 2007, Davis et al 2008), while others explore the potential of collaborating with consumers across the spectrum of care from prevention of errors to their investigation (Mansell et al 2005). A further example is the UK Citizens Council established by the National Institute for Clinical Excellence (NICE), which seeks input from citizens on issues of clinical need. As well as Canada and the UK, other countries are also undertaking activity in SDM to varying degrees including Italy, Germany, France and the Netherlands (Evans et al 2007, Goss & Renzi 2007, Legare et al 2007, Loh et al 2007, Moumjid et al 2007, van der Weijden et al 2007).

On a broader front, identifying ways in which patients and the public can be more involved in decision making has produced a large body of literature that covers every-thing from the micro-medical encounter to macro-health-system-related policymak-ing. Loh et al (2007a) categorised public participation as occurring at three levels: the micro (medical encounter) level, the meso (service/program) level and macro (system) level. Loh et al report that the members of the public they surveyed see their contribu-tion as applying to the macro and meso levels and that the micro level is one where patients themselves should be involved.

Addressing SDM at the macro level, Litva et al (2002) identified a range of 'impulses' that projected public participation into the healthcare debate in the UK. These impulses are instrumental, communitarian, educative, expressive and accountability related. The authors described these impulses as promoting or defending the interests and goals of the public in healthcare decisions (instrumentalist), involving communities with com-mon interests and expertise in local healthcare services (communitarian), developing citizens' sense of competence and responsibility (educative), expressing political iden-tity and belonging (expressive) and the desire for local accountability for a publicly funded service (accountability). Litva et al (2002) further noted that little work had occurred to systematically examine public preferences for being involved in health-care decision making, including health service rationing, the Oregon experiments (see Sorensen & Iedema, Chapter 1) with public involvement in health resource alloca-tion notwithstanding (Litva et al 2002). The importance of this work is that it showed variations in the willingness of members of the public to be involved. Specifically, the public had a strong desire to be involved in decision making at the system and program levels, preferably through consultation, but without always being prepared to accept responsibility for such decisions. Moreover, the public's participation was seen to be contingent on a guarantee that their contributions were fully heard and that decisions taken following consultation were explained.

Commenting on meso-level involvement, McGurk et al (in press) suggest that ser-vice users have a role to play in service development as well as to support the provision of care. Equally, Gagliardi et al (2008) believe that the public should be involved in service planning and evaluation. These proposals echo Mansell and colleagues' work on initiating collaborations with consumers around service redesign in the interest of patient safety (Mansell et al 2005). In this respect, the New South Wales (NSW) Health Clinical Services Redesign Program (CSRP) has developed a method for capturing and analysing patient and carer experiences to improve the 'patient journey' through the NSW health system. A patient journey refers to the process or progressive steps taken by a patient as they received healthcare. The project is based on research from the Picker Institute UK that found that patients and carers value:

- access to care
- respect for patient values, preferences and expressed needs
- coordination and integration of care
- information and education
- transition and continuity
- physical comfort
- emotional support and alleviation of fear and anxiety
- involvement of family and friends.

Initiatives are also occurring at the patient advisory level. In the UK, the recent *Local Government and Public Involvement in Health Act 2007* established local government networks to consider, among other things, the commissioning, provision and scrutinising of local healthcare services. For its part, the NSW Clinical Excellence Commission (CEC) has established the Citizen Engagement Advisory Council to advise the CEC in relation to systemic safety and quality issues. In this context, 'citizens' are those who have experience in the provision of safety and quality in high-risk industries such as the airline and mining industries. This citizen input is supplemented with user input from patients and former patients who have used the NSW health system as well as from interest groups. An important finding about patient experience is that it includes insights into what happens during the 'gaps' between the episodes of clinical care – time spent waiting at home for an appointment or time spent recovering in a ward, for example. Strong perceptions of the health system are created during these gaps – usually as a result of the interactions (or lack of interactions) between the patient and carer and healthcare professionals (refer to www.archi.net.au/e-library/build/ stories; see also Berding, Resources). Davis and colleagues' investigation into involving consumers in meso-level collaborations over the shape of services concludes that

> … in order to achieve effective and sustainable outcomes for the active involvement of the patient in patient safety, it is important to foster a working partnership between patients and health care professionals. This requires that patient involvement in safety-related behaviours be perceived by all (i.e. hospital staff (e.g. nurses, doctors) and patients) as beneficial to the medical encounter rather than challenging the health care professionals' clinical skills and abilities.

> (Davis et al 2007:265)

Early work at the micro level investigated the views of nurses, doctors and members of the public on behaviour to effectively involve patients in their own healthcare, Weiss (1986) found a number of key norms in six core clusters. Some 20 years ago, Weiss found that developing overt contracts in health relationships, forming egalitarian communication between patient and professional, giving patient access to broad-based information, tailoring of treatment programs, self-care and lifestyle modification activities were beneficial to healthcare outcomes (Weiss 1986). These principles, especially the first three, are of importance to realising initiatives centring on the disclosure of and organised response to unexpected outcomes, a collaborative approach to investigating incidents, and the broadening of informed consent.

The literature just reviewed opens up the notion that not everyone wants to participate in healthcare decision making, or does not want to participate in the same way. Recognising this, Flynn et al (2006) have developed a typology of participation preferences. Clearly, categorising patients as either 'active' or 'passive' has been unhelpful in the effort to understand those more likely to participate and how they might do so. Instead, the desire to participate can be distinguished based on consumers' desired roles in decision making. The majority of older adults wanted to be given treatment options, but there are substantial differences in how they wanted to be involved in discussing and selecting particular treatments. Specifically, being female, with higher education, a better self-rated health status, fewer prescription medications and a shorter duration at a usual place of care predicted a higher probability of highly active involvement (Flynn et al 2006, Gaston & Mitchell 2005). Others suggest that much more research still needs to be done on the role that patients themselves wish to play, as well as on the conceptual meanings of 'involvement' and 'participation' (Thompson 2007). Significantly, Thompson found empirical evidence from a large-scale qualitative study that participation was co-determined by both patients and professionals through reciprocal relationships of dialogue and SDM. Further, involvement depended on the type and seriousness of illness, patients' personal characteristics and their relationships with professionals. What is emerging here, Thompson believes, are ideas for the basic building blocks of a more sophisticated understanding of involvement within and between different contexts.

In their exploration, Davis and colleagues propose a five-fold taxonomy as an attempt to map the factors that affect patient involvement (Davis et al 2007). Targeting the involvement of consumers in service design and the improvement of patient safety, their framework captures 'the likely determinants of patient participation in safety-related behaviours'. They propose five determinants affecting consumers' willingness to become involved:

1. *'Patient-related*: patients' knowledge and beliefs about safety; emotional experiences with health care delivery and relevant coping styles; and demographic characteristics
2. *Illness-related*: stage and the severity of the patients' illness(es); symptoms; treatment plan; patients' health outcomes; and prior experience of illness (and prior experience of patient safety incidents)
3. *Health care professional (HCP)-related*: health care professionals' knowledge and beliefs about safety and patients' involvement in it; and the way in which health care professionals interact with patients
4. *Health care setting (HCS)-related*: type of health care setting – primary, secondary or tertiary care setting; and admission process – emergency or elective
5. *Task-related*: the specific patient actions/behaviours required for involvement in safety.' (Davis et al 2007:260–1)

Not surprisingly, one of the problems in researching patient participation in decision making is measuring results. Such measurement is made difficult by the complex ways in which consumers can become involved. Patient satisfaction has been a common measure for some time, but Draper & Hill (1996) recommend a more robust approach, including a government mandate on consumer feedback and resourcing the development of expertise in feedback by: trialling and evaluating approaches and technologies for obtaining feedback; disseminating research and effective models; and resourcing consumer organisations to be participants at all stages (Draper & Hill 1996). In Simon et al's (2007) view the problem remains, however, especially in comparing the outcomes of different studies. They point to the likelihood of inconsistent measurement given the complexity of SDM being reflected in how its outcomes are measured (Simon et al 2007), although in Australia, the Australian Council for Health Care Standards (ACHS) is attempting to measure results more consistently by including a consumer participation measure in their EQuIP accreditation standards (refer to www.achs.org.au/EQUIP4).

A range of strategies have been proposed to close the gap between evidence that consumer involvement is needed and the practice of consumer involvement. Studies of processes involving patients with specific conditions have been productive in identifying the types of intervention strategies most likely to encourage positive participation by both patients and professionals. These studies also serve to make the benefits of patient participation clearer. In relation to asthma patients, Schneider et al (2007) found that patient participation led to better patient outcomes. For their part, Irwin & Richardson (2006) found that patient-focused care improved physicians' performance, patient satisfaction and health outcomes without additional investment of time and resources. Irwin & Richardson also found better medication compliance an issue in asthma care, although Schneider reports an association between higher participation and medication discontinuation when the patient felt either better or worse. That is, patients appeared to be undergoing an internal negotiating process and coming to decisions for action based on their personal evaluation of their own particular circumstances. Loh (2007) reports similar findings in relation to the primary care of depression.

In relation to cancer care, Gaston & Mitchell (2005) found that all patients with advanced non-curable cancer wanted full information, although only two-thirds wanted to participate actively in decision making. They also found that active decision making was more common in patients with certain cancers. Improvements in the verbal communicative skills of cancer clinicians, and involvement of patients in decision making both generally improve patients' assessments of their quality of life (Arora 2003). Gattellari et al (2001) found that cancer patients who reported a shared role in decision making were most satisfied with the consultation, information about treatment and emotional support. Importantly, they found that patients were least satisfied when decisions were made exclusively by either party – the patient or the doctor (Gaston & Mitchell 2005, Gattellari et al 2001). Simple interventions such as question prompt sheets, audio taping of consultations and patient decision aids facilitated involvement (Gaston & Mitchell 2005). Variation in patient involvement in decision making may be a hitherto unrecognised cause of practice variation (Sepucha et al 2004).

Donovan & Blake (1992) examined the concept of compliance, and found that patients weighed up costs and risks against benefits as they perceived them and made rational choices based on their perceptions, personal and social circumstances, as Thompson suggested above with asthma patients. Thus, rather than a focus on non-compliance as a factor that plays a role in the (mis)utilisation of resources, a focus on more open and cooperative clinician–patient relationships may be more revealing of both 'compliance' and resource utilisation (Donovan & Blake 1992). In relation to Parkinson's disease, Cohen et al (2007:537) sum up the patient perspective in describing the outcomes of the Parkinson's pipeline project as 'authentic voices of patients as collaborators' and 'an example of a new breed of knowledgeable consumers armed with first-hand access to research findings and reinforced by online connections to like-minded peers throughout the world'. This type of patient-driven activity reinforces McCaffery et al's (2007) exhortation that to encourage patient participation, activity needs to move from supply-side to demand-side strategies.

A number of constraints have been identified as limiting patient participation and collaboration. These are outlined below.

1. Friction between professionals in their healthcare roles that can bring conflict that negatively influences patient outcomes and the general work environment (Attaberry 2007). Attaberry (2007) proposes shared governance to promote team building, role understanding, autonomy and employee retention. Clinicians may initially need to develop this model within their own community of practice given the differences that exist within professions as well as between them (Sorensen & Iedema 2007).

2. Burnout from this type of 'emotional work' (Strauss et al 1982) has been noted by a number of authors (Sorensen & Iedema in press, Zapf et al 2001). Initiatives such as open disclosure and root cause analysis demand much 'emotional labour' (Hochschild 1983) even before contact is made with consumers. Practitioners do report however that emotional labour with colleagues and with consumers, while taxing, can result in greater work satisfaction and better relationships (Iedema et al 2007).

3. Family requests for deception to protect a patient from bad news and doctor compliance can have a cascading effect. As Capozzi & Rhodes (2006) assert, when something is concealed, people avoid situations where the issue might arise. Avoidance, in turn, results in distancing between the clinician and the patient (and family) precisely when attention and intimacy might be needed. Complicating this as well, when truths are ultimately revealed, trust deteriorates still further. Hence, serious harm and emotional abandonment are the likely outcomes of non-openness, even in cases where the deception is initiated for the patient's good (Capozzi & Rhodes 2006).

4. In a study in psychiatry, Goossensen et al (2007) found that clinicians did not explicitly ask meta-questions, such as checking the preferred approach of the patient to receive information or the preferred level of involvement in decision making, but rather choose to rely on an intuitive 'feel' as to whether the patient wanted to be involved or not. The authors concluded that physicians should be able to take part in SDM even if the patient is not asking them to.

5. The discourse of the patient as an active agent in managing their illness and healthcare may become a means through which clinicians can withdraw from responsibility for areas of patient need that are problematic, for example unexplained symptoms, chronic disease and pain (Salmon & Hall 2003). Thus, Salmon & Hall (2003) suggest that the patient involvement discourse can affect the boundaries of medical responsibility in a way that advantages medicine. In this regard, Anderson (1996) believes that the unreflexive use of consumer empowerment can deflect attention away from economic and social structures that perpetuate inequalities, for instance among people who are marginalised and disadvantaged.

Linked in with this last point, Allsop & Mulcahy (1998) found that physicians regarded complaints as a challenge to their expertise and technical competence. Complaints were therefore seen to threaten professional identity. Berlinger (2003) suggests that the rift between patients who suffer medical error and doctors who commit them may occur because physicians or hospitals fear exposure for legal and insurance reasons (Berlinger 2003). There is evidence emerging to suggest however that 'radical openness' may pre-empt consumers' intention to file complaints and lawsuits (Kraman & Hamm 1999, Lamb 2004, Wojcieszak et al 2006). In the following section we explore what this new policy of openness means for consumers.

The experience of open disclosure

Clearly, the factors that inhibit openness and participation are complex, personal, professional, organisational, legal and financial. Complicating this further is that goal setting and treatment processes in clinical medicine are complex, and the potential for unexpected changes as well as disagreements regarding these goals and processes are substantial (Bradley et al 1999). But there are factors that can mitigate this complexity. In looking at what influences physician communication and perceptions, Street Jr et al (2007) found that physicians' inclination to be patient-centred depended on patients' willingness to be involved, although the question arises whether patients' willingness indeed determines physicians' inclination, and to what extent the obverse is true. One would expect involvement to be co-constructed, with reciprocity and mutual influence playing a prominent role in patient–physician interactions.

Other commentators have pointed to readiness as a factor determining involvement. In reviewing research on patient participation in decision making, Guadagnoli & Ward (1998) concluded that the patient's level of readiness to participate in decision making must be assessed and methods to engage patients should be developed based on their level of readiness. Nevertheless, the same might be true for clinicians who themselves may need to have reached a level of readiness in their personal and professional attitudes to patient care before they are capable of realising adequate consumer involvement. Cancer patients who were given a booklet that included a question prompt sheet and booklets on clinical decision making and patient rights were more anxious and significantly less likely to achieve their preferred involvement in decision making (Butow et al 2004). The authors described their causal view in the article titled: 'Changing patients but not physicians is not enough'. The organisation must also be supportive. In one study consumers ceased proffering a patient-held record when they perceived that they were imposing extra 'paperwork' on stretched NHS staff (Williams et al 2001).

Currently, a fear of legal and insurance implications and uncertainty about personal ramifications on the part of professionals are preventing not just formal disclosure of and apology for unexpected outcomes, but also consumers' involvement in service improvement and patient safety (Iedema et al 2007). The evaluation just cited does nevertheless suggest that health professionals respond positively to the principles and practices of open disclosure, and that it 'is met with approval and relief on the part of health professionals and consumers' (Iedema et al 2007:4). Not all clinicians respond in this way. In addition to the group of interviewees who expressed relief about being mandated to disclose unexpected outcomes, another group claimed that 'they were already doing open disclosure' and had been doing it 'for quite some time'. Interviews with consumers about how their unexpected outcomes were handled suggested, however, that in surprisingly few instances adequate open disclosure procedures were followed. This calls into question clinicians' confidence about the effectiveness of their disclosures, and the representativeness of their views about the adequacy of their communications with patients (and their families).

We feature five excerpts that illustrate how clinicians and clinical managers are changing their attitudes to patient engagement and their manner of practice in relation to open disclosure, and how patients are enabled and encouraged to take on a co-productive role in (re)defining the type of healthcare they wish to receive. The first excerpt features a clinician who has attended an intensive open disclosure training program. Here, this interviewee talks about advising colleagues about what is necessary for open disclosure to succeed.

Excerpt 1: Clinician A
As soon as you say open disclosure I think everyone feels more comfortable anyway
… And it might just be a personal feeling. I am a person who feels quite uncomfortable
when everything is to be too confidential (e.g. in root cause analysis processes) rather
than everything is going to be open … I think it is probably the fact that you can go to
them (other clinicians) and say, 'Look, there is actually a really good way of dealing with
this. It is very simple. I've done the [open disclosure] course and this is what it teaches
you and you really think this really does work very well.' And I told them what to expect:
'When we walk in there, the patient will be angry. The body language will be angry. The
eyes will be angry, the words will be angry.' And what happened of all the things I have
said will happen, happened … I talked about it in theory before we got there and said,
'The most important thing upfront is this, do such and such. We are going to say sorry
and then we are going to sit down and shut up.' Because basically you can put it down
into: 'Say sorry, shut up and listen.' And then explain if you need to. But explain it at the
patient's pace, not your own. And everything just went from there really …

(14 June 2007)

The way in which this clinician achieved this ability to 'listen to patients' is recounted
in the second extract below.

Excerpt 2: Clinician A
And one of the good things about the course we did was that they had actors who did it.
And it is one thing to say, 'Oh, yes, I do this.' It is one thing to verbalise what you do
but it is a very different thing to actually do it … However little experience you've got
even with a single course, I have done this once, but just having had that course I felt
Yes, I think I know how to do this and I went in there and it worked. And it was one of
the most useful things I learnt to do.

(14 June 2007)

For their part, patients often have clear care expectations, and this is particularly the
case with childbirth. The following excerpt is a dialogue from an interview with a patient
whose delivery went seriously wrong. This patient and her husband had prepared a specific plan for the birth of their child. This plan was discussed and agreed on with the delivering clinicians beforehand. In response to a question from the interviewer about whether
the patient was told and knew of the risks before she delivered her baby, she responded:

Excerpt 3: Patient A
No. I mean, I'm overweight, and obviously that's always a risk factor but I wouldn't have
thought that would be a risk factor for tearing, but even if it is, I had a second degree tear
with my first daughter, so I did expect that there would be some tearing. When I sort of
found a position for delivery that I was comfortable with I asked whether it was suitable.
I did ask whether they'd like me on the bed and they said, 'No, wherever you're comfortable.' And I thought okay, let's do it … and I'm very lucky; the labour for me was
perfect – the tear hasn't affected the way I feel about the delivery … My daughter was
facing the wrong way; they never picked that up and … I was mentioning to them that
my stomach felt like she was facing the wrong way and they didn't take that into account
and I feel that they didn't really listen to me from the very beginning. I had to force them
to read my … plan … My husband and I had a … plan …very, very definite feelings on
childbirth and we had to really encourage them to read that and take it seriously. They're
all things that didn't bother me at the time but in hindsight it's very distressing.

(6 July 2007)

The role of clinical managers is pivotal in engaging with patient-centred policies such as open disclosure, in promoting disclosure in clinical circles and in managing the appropriate enactment of this innovative policy. In the excerpt that follows the clinical manager, the deputy director of the clinical division in which the standard was being implemented, indicates the level of support that implementation received in the organisation, a large metropolitan tertiary teaching hospital.

Excerpt 4: Clinical manager A
The organisation, and the leaders in our division see it as a very good idea and feel committed to it, but it's the individual senior clinicians [who] have to be won over. I reckon if they got exposed to it, to understand, to have the opportunity to do the training on a widespread basis I'm sure they could, you know, I'm sure they'd actually feel a lot more committed to it.

(13 June 2007)

In relation to a question about how to get doctors involved in the process, he went on to say the following.

Excerpt 5: Clinical manager A
Oh, I think all doctors are a bit, I mean, anything that forces you to confront people when the outcome has been bad is quite threatening and furthermore, threatening because doctors have to admit that they have something to learn before they'll go for it, um, and finally, I think even though intellectually you can say, *Oh, this is a really good idea*, there's still a slight fear about revealing the details of things, particularly when it hasn't been handled very well with people, and that's pretty threatening too, to actually find yourself in a situation where you're admitting something's gone wrong because it just hasn't been the way medicine has been.

(13 June 2007)

In effect, open disclosure is a policy that mandates co-production of care, albeit only in cases of unexpected outcome. But the success of open disclosure is to a large extent contingent on the way clinicians have shaped their relationships with consumers in the course of the treatment trajectory. These relationships, in turn, are forged in an important sense upon admission. An important part of this forging includes informed consent, a topic that warrants separate detailed examination in this regard. In this sense, the pressure to disclose has ramifications for all dimensions of professionals' communications with consumers. Equally, open disclosure represents an important driver towards acknowledging the consumer as prosumer.

The implications for practice of co-production

We take the three levels of participation outlined by Loh et al (2007) above and consider the foregoing information in terms of its applicability at the macro (system), meso (service/program) and micro (medical encounter) levels of practice. Table 7.1 sets out the levels of participation and the kinds of activities that might be associated with practice at each level, from a co-production perspective.

The information in Table 7.1 indicates that co-producing care at each of these three levels is not a matter for one stakeholder alone, but is an organisation-wide and health systemic endeavour. At the system level, it will involve senior managers engaging with the public as citizens, in envisioning the values of healthcare, in allocating scarce resources, in developing standards of care, and in assessing accountability for the outcomes of the system. At the service level, it will involve senior administrative and clinical managers engaging with the public as citizens to plan services and to evaluate program outcomes, tailoring care to individual patients within a standard case type of care, developing and agreeing feedback mechanisms, indicators of service performance and strategies for improvement. At the medical encounter level, it will involve structuring care options with and for patients, outlining the probable risks and outcomes of care and, together with other members of the multidisciplinary team, developing an agreed patient care plan, reviewing the outcomes of care, including where appropriate, the status of the patient's health, any errors that may have occurred and strategies to remediate those errors. Increasingly, at each of these levels consumers will need to have their say in recognition of the validity of their experiences, their insights, and their right to know about and co-determine healthcare processes.

Table 7.1 Associated practices at each level of participation

Level of participation	Associated practice
Co-producing quality at the micro (medical encounter) level	• Informed consent to treatment options with disclosure of probable risks and outcomes • Collective, inclusive multidisciplinary team collaboration, pooling information and generating consensus, that includes the patient to develop an agreed plan of care (see Kerosuo, Chapter 5) • Reviewing care outcomes, including disclosing information about patient status such as where errors are made and their remediation (see Willis, Dwyer & Dunn, Chapter 6)
Co-producing service at the meso (service/program) level	• Planning services and evaluating service outcomes • Linking population and patient-based care, e.g. through mass customisation methods (see Berg, Schellekens & Bergen, Chapter 8) • Obtaining feedback and incorporating consumer groups' expertise in particular conditions
Co-producing the vision at the macro (system) level	• Allocating scarce resources • Governing standards and assessing accountability for system outcomes • Deliberation about what the system should achieve such as the moral and ethical underpinning of healthcare, e.g. through citizen's juries (see Mooney, Chapter 13)

Conclusion

Public participation in producing healthcare will be predicated on a changing orientation to healthcare practice by all stakeholder groups. This reorientation is already occurring, evidenced by the observations made by the clinician and the clinical manager featured in the excerpts above. The changes they comment on as having happened to them, to the relationships they have with colleagues, and to their relationships with patients point to important changes in healthcare, in particular that:

- new kinds of people will deliver and shape the healthcare of the future
- new kinds of workers who embody new and different relationships will plan and deliver care, in conjunction with prosumers who have knowledges and discourses enabling them to make their lifeworld experiences relevant, audible and visible to healthcare staff, over and beyond the confines of 'history taking', explanations of 'known risks', and expressions of care preferences
- new kinds of expertise will develop that includes the clinicians' ability to enhance the exercise of technical skills and knowledge to collaboratively produce care.

These new workers and prosumers will find ways to collaborate in the construction of healthcare processes, ranging from chronically ill patients taking charge of their disease as part of their role in their 'year of care' contract (Degeling et al 2006) to victims of harm being invited to participate in incident investigations and practice redesign (Iedema et al 2007).

Finally, while profoundly significant in itself, involving the public in healthcare is also important in that it extends beyond making sure that individuals' and issue groups' views and experiences are taken into account in the enactment of healthcare treatments, the planning of services, and in the determination of policy. For healthcare organisations and health departments to retain public respect and support, the absence of deliberative space that has thus far characterised relationships and practices in health needs to give way to processes, intensities and dynamics that retrieve healthcare's legitimacy, or its 'public value' (Horner et al 2006, Moore 1995). Policies like open disclosure, and trends like patient centredness and consumer involvement, are, in that sense, crucial resources by means of which state governments need to reconcile the growing gap between healthcare promise and healthcare performance. The health of healthcare was once thought to depend on the invention of new medical technologies and drugs on the one hand, and on the eradication of under-performing individuals on the other hand. We suggest we have entered a new era, where neither of these kinds of blunt strategies will carry much weight. Simple transparency of process can erode trust (Taylor-Gooby & Zinn 2005), however, if the consequences of the manner in which healthcare services are planned, produced and delivered are not addressed. A discerning public will expect to be informed in less simplistic ways about the future options of healthcare practice. In sum, the public value of health is now conditional upon health practitioners and policymakers capitalising on the emergence of the health prosumer.

References

Allsop J, Mulcahy L 1998 Maintaining professional identities: doctors' responses to complaints. Sociology of Health and Illness 20(6):802–824

Anderson J M 1996 Empowering patients: Issues and strategies. Social Science & Medicine 43(5):697–705

Arora N 2003 Interacting with cancer patients: the significance of physicians' communication behaviour. Social Science & Medicine 43(5):697–705

Attaberry N E 2007 Multidisciplinary team building in radiology through use of shared governance principles. Journal of Radiology Nursing 26(3):99–101

Bauman A E, Fardy H J, Harris P G 2003 Getting it right: why bother with patient-centred care? Medical Journal of Australia 179:253–256

Berlinger N 2003 Broken stories; patient, families, clinicians after medical error. Literature and Medicine 22(2):230–240

Bradley E H, Bogardus S T, Tinetti M E et al 1999 Goal-setting in clinical medicine. Social Science & Medicine 49(2):267–278

Butow P, Devine R, Boyer M et al 2004 Cancer consultation preparation package: changing patients but not physicians is not enough. Journal of Clinical Oncology 22(21):4401–4409

Capozzi J D, Rhodes R 2006 A family's request for deception. Journal of Bone & Joint Surgery, American Volume 88(4):906–908

Carey-Hazell K 2005 Improving patient information and decision making. The Australian Health Consumer 2005–6(1):2

Charles C A, Whelan T, Gafni A et al 2003 Shared treatment decision making: What does it mean to physicians? Journal of Clinical Oncology 21(5):932–936

Cohen P D, Herman L, Jedlinski S et al 2007 Ethical issues in clinical neuroscience research: A patient's perspective. Neurotherapeutics 4(3):537–544

Davis R, Jacklin R, Sevdalis N et al 2007 Patient involvement in patient safety: What factors influence patient participation and engagement? Health Expectations 10(2007):259–267

Davis R, Koutantji M, Vincent C 2008 How willing are patients to question health care staff on issues related to the quality and safety of their healthcare? Quality and Safety in Health Care 17:90–96

Degeling P, Close H, Degeling D 2006 Re-thinking long term conditions: a report on the development and implemenaiton of co-produced, year-based integrated care pathways to improve service provision to people with long term conditions. Durham Centre for Clinical Management Development, Durham

Donovan J L, Blake D R 1992 Patient non-compliance: Deviance or reasoned decision-making? Social Science & Medicine 34(5):507–513

Draper M, Hill S 1996 Feasibility of National Benchmarking of Patient Satisfaction with Australian Hospitals. Int J Qual Health Care 8(5):457–466

Evans R, Edwards A, Coulter A et al 2007 Prominent strategy but rare in practice shared decision-making and patient decision support technologies in the UK. German Journal for Quality in Health Care 101(4):247–253

Flynn K E, Smith M A, Vanness D 2006 A typology of preferences for participation in healthcare decision making. Social Science & Medicine 63(5):1158–1169

Gagliardi A R, Lemieux-Charles L, Brown A D et al 2008 Barriers to patient involvement in health service planning and evaluation: An exploratory study. Patient Education and Counselling 70(2):234–41

Gaston C M, Mitchell G 2005 Information giving and decision-making in patients with cancer: A systematic review. Social Science & Medicine 61(10):2252–2264

Gattellari M, Butow P N, Tattersall M H 2001 Sharing decisions in cancer care. Social Science & Medicine 52(12):1865–1878

Goossensen A, Zijlstra P, Koopmanschap M 2007 Measuring shared decision making processes in psychiatry: Skills versus patient satisfaction. Patient Education and Counseling 67(1–2):50–56

Goss C, Renzi C 2007 Patient and citizen participation in healthcare decisons in Italy. German Journal for Quality in Health Care 101:236–240

Guadagnoli E, Ward P 1998 Patient participation in decision-making. Social Science & Medicine 47(3):329–339

Hochschild A R 1983 The Managed Heart: Commercialisation of Human Feeling. University of California Press, Berkeley

Horner L, Lekhi R, Blaug R 2006 Deliberative democracy and the role of public managers: Final report of The Work Foundation's public value consortium. The Work Foundation, London

Iedema R, Mallock N, Sorensen R et al 2007 Final Report: Evaluation of the National Open Disclosure Program. University of Technology, Sydney

Iedema R, Jorm C, Wakefield J et al submitted A New Structure of Attention? Open Disclosure of Clinical Errors to Patients and Families. Journal of Language & Social Psychology

Iedema R, Jorm C M, Braithwaite J et al 2006 A root cause analysis of clinical error: Confronting the disjunction between formal rules and situated clinical activity. Social Science & Medicine 63(5):1201–1212

Irwin R, Richardson N 2006 Patient-focused care: Using the right tools. Chest 130(1): 73S–82S

Kraman S S, Hamm G 1999. Risk management: Extreme honesty may be the best policy. Annals of Internal Medicine 131(12):963–967

Lamb R 2004 Open disclosure: the only approach to medical error. Qual Saf Health Care 13(1):3–5

Legare F, Stacey D, Forest P-G 2007 Shared decision-making in Canada: update, challenges and where next! German Journal for Quality in Health Care 101(4):213–221

Litva A, Coast J, Donovan J et al 2002 'The public is too subjective': public involvement at different levels of health-care decision making. Social Science & Medicine 54(12): 1825–1837

Loh A, Simon D, Wills C E et al 2007 The effects of a shared decision-making intervention in primary care of depression: a cluster-randomized controlled trial. Patient Education and Counselling 67(3):324–332

Madden B, Cockburn T 2007 Bundaberg and beyond: Duty to disclose adverse events to patients. Journal of Law and Medicine 14:501–527

Mansell P, Harris W, Carthey J et al 2005 Patient and public involvement in patient safety: the role of the National Patient Safety Agency. National Patient Safety Agency, London

McCaffery K J, Shepherd H L, Trevena L et al 2007 Shared decision-making in Australia. German Journal for Quality in Health Care 101(4):205–211

McGurk V, Bean D, Gooney T et al in press Treating patients well: Improving the patient experience. Journal of Neonatal Nursing

Moore M 1995 Creating Public Value: Strategic management in government. Harvard University Press, Cambridge

Moumjid N, Bremond A, Mignotte H et al 2007 Shared decision-making in the physician-patient encounter in France: a general overview. German Journal for Quality in Health Care 101:223–228

Salmon P, Hall G M 2003 Patient empowerment and control: a psychological discourse in the service of medicine. Social Science & Medicine 57(10):1969–1980

Sepucha K F, Fowler J F, Mulley Jr A G 2004 Policy Support for Patient-Centred Care: The Need for Measurable Improvements in Decision Quality. Health Affairs 54:1–9

Schneider A, Wensing M, Quinzler R et al 2007 Higher preference for participation in treatment decisions is associated with lower medication adherence in asthma patients. Patient Education and Counselling 67:57–62

Simon D, Loh A, Harter M 2007 Measuring (shared) decision-making – a review of psychometric instruments. German Journal for Quality in Health Care 101(4):259–267

Sorensen R, Iedema R 2007 Advocacy at end-of-life. Research design: An ethnographic study of an ICU. International Journal of Nursing Studies 44(8):1343–1353

Sorensen R, Iedema R in press Emotional labour: clinicians' attitudes to death and dying. Journal of Health Organization and Management

Strauss A L, Fagerhaugh S, Suczek B N et al 1982 The work of hospitalized patients. Social Science & Medicine 16(9):977–986

Street Jr R L, Gordon H, Haidet P 2007 Physicians' communication and perceptions of patients: Is it how they look, how they talk, or is it just the doctor? Social Science & Medicine 65(3):586–598

Taylor-Gooby P, Zinn J 2005 Social contexts and responses to risk network (SCARR) Canterbury, Kent, UK: School of Social Policy, Sociology and Social Research, University of Kent, Canterbury

Thompson A G 2007 The meaning of patient involvement and participation in health care consultations: a taxonomy. Social Science & Medicine 64(6):1297–1310

van der Weijden T, van Veenendaal H, Timmermans D 2007 Shared decision-making in the Netherlands – current state and future perspectives. German Journal for Quality in Health Care 101:241–246

Vines P 2005 Apologising to avoid liability: Cynical civility or practical morality? Sydney Law Review 27(3):483–505

Weiss S J 1986 Consensual norms regarding patient involvement. Social Science & Medicine 22(4):489–496

Williams J G, Cheung W Y, Chetwynd N et al 2001 Pragmatic randomised trial to evaluate the use of patient held records for the continuing care of patients with cancer. Quality in Health Care 10(3):159–165

Wojcieszak D, Banja J, Houk C 2006 The sorry works! Coalition: making the case for full disclosure. Journal on Quality and Patient Safety 32(6):344–350

Zapf D, Seifert C, Schmutte B et al 2001 Emotion work and job stressors and their effect on burnout. Psychology & Health 16:527

Integrating performance: linking healthcare domains

Marc Berg, Wim Schellekens & Cé Bergen

Introduction

The US Institute of Medicine reports 'To Err is Human' and 'Crossing the Quality Chasm' have had repercussions throughout Western medicine (Committee on Quality of Healthcare in America 2000, 2001). Given the resources spent and the qualifications of its professionals, the reports argue, there is a chasm between what the overall quality delivered by the system should be and what it actually is. The US healthcare system is fragmented and 'wasteful'. Any journey through it includes many 'steps and handoffs that slow down the care process and decrease rather than improve safety' (Committee on Quality of Healthcare in America 2001:28).

As the earlier chapters in this book also testify, the reports' insights are applicable to most Western countries, and the demands on the healthcare system in the near future will only increase. The safety, effectiveness, patient centredness and timeliness of care have to be improved, while keeping costs from rising further. How can we align these targets? Small, local improvement initiatives will not do the job. Nor will large, sweeping 'quality-improvement initiatives' have a lasting impact if the improvements do not become embedded in a more fundamental redesign of the operations of healthcare work.

In this chapter, we take up this challenge. We do not discuss the (country-specific) payment and regulatory systems that stimulate or obstruct change at the level of the care process. We will, rather, describe a series of less country-specific, interrelated design principles that depict how healthcare delivery could be organised. This vision is futuristic: no healthcare practice has fully achieved it. Yet it is simultaneously realistic, in that it builds upon elements that are broadly accepted and proven – both theoretically and practically.

The design principles pivot around the notion of *care programs*: work routines based on multidisciplinary protocols that encompass tasks, decision criteria and work procedures for the care professionals involved in the care of a patient category. Such care programs touch upon all levels of the organisation: operational, tactical and strategic. On the operational level, they streamline work processes and, when designed properly, increase efficiency, patient safety, effectiveness and patient centredness simultaneously. Yet these operational characteristics may ultimately not be the most important ones. On the tactical and strategic level, we will argue, care programs will be the organisational building blocks around which the healthcare organisations of the future will be shaped. Care programs will bring together teams of professionals producing optimal quality care for patients with a given condition or problem. In line with current trends in healthcare financing and regulation, the teams running these care programs will become self-steering – responsible for their own clinical and financial results.

Integrating professional and organisational quality

In current healthcare practices, many individuals are working to improve the different dimensions of 'quality'. Through guidelines and audits, professionals attempt to enhance the evidence-based nature of their work (Grol 2000). Quality managers organise the certification or accreditation of their organisation, information managers develop the information technology infrastructure, and unit managers worry about the optimal planning of scarce resources such as personnel and expensive technologies (Klazinga 2000, Berg 2004). Usually, however, these activities are organisationally separate and the responsible individuals, including professionals, information managers and quality managers, interact more with their peers in other organisations than with each other (Berwick 1998). In addition, they focus on different quality dimensions: professionals mainly focus on effectiveness and safety, line managers on efficiency, and so forth. At heart, the deepest dividing line runs between the professionals 'owning' and improving the *content* of healthcare work and the managers 'owning' and improving the *organisation* of that work.

To overcome the quality chasm, these separate activities have to become integrated. This is partly a matter of organisation: rethinking the composition of a project's steering group, for example, or organising 'integrated quality meetings' at board level (Leape et al 2000, Murray & Berwick 2003). Yet the true integration of these activities requires a *conceptual* innovation: a vision on *how* these different activities are part and parcel of the same enterprise. To overcome the quality chasm, to improve the *different* dimensions of 'quality' simultaneously, we need to join state-of-the-art insights from different fields into a single integrated approach. In other words, we need to learn to simultaneously think about *content* and *organisation* of healthcare work for radical change to become possible.

Standardisation – creating care programs

The heart of fundamental care delivery innovation lies in the standardisation of care into 'care programs' (see Figure 8.1). Currently, the archetypal mode of organising healthcare delivery is the *ad hoc step-by-step approach*. Since every patient trajectory is unpredictable, the care professional requires the freedom to 'pick' what this unique patient requires next from the palette of their professional knowledge base. Every patient follows his own trajectory and in these trajectories each next step is decided upon the step before (de Vries & Hiddema 2001, Strauss et al 1985).

One-hundred years ago, before the times of medical specialisation, physicians could handle most of what any patient could bring to their attention, and few diagnostic and therapeutic options were available (Howell 1989). At that time, the step-by-step mode of care delivery was both patient centred and efficient. In our times, however, the theory and practice of medicine have become highly complex. Healthcare institutions are populated by many different professions and specialists, handling patients that often require the attention of several of these. Yet most of our care delivery is still organised according to this archetypal form. Every *next* step (e.g. a surgical operation) is only conceived and planned at the completion of the *previous* step (e.g. obtaining diagnostic test results), resulting in frequent waits and, more often than not, very ad hoc and variably shaped patient trajectories. The result is a care process that is fragmented (not patient centred), unsafe and inefficient (see Claridge & Cook, Chapter 4).

Yet is patient care not in principle organised this way because individual patients have individual histories and needs (Strauss et al 1985, Timmermans & Berg 2003)? The individual trajectory of a patient suffering from heart failure, for example, is indeed unpredictable. A patient's personal and medical history will shape his and his physician's preferences in unique ways, and symptoms and reactions to therapeutic interventions never quite behave according to textbook definitions. Yet at an aggregated level, much of this individual variation disappears. For the category of heart failure patients, the steps that are mostly taken, or that should be taken, can be predicted.

For the major categories of patients that an organisation deals with care programs can be developed. As stated, care programs are work routines based upon multidisciplinary protocols that encompass tasks, decision criteria and work procedures for the care professionals involved in the care of such a patient category (see Box 8.1). Care programs can be limited to a hospital or a department, but they should ideally include all providers having a role in the care of a category of patients. The different professionals jointly develop these protocols, drawing upon evidence-based guidelines wherever possible.

Figure 8.1 Care program model

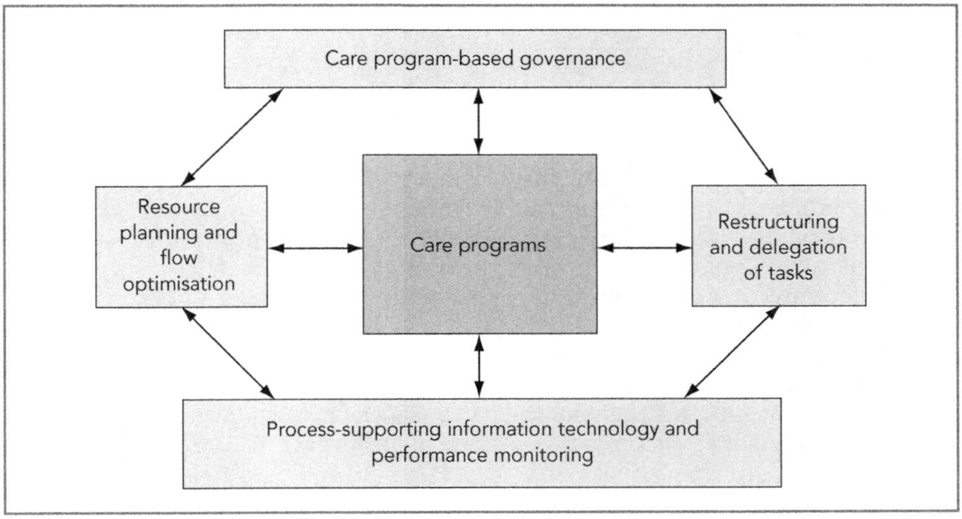

Care program-based governance

Resource planning and flow optimisation

Care programs

Restructuring and delegation of tasks

Process-supporting information technology and performance monitoring

Most of the benefits of care programs are well known: care delivery becomes more evidence based, and colleagues, patients and payers know what care to expect. Time after time, it has been shown that following smart guidelines meticulously yet non-dogmatically saves lives (Berenholtz et al 2004, Luthi et al 2003, Schiele et al 2005). Also, care programs afford safer care. Every safety expert knows that there is nothing more lethal than unwarranted variation in critical processes. Uncontrolled variation obstructs flow, unnecessarily burdens the cognitive processes of those involved in the process check and prohibits learning (because the process outcomes cannot be compared to each other) (Carroll & Rudolph 2006, McManus et al 2003, Rozich et al 2004).

Care programs also afford a *reduction of coordination work*. Working step-by-step requires each next step to be organised and planned anew, including all the ad hoc phone calls and form filling that comes with that. In organisations that work under pressures of time and resources (and most healthcare organisations do), this implies stress and loss of professionals' and patients' time. With care programs, the sequence of activities to pursue and professionals to see is already established. Rather than establishing this anew every time a patient comes in with 'heart failure', this care program is made beforehand by the professionals involved. Since everyone knows what to expect in the next, and previous, steps, coordination work is reduced (Mintzberg 1979, Timmermans & Berg 2003).

Finally, well-designed care programs are patient friendly. Those who mistake this call for standardisation for a call to quench the 'art' of medicine cannot be more mistaken. There is nothing 'patient friendly' in unnecessary waiting times and unnecessary safety risks. There is, on the other hand, nothing more patient friendly than a well-organised, smooth trajectory, in which everyone involved knows what is expected of them, is optimally informed, and can give their full attention to the patient (Millenson 1997).

Box 8.1 Care program – A note on terminology

The term 'care program' is used to emphasise the patient-centred *organisation* of care around the major patient categories the organisation(s) involved deals with. We do not use the term 'critical pathway', or 'carepath' because these terms usually refer to a detailed protocol, sometimes used in the form of a time-oriented recording sheet. Usually, 'critical carepaths' are predominantly about increased *effectiveness*, although sometimes an increase in efficiency (such as through reducing length of stay) is included. Also, the 'critical pathway' literature is largely nursing oriented, while we emphasise the multidisciplinary nature of the care program.

A care program is typified by the integration of activities between disciplines, professions, departments and, in the case of a multi-organisational care path, organisations. Also, care programs are about tackling professional and organisational quality simultaneously: optimising effectiveness, efficiency, patient centredness and safety through *integrating* (*not* running side by side) professional and organisational 'best practices'. Finally, with the notion of 'care program' we explicitly refer to both the operational *and* the tactical/strategic impact of redesigning care processes in such a way.

At the same time, a terminological battle is meaningless: much current 'carepath' work comes close to what we address in this paper.

For this to work, it is crucial that care programs are not just written guidelines. They should be concretely 'anchored' in the organisation through working arrangements between professionals and departments, special outpatient and inpatient facilities, the information technologies and forms used, material affordances and constraints, and so forth. For example, charts may be prestructured to indicate the steps to take next, or an outpatient clinic designed for optimal breast cancer care may be put in place. Likewise, the sterilised instrument baskets used in operating rooms can be standardised to ensure that the right tools for the job will be at hand, and checklists can be put in place that *must* be followed before a high-risk procedure is started (Committee on Quality of Healthcare in America 2000, Norman 1988, Parker 1997). (See Box 8.3 for the importance of 'flexible standardisation' in making care programs work.)

> **Pause for reflection**
>
> The call for more 'standardisation' in healthcare practice is not new. In what forms has this call been heard in earlier years? Why has it been mostly ignored, until recently? What are the factors that might make it heard this time around.

Restructuring and delegating tasks

When developing care programs, the individual tasks, decision moments and work procedures should be critically reconsidered as to their organisational safety, patient centredness and efficiency. Can blood tests not be performed on the same day as the next visit? Can the variety in surgical techniques used by different surgeons be limited (Bell et al 2006, Committee on Quality of Healthcare in America 2000, Dy et al 2003)? This redesign starts by considering the four different components that constitute every care program: triage, intake, the core activities of the care program, and follow-up. Not all care programs will require these steps to be separated, but any care program requires:

- the decision whether the patient belongs here (triage)
- the selection of the optimal care program (including (further) diagnostic workup) (intake)
- a limited set of core diagnostic and/or therapeutic activities (core)
- follow-up activities (follow-up).

Triage and intake are often necessarily entwined. In emergency situations the intake and the core activities are often inseparable. In chronic care the 'core' of the care program can extend for years. In acute care situations it may last only briefly. In general, however, disentangling these components helps in designing subtasks that can be delegated, or executed in a more effective, patient-friendly and efficient way. In current practices, every individual patient encounter seems unique because every patient comes to that encounter through a different route, with different diagnostic and therapeutic activities being done. In current healthcare practices, *every single patient encounter is unique partially because there is no conscious attempt to streamline these encounters*. By separating 'triage' and 'intake', and by organising the care delivery process accordingly, patient flows become more predictable. Patients remain unique, but not in the sense of varyingly incomplete diagnostic histories, or large differences in therapeutic steps already taken.

Often, (specialised) nurses can do (part of the) intake, so that the physician is freed from tasks that do not require their expertise. Ensuring a complete work-up before the consultation with a medical specialist, for example, can save many unnecessary outpatient visits. Given shortages in qualified personnel, such a redistribution of tasks is essential to managing the increasing demand for care. Retinopathy screening for diabetes patients, medication optimisation in heart failure patients (see Box 8.2) and glaucoma treatment are some of the examples where a redistribution of tasks between doctors, nurses and/or paramedics can provide optimal care for more patients (Johnson et al 2003).

Care programs and restructuring and delegating tasks are mutually dependent (see the arrows in Figure 8.1). On the one hand, restructuring and delegating tasks makes standardisation feasible: without this, one could not achieve as much quality gain with care programs. Again, multiple dimensions can now be optimised simultaneously: efficiency (optimal use of expensive capacity), timeliness (reduced throughput times), effectiveness (appropriate combinations of expertise at the right time and place) and patient centredness (a care program organises the care delivery resources around the patient rather than vice versa).

On the other hand, care programs are a necessary element of redesign and task delegation. Care programs can ensure both (a) the quality of the work delivered by the different care professionals involved and (b) the coordination of their work tasks. Both require standardisation of decision criteria (which patients may be handled by the nurse; what to do in case of doubt), data (what to register, terminology to use) and work procedures (what actions that should be done by whom). In the example of heart failure care (see Box 8.2), the nurse practitioner is supported by simple computer-based decision support systems that have been made by the physicians who hold final responsibility. In addition, the chance of errors is minimised: whenever uncertainty arises, the patient drops out of the 'standard' category, and is seen by a cardiologist immediately.

> **Box 8.2** Example – Software-assisted nurse care program for heart failure care
>
> In the Martini Hospital in Groningen, the Netherlands, patients suffering from heart failure used to occupy some 40% of the hospital's cardiology beds. Most of these patients had been admitted because their conditions had slowly deteriorated to the point that admission was necessary. They had usually been under 'standard' care: regular consultations with the cardiologist or visits to the general practitioner had not prevented their hearts from decompensating. A combination of factors appeared to be at work: primarily suboptimal medication (Bouvy et al 2003), but also poor lifestyle education and poor compliance of patients with the medication and lifestyle rules. Working under time pressure, and having many other patients with acutely pressing problems, cardiologists and practitioners often spent too little time on medication finetuning and lifestyle education.
>
> Nowadays, patients with heart failure visit a special outpatient clinic, run by cardiologists and nurse practitioners. After an initial joint consultation with a cardiologist and nurse, the nurse, supported by a computerised decision-support tool, monitors the patient's blood pressure, weight, renal function and so forth, and finetunes the medication prescribed by the cardiologist over some five to six sessions. Based upon evidence-based guidelines, the computer similarly helps the nurse to counsel the patient on required lifestyle changes. The cardiologist only comes into play during the first session (unless unexpected reactions to treatment, for example, lead the nurse to consult the cardiologist on an ad hoc basis) (de Vries et al 2002).
>
> In this way, the outpatient cardiology clinic has liberated 6–8% of overall capacity, because patients are now handled by the nurse practitioner, and because patients suffer less from unnecessary deterioration of their condition. Overall, 80% of heart failure patients now receive optimal medication treatment, the average patient's ejection fraction (a core effectiveness indicator) has improved by 60%, and heart failure readmissions have reduced by 30%. The software application is now in use in over 40 Dutch hospitals (de Vries et al 2002).

Resource planning and flow optimisation

The current step-by-step approach in care delivery comes with a significant level of autonomy of the individual professionals, departments or organisations 'processing' each step. The operating room, outpatient clinics, hospital pharmacy, radiology and pathology departments generally run 'their own ship', having their own lines of accountability with organisational management. Making links between units (such as booking a CT scan or requesting a consultation) take place on an ad hoc basis.

When qualified staff, expensive technologies, investigation rooms and beds are abundant, the patient's trajectory through such a loosely coupled system may be smooth (see Figure 8.2A, Patient A). When such resources are not abundant, it is unlikely that they are available when the patient's care demands it. As a result, the patient's trajectory will look like Patient B (see Figure 8.2A): after having waited for a first appointment, the patient waits for a slot in the diagnostic facility, then returns to the consultant and waits for a place in the operating room schedule. For the patient and the care institution(s), time is wasted, during which unnecessary coordination work has to be performed and additional costs are incurred.

In Figure 8.2A the straight trajectory of Patient A signifies a smooth handling of the patient, including at the interfaces between units (e.g. outpatient clinic, diagnostic facilities, inpatient ward). The shaded box below the Patient B trajectory is the time lost due to waiting times between Units 2 and 3. Such waiting times are often not noticed at the level of the management of the whole organisation, since units generally each report about their own performance, not about the performance of the 'transfer' moments between units.

Figure 8.2A Units as the central organising principle

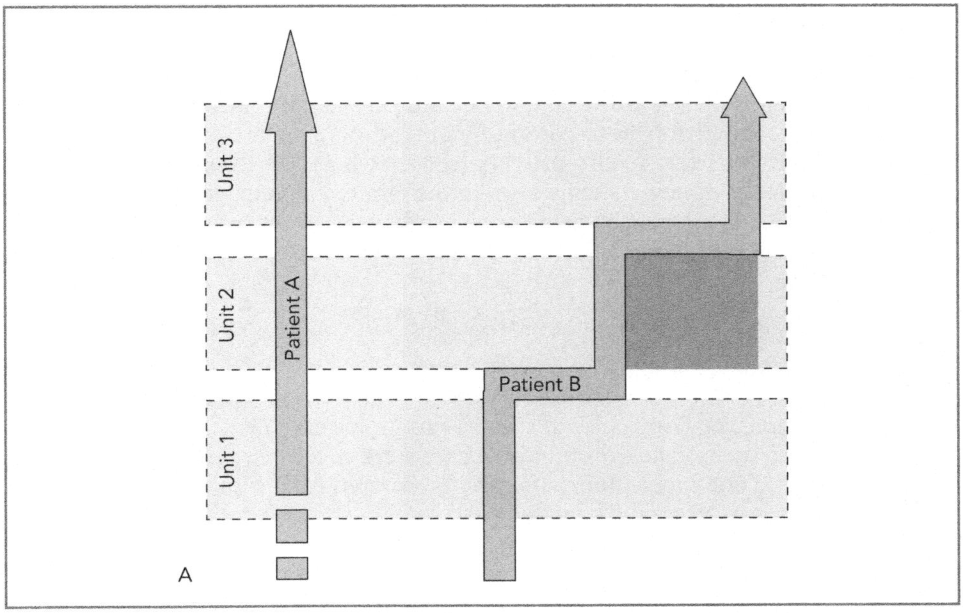

In Figure 8.2B the care programs X, Y, Z are now leading; the organisation and internal management of the units is now dependent on the care program that the organisation has decided upon. The smooth arrows indicate smooth handling. 'Patients X and Y' indicate that not all patients fit care programs; these patients can and should also be anticipated and planned for separately. As the diagram indicates, both types of patients can be managed in parallel.

Figure 8.2B The patient as the central organising principle

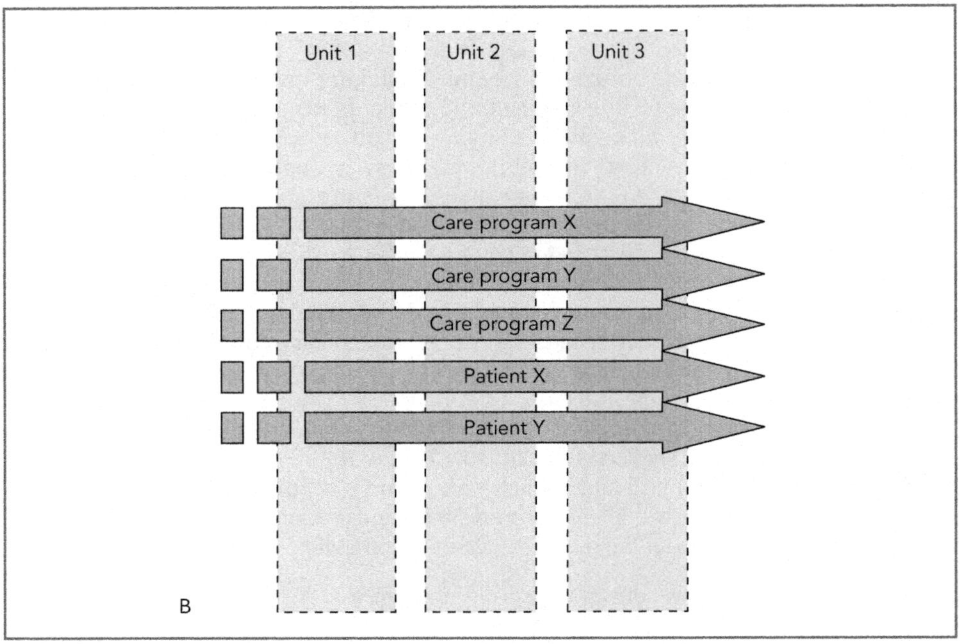

Through care programs, optimising the planning of scarce resources becomes possible. When it is made clear what the standard paths are for the majority of patients, the resources required for those care programs become apparent. By organising an outpatient clinic for heart failure patients (see Box 8.3), for example, and knowing the average number of new patients visiting the clinic, the number of nurse practitioners and consultancy rooms can be planned in advance. If, for example, 25% of cases require additional cardiological testing, this can be planned for as well.

Box 8.3 Flexible standardisation – Integrating standardisation and flexibilisation

The term 'standardisation' is often associated with 'Taylorism' or 'managed care', and thus carries many predominantly negative associations: bureaucracy, over-regulation, standardisation for standardisation's sake (Wiener 2000). Yet as we emphasise here, standardisation – of core steps in a care program, of techniques used, of communication patterns – is a prerequisite for the ambitions set by the Institute of Medicine's reports.

Importantly, however, standardisation should remain flexible. The care program is no 'assembly line'. At each individual step, the care professional can choose to not take the next step planned, and plan an alternative action in the traditional step-by-step approach. In addition, standardisation should not be pursued for its own sake (as it often is); only when standardisation of a step in a care program will lead to an improvement on one or more of the dimensions of quality should it be undertaken.

> **Box 8.3** Flexible standardisation – Integrating standardisation
> and flexibilisation – cont'd
>
> In many instances, the professional knowledge and motivation of healthcare
> workers can be most optimally drawn upon by *not* attempting to standardise it.
> This is true for those patients that do not fit the care programs, but it is also true
> for many steps *within* care programs. The activity of triage, for example, will
> always contain a large part of clinical judgment, which is most effectively dealt
> with by a highly experienced healthcare professional. In fact, bureaucratic regu-
> lations and inherited 'standard operating procedures' often have to be undone
> to fully profit from the professionals' skills (flexibilisation). Doing away with
> complicated schedule systems for outpatient visits (having fixed times for sepa-
> rate types of patients, attempting to spread new patients over the week, etc), for
> example, and leaving proper scheduling to the scheduler in charge, has proven
> to be very effective in reducing waiting lists (Murray & Berwick 2003).
>
> Flexible standardisation, then, is about *enhancing* competencies of profes-
> sionals. Supported by physician-developed protocols, heart failure nurses are
> now responsible for therapeutic activities that traditionally would have been
> seen as restricted to physicians. Standardisation is only about 'cookbook medi-
> cine' when one confuses the standardisation of the overall care program with
> the standardisation of the care of an individual patient. Working with care pro-
> grams is highly skilful work; it implies judging, at every step, whether the next
> planned step is indeed appropriate for this individual case (Timmermans &
> Berg 2003). This requires knowledge about the care programs' purposes, and
> clinical skills to realise its (in)appropriateness.

Given adequate numbers, even the emergency consultation or admission is predictable at aggregate level, and can thus be planned for. It can be predicted how many
patients will visit an outpatient clinic without a scheduled appointment each day, or
how many emergency surgeries come to the hospital daily. Separating these patients
from the 'usual' workflow drastically reduces the interruptions hindering this work,
and improves the handling of the emergency cases both in the emergency department
and on admission (Litvak & Long 2000).

This should not imply that every individual patient is 'planned' in a sequence of
individual and dedicated 'slots' per unit. Planning every individual patient trajectory
ahead in this way would require a substantial planning effort and constant rescheduling activities when plans have to be changed. Unused slots cost time, and match-
ing individual slots to individual patient trajectories, while keeping waiting times at
a minimum *and* optimising resource use, is difficult to achieve. Only for those care
trajectories where all individual steps can be predicted 95% of the time may such
detailed pre-planning be feasible. Outside of these so called 'focused factories', such a
'solution' would make matters worse (see Leggat, Chapter 2).

A smarter strategy is to use 'advanced access' (Murray & Berwick 2003) principles
for all but the most scarce and/or expensive resource. That is to say: services, that is,
clinic, ward, and also radiology, lab and operating room, keep their waiting lines very
short, so that everybody can be served (almost) immediately when the need arises and
no planning of individual slots is necessary. Because demand is predictable, resources
can be planned to be available when needed. This is a planning task at the aggregated
level of the program: so much MRI capacity is available at day X, so many bloodtests
can be done, so many outpatient visits or beds are required. Each individual patient

falls in line behind the resource s/he happens to require, and is served in turn. This can be done for diagnostics such as MRI, echo and blood tests, but also for outpatient visits or basic therapeutic interventions.

As said, care programs can properly estimate the amount of resources required at any given time. For advanced access principles to work at all or at most steps along the patient trajectory, however, the variability in patient numbers arriving at any step at the same time also needs to be minimised. Even when 'demand' and 'capacity' are seemingly optimised at the aggregated level, small variations in the 'input' have large consequences for resource use: small peaks leading to rapidly lengthening waiting times, for example, and small dips leading to resource underuse (McManus et al 2003). Care programs also help in this regard. By organisationally separating the distinctive building blocks of a care program (see Box 8.2), the variability of the demands posed on the resources by the incoming patient flow is reduced.

Resource planning is optimised for the individual service capacities 'handling' the individual patient's trajectory, and variations are reduced in the 'input' and 'output' of the individual process steps. It therefore becomes possible to combine optimal throughput times for the patient with high efficiency for the required service capacities. Planning individual patients for individual slots is only necessary for the most expensive resources, such as operating room time. Of course, we 'buy' such overall *system* efficiency by allowing slight inefficiency at the *subsystem* level: individual service capabilities will inevitably run at 80–90% occupancy rate, rather than the 100% that could theoretically be achieved by planning every slot. Aiming for 100% optimisation for individual services capabilities would lead to sub-optimisation at the system level: increased throughput times and exponential increase in 'coordination work' to push patients through the overcrowded services (Goldratt & Cox 1984). Units that attempt this in practice usually end up realising occupation rates of far below 80% because of all the unfilled slots and time wasted 'repairing' the obstructions they themselves cause. Working this way is patient friendly and effective (the likelihood of errors is reduced because of faster and better organised 'processing'), and the reduction of ad hoc coordination tasks is inevitably a relief for all professionals involved.

Process-supporting information technology and performance monitoring

For professionals to take up responsibility for 'their' care program, balanced steering information is a prerequisite. A well-designed system of monitoring of, and feedback on, the outcomes of a particular care process is a core building block of high-quality care (Committee on Quality of Healthcare in America 2001). Yet generating such information appears difficult in practice. Record keeping habits are usually well suited to getting the actual work done, but not for secondary purposes such as using this information for quality improvement monitoring, or, even more challenging, for research (Solberg et al 1997). Information capabilities for multiple uses requires more detailed and precise record-keeping habits, which cannot be simply added on to the professionals' current, and often already overburdened, workloads.

Well-designed care programs solve this problem. The delivery process can be organised so that the secretaries, clerks, nurse practitioners (or patients themselves) enter information in standard formats, so that a more complete record, with comparable and 'exportable' data, becomes feasible. Simultaneously, the most expensive care professionals will be less burdened with administrative tasks (Massaro 1993). The care programs form a natural background for this data gathering and analysis. The guidelines underlying the care program form the framework that connects the otherwise isolated data items, giving more insight into the reasons *why* specific steps were taken or decisions made.

Finally, these guidelines allow the relevant outcomes for monitoring and steering the care program to be deduced. When fed back to the professionals 'owning' the care program, a professional-oriented quality system comes into being: measuring, improving and consolidating. By constantly monitoring the impact of the care program on all dimensions of quality, continuous quality improvement can thus become part of everyday work practice. The care programs can be constantly improved and updated when new scientific or practice-derived insights arise.

Information technology is crucial for realising not only this continuous monitoring of performance, but also the whole interplay of working with care programs, re-delegating tasks, optimising flow and resource planning, and measuring performance. Important first steps can be made with all these topics without dedicated IT support, but progress will remain limited. One professional's information has to be at the other professional's desk speedily and in a structured way for care programs and task restructuring to function, and information gathered in the care process has to be aggregated to become performance information about the care program. For this, electronic patient record functionalities are required to share information, and order-communication, triage-supporting decision technologies and basic workflow techniques are needed to initiate, support and monitor care programs.

Interestingly, process-supporting information technology is dependent on care programs to succeed. Information technology can only fulfil its potential in a workplace when decision criteria, terminologies and work processes in that workplace are sufficiently standardised. To have a useful electronic patient record, professionals need to use that record in similar ways; to work with order entry, they have to heed the agreements assumed by the application. When such standardisation is not explicitly set as a goal for an information technology implementation project, and when this is not beneficial to the practitioners involved (see also above), the implementation will fail. Working with care programs, therefore, is the optimal way to start to work with information technology in healthcare. The care programs bring the standardisation that information technology requires, and, in its turn, information technology can further improve the cooperation, data management and planning possibilities brought by the care program.[9]

> **Pause for reflection**
>
> Information technology implementation in the primary care process has a poor track record. Think of examples where information technology failed, and see if you can find examples of 'unreflexive standardisation' in these attempts. Think also of successful implementations. Can you discern how standardisation improved the work process in ways deemed relevant by the users?

Care program-based governance

Behind this operational restructuring of the healthcare enterprise lies a development that changes the way this enterprise is structured and governed. In addition to being intimately linked to IT development, performance measurement and resource planning, care programs are simultaneously, and perhaps more importantly, the organisational building blocks around which the healthcare organisations of the future will be shaped.

---

[9] For more on process-supporting information technology in healthcare, see e.g. Coiera 2003 & Berg 2004

Here, societal developments meet and strengthen the 'logic' of enhancing quality and efficiency described above. More and more, payers and patients will demand that the service and technical quality of the care they receive is of the same or higher level as other goods and services they are used to. Long waits, poor service coordination, and high levels of error will no longer be accepted now that the public is learning just how avoidable these problems are. Costs of care delivery will need to be kept in check as the demand for care can potentially outstrip the gross domestic product (GDP) of most countries.

In many countries, one of the ways in which the pursuit of quality and cost control is engineered at the system level is by introducing product-based payment, that is, paying providers a fixed sum for the integrated care of a patient with diagnosis X. The fixed (and ideally severity-adjusted) price should cover all care activities and materials required for the complete care trajectory for patients with this condition. A provider that succeeds in delivering this care at a lower cost per patient can keep the difference; a provider that has higher expenses (maybe because of a higher surgical wound infection rate) loses out on this patient category.

When public performance reporting is linked to product-based payment, a system emerges in which high-quality care is recognised and rewarded, and providers that manage to combine high quality with low cost care thrive. Of course, there is still a gap between the way systems such as diagnosis-related groups (DRGs) are currently being used and introduced throughout the world, and this optimal way of implementing product-based payment.[10] Yet the convergence of 'pay for performance' (P4P) schemes with the fundamentals of healthcare financing is clearly under way (Berg et al 2006, Lindenauer et al 2007).

As we argue above, achieving high-quality and efficient care for a given patient category, and doing so constantly and predictably, is only possible through introducing care programs. By juxtaposing this conclusion with the societal development we describe, we can start to understand why there is such a clear drive to restructure managerial control and governance at this same level. It is at this level, the integrated care around a patient's diabetes, or liver disease, or hip arthrosis, that the value of the care (the quality bought per dollar/euro spent) is determined – not at the level of the hospital, nor at the level of the individual professional – but at the level of teams of professionals, supporting and managing staff cooperating around specific patient conditions (Porter & Teisberg 2006, Sutton & McLean 2006).

Making these teams responsible for their own clinical and financial results, allowing them to become (more) self-steering can optimise their commitment and motivation to this delivery of value. Rather than drowning in perverse incentives (cost constraints that are unrelated to patient needs, financial rewards irrespective of quality delivered, and so forth) professional motivation is then fully aligned with financial compensation. The teams set and maintain the care programs, and are responsible for measuring, continuously improving and accounting for their (quality and financial) results to patients and payers. They re-delegate tasks among themselves, and are directly responsible for smooth patient flow and the optimally efficient use of resources.

This transition, of course, is not painless. Yet the pain should not run deep. After all, this is ultimately not a loss but a transformation of autonomy: executing autonomy at the level of the individual patient program (resulting in all the problems discussed above) is traded for executing autonomy with the other professionals involved in

---

[10] The care trajectories paid for are often circumscribed by boundaries that are more determined by institutional boundaries (between hospitals and primary care, for example) than by the clinical course of these trajectories and the patient's experience. In addition, DRG payments seldom pay for the *integral* costs of care delivery. Often, specialists' payments or medication costs are separated, and so forth. See for discussions e.g. Porter & Teisberg 2006, Reinhardt 2006.

deciding what an integrated care program should look like. In most current healthcare settings, departments and specialists rule their turf, regardless of how the delineation of that territory links to achieving optimal patient outcomes. Working with integrated care programs implies a radical break from this history. First of all, starting to measure performance and sharing the results with the other professionals and managers involved in the care program is, at least for most professionals, a fundamental break from the past. Whereas high status and financial rewards used to come with just the position of a medical specialist, now one's actual performance is being measured and discussed by other specialists and managers.

In addition, professionals and departments have to give up part of their individual autonomy in another way. They no longer freely decide how to handle patients, or control input, throughput and output through their clinics, operating room or outpatient offices: the integrated care programs do so. While still in charge of the precise path individual patients will take, the care program does determine the outlines and core steps. Also, the care programs determine the organisation and planning of resources (see Figure 8.2B). This 'loss' of autonomy affects everyone: each individual professional in the care program has to be able to work from the assumption that everyone else follows the predetermined path. Also, specialists will get to plan radiology's timeslots, but through creating the care programs, radiologists will also get a say in defining the indications for which these 'blocks' can be used.

There is no blueprint for what this 'pathway-based model of clinical governance' (Degeling et al 2004a, Degeling et al 2004b) should look like in any particular case. Much is dependent on the particular financial and regulatory context, on the volumes of patients per patient category, on the aims and ambitions of the teams involved and on the vision of the services in which they work. Some facilities and professionals core to a care program may be an integral part of this self-steering group; others may be contracted to provide high-level services (diagnostic, consulting) only when required. In some cases, such new organisational arrangements will be clustered around traditional specialties (cardiological and cardio-surgical care programs or ophthalmological care programs that tend to cluster together in logical wholes). In other cases, organisational arrangements will tie together different medical specialties around a given condition, creating new boundaries within specialties (oncological conditions are a case in point).

Conclusion

A careful and 'flexible' standardisation of care programs, we argue, is central to any viable healthcare delivery system of the future. Yet such standardisation is not possible without a thorough restructuring and delegation of tasks, resource planning and flow optimisation, and implementing process-supporting information technology (including performance monitoring). Vice versa, these additional principles can only function properly when integrated with a proper standardisation of care programs. The latter step is crucial, since more often than not, continuous quality improvement (CQI) programs and IT development programs are independently managed, and lack a common focus. Without this, the individual CQI projects remain just that, and the IT implementation is bound to yield disappointing results (Berg 2004).

The vision described here can only be achieved gradually. Healthcare is a complex system (Committee on Quality of Healthcare in America 2001) and changing one part, such as the introduction of a part of a care program, can have unexpected consequences. Redesigning care processes to overcome waiting times can lead to increased waiting times when patients become attracted to this innovative practice, for example. A 'blueprint approach' to care innovation, then, can only fail. Rather, care organisations will need to select their own priorities, building upon an analysis of their own resources and advances within the individual elements of the vision described above. Likewise, a care program does not have to be 'finished' (if that is at all possible) in one single step. The most urgent quality problems of a certain unit may be solved by standardising only a small part of the care program. Building *towards* this vision, then, in an iterative, step-by-step way, and learning from all the mistakes made, is the only way to proceed. In this learning process, the vision itself will certainly evolve and, simultaneously, will become part of the organisation's culture (Ciborra et al 2000).

Acknowledgements

This paper is built upon an earlier publication in the *International Journal of Quality in Healthcare* (Berg et al 2005).

References

Bell D, Mcnaney N, Jones M 2006 Improving healthcare through redesign. BMJ 332: 1286–1287

Berenholtz S M, Milanovich S, Faircloth A et al 2004 Improving care for the ventilated patient. Jt Comm J Qual Saf 30:195–204

Berg M (ed) 2004 Health Information Management: Integrating Information and Communication Technology in Healthcare Work. Routledge, London

Berg M, De Brantes F, Schellekens W 2006 The right incentives for high-quality, affordable care: a new form of regulated competition. Int J Qual Healthcare 18:261–3

Berg M, Schellekens W, Bergen C 2005 Bridging the Quality Chasm: Integrating Professional and Organisational Quality. International Journal of Quality in Healthcare17:75–82

Berwick D M 1998 Crossing the boundary: changing mental models in the service of improvement. Int J Qual Healthcare 10:435–41

Bouvy M L, Heerdink E R, Urquhart J et al 2003 Effect of a pharmacist-led intervention on diuretic compliance in heart failure patients: a randomized controlled study. J Card Fail 9:404–11

Carroll J S, Rudolph J W 2006 Design of high reliability organisations in healthcare. Qual Saf Healthcare 15:i4–i9

Ciborra C U, Braa K, Cordella A (eds) 2000 From control to drift: The dynamics of corporate information infrastructures. Oxford University Press, Oxford

Coiera E 2003 Guide to Health Informatics. Arnold, London

Committee on Quality of Healthcare in America 2000 To Err is Human: Building a Safer Health System. National Academy Press, Washington

Committee on Quality of Healthcare in America 2001 Crossing the quality chasm: a new health system for the 21st century. National Academy Press, Washington

de Vries A, Van Dijk R, Hendriks M et al 2002 Medical nurses and the use of expert software in the treatment of patients with congestive heart failure: first year experience. Eur J of Heart Failure Supplement I:29

de Vries G, Hiddema U F 2001 Management van patiëntenstromen. Bohn Stafleu Van Loghum, Houten

Degeling P J, Maxwell S, Iedema R 2004a Restructuring clinical governance to maximize its developmental potential. In: Gray A, Harrison S (eds) Governing Medicine: Theory and Practice. Open University Press, Maidenhead, UK

Degeling P J, Maxwell S, Iedema R et al 2004b Making clinical governance work. BMJ 329:679–81

Dy S M, Garg P P, Nyberg D et al 2003 Are critical pathways effective for reducing postoperative length of stay? Medical Care 41:637–48

Goldratt E M, Cox J 1984 The Goal. A Process of Ongoing Improvement. Gower, Aldershot

Grol R 2000 Between evidence-based practice and total quality management: the implementation of cost-effective care. Int J Qual Healthcare12:297–304

Howell J D 1989 Machines and medicine: technology transforms the American Hospital. In: Long D E, Golden J (eds) 1989 The American General Hospital. Cornell University Press, Ithaca and London

Johnson Z K, Griffiths P G, Birch M K 2003 Nurse prescribing in glaucoma. Eye 17:47-52

Klazinga N 2000 Re-engineering trust: the adoption and adaption of four models for external quality assurance of healthcare services in western European healthcare systems. Int J Qual Healthcare 12:183–9

Leape L L, Kabcenell A I, Gandhi T K et al 2000 Reducing adverse drug events: lessons from a breakthrough series collaborative. Jt Comm J Qual Improv 26:321–31

Lindenauer P K, Remus D, Roman S et al 2007 Public Reporting and Pay for Performance in Hospital Quality Improvement. N Engl J Med, NEJMsa064964

Litvak E, Long M C 2000 Cost and quality under managed care: irreconcilable differences? Am J Manag Care 6:305–12

Luthi J C, Lund M J, Sampietro-Colom L et al 2003 Readmissions and the quality of care in patients hospitalized with heart failure. Int J Qual Healthcare 15:413–21

Massaro T A 1993 Introducing Physician Order Entry at a Major Academic Medical Centre: I. Impact on Organisational Culture and Behavior. Academic Medicine 68:20–25

McManus M L, Long M C, Cooper A et al 2003 Variability in Surgical Caseload and Access to Intensive Care Services. Anesthesiology 98:1491–6

Millenson M L 1997 Demanding medical excellence. Doctors and accountability in the information age. University of Chicago Press, Chicago

Mintzberg H 1979 The Structuring of Organisation. Prentice Hall, Englewood Cliffs

Murray M, Berwick D M 2003 Advanced access: reducing waiting and delays in primary care. JAMA 289:1035–40

Norman D A 1988 The psychology of everyday things. Basic Books, New York

Parker C S 1997 Charting by exception. Caring 16:36–40, 42–4

Porter M E, Teisberg E O 2006 Redefining Healthcare. Creating Value-Based Competition on Results. Harvard Business School Press, Boston

Reinhardt U E 2006 The Pricing Of U.S. Hospital Services: Chaos Behind A Veil Of Secrecy. Health Aff 25:57–69

Rozich J D, Howard R J, Justeson J M et al 2004 Standardisation as a mechanism to improve safety in healthcare. Jt Comm J Qual Saf 30:5–14

Schiele F, Meneveau N, Seronde M F et al 2005 Compliance with guidelines and 1-year mortality in patients with acute myocardial infarction: a prospective study. Eur Heart J 26: 873–880

Solberg L I, Mosser G, Mcdonald S 1997 The three faces of performance measurement: improvement, accountability, and research. Joint Commission Journal on Quality Improvement 23:135–47

Strauss A, Fagerhaugh S, Suczek B et al 1985 Social Organisation of Medical Work. University of Chicago Press, Chicago

Sutton M, McLean G 2006 Determinants of primary medical care quality measured under the new UK contract: cross sectional study. BMJ 332:389–90

Timmermans S, Berg M 2003 The Gold Standard: An Exploration of Evidence-Based Medicine and Standardisation in Healthcare. Temple University Press, Philadelphia

Wiener C L 2000 The Elusive Quest. Accountability in Hospitals. Aldine de Gruyter, New York

PART 3

Accounting for outcomes

A viable health system that achieves cost effectiveness objectives is dependent on good direction and practical implementation strategies. What role should policy play in this endeavour? Who should be involved in developing it? As with clinicians, policymakers are expected to do no harm. Does present policy achieve this aim? Is the process of policy development effective? How is policy implementation managed and to what extent does policy support clinical practice on the ground? Has it brought improvements? Are health services accountable for their performance? To what extent does policy and practice support services to achieve desired outcomes? These questions and others will help us to understand the environment within which health services operate, clinical practice improvement occurs and clinicians and managers are accountable for service outcomes.

In accounting for outcomes, integrating clinical and managerial systems of process management and practice improvement to achieve health service outcomes of quality, efficiency and safety is an essential step. Improving quality is a multidimensional concept that includes having the right structures and processes to produce the desired outcomes. In doing so, a challenge for health services is to reorient the goals of the professions to move beyond the immediate sphere of clinical knowledge and expertise to engage with the technical, organising and social dimensions of care and quality improvement, just as it will require lay managers to also engage with these dimensions. This will involve acquiring a different and particular set of skills appropriate to healthcare organisation and applying them. How will this reorientation be accomplished? How will it be supported and evaluated? Can research findings help improve health policy development, implementation and practice and improve safety and quality?

The relationship between safety and quality is a current issue of debate in healthcare. Is safety a unique outcome in its own right, for instance, or a subset of quality? If it is a unique element, how can it be managed independently? If it is a subset, how can it be incorporated into a broader quality agenda? A related question is: How much quality and safety is enough? If not all quality and safety can be achieved, what is the optimum balance? How can risk be reduced in clinical workplaces and how can lay managers assure themselves that appropriate and safe practices are in place? This is a particular issue in health services with their high levels of fragmentation, complexity, diversity, uncertainty and autonomy. The system is not perfect, but how can it be improved?

We take up these issues in the following chapters. We outline a model for evaluating quality and safety initiatives and how to prioritise them; we consider the organisation needed to implement quality and safety initiatives; we discuss methods to manage patient safety in clinical units; we explore the changing dynamic of policy and practice; and we propose ways to involve communities in healthcare decision making. Finally, we sum up the main issues arising from the theory and practice encompassed in this book to draw conclusions about the implications for health services, and offer resources for those who wish to read more widely on the subject of clinical process management.

Chapter 9

Quality and patient safety: How do we get there from here?

Rebecca Warburton

Introduction

This chapter is about prioritising action to improve quality and safety in healthcare. The evidence is now overwhelming that 'the way we've always done things' in healthcare is no longer good enough. The issue is out of the closet and no one can be complacent about patient safety. Unacceptable levels of patient harm from care are forcing all healthcare organisations to try new ways of doing things with a view to improving safety.

The journey is turning out to be more complicated than many hoped. There are no 'quick fixes', simply pointing out the problem has not changed things. Insights into the reasons why this is so are coming from many other fields including from complex systems, human factors engineering, high-risk industries such as aviation and nuclear power, and from studies into organisational culture and change.

Most healthcare organisations still lack basic measurements of the scope of the safety problem in their own settings. While the previously common 'don't ask, don't tell' code of silence is fading, recent infant heart surgery scandals in Winnipeg and Bristol (Gillies & Howard 2005) show that it isn't gone. Similarly, the blame–shame–name culture that focused on weeding out the 'bad apples' (the person approach) is giving way to the systems approach (where it is recognised that systems, not careless individuals, create most patient harm) but the shift is far from complete. There is cause for hope, but also a great deal that needs to be done for healthcare to realise its full potential of creating benefit for patients and avoiding harm.

Awareness of the need for improvement now extends well beyond the services that deliver healthcare. Quality and safety recommendations and requirements from accreditation agencies, government departments, drug and equipment vendors and improvement organisations regularly inundate hospitals and other healthcare provider organisations. Yet a key problem for administrators and clinicians is that little guidance is available about the relative priority of desired changes. Other chapters in this book consider quality and safety improvements from the perspective of those working in the organisation that are charged with the responsibility to improve performance. This chapter proposes an economic model to prioritise improvement, recognising that not everything can be done immediately, and that solid research evidence does not yet exist on the costs and effects of many potential improvements.

The chapter argues that if we are to gain the maximum reduction in harm for the resources that hospitals have available to improve safety, we need to collect and use cost-effectiveness evidence both to prioritise proposed safety improvements and to target new research. The chapter:

- explains the rationale for the need to prioritise quality and safety initiatives
- describes the methods needed to produce evidence of cost effectiveness
- suggests a number of promising starting points to improve healthcare safety in the absence of good evidence.

How much safety is enough?

The dictum of 'first, do no harm' drives healthcare providers to seek perfect, harm-free performance. Yet modern medicine, like modern life generally, cannot always be made perfectly safe. Holding perfection as an ideal is inspiring and perhaps necessary to discourage complacency (Berwick 2001), but there can be great harm in trying to achieve perfection because near-perfection often imposes near-infinite costs. The closer we get to perfection in any particular area, the more likely it becomes that we could have achieved 'a better bang for our preventive buck' somewhere else (Warburton 2003). Therefore actions must be prioritised, and evidence of benefit and cost is needed to do so.

Economists count as a cost anything of value that any person gives up, including money, time or pleasure. Leading advocates of evidence-based medicine have adopted this approach, and suggest that physicians think of costs as 'other treatments you can't afford to do if you use your scarce resources to do this one', noting that 'when internists borrow a bed from their surgical colleagues in order to admit a medical emergency tonight, the opportunity cost includes tomorrow's cancelled surgery' (Sackett et al 1997:100).

In healthcare terms, the costs of preventable adverse events are the value of the lost quality-adjusted life years (QALYs) of patients harmed *plus* the QALYs and lifetime productivity lost by health professionals unfairly blamed for 'committing'[11] an error *plus* the value of the time and resources used trying to mitigate or reverse harm, analyse the error and order compensation (i.e. treatment, risk analysis, legal and court costs).[12] The costs of preventing these events include the direct costs of resources put into safety-improving initiatives, which could otherwise have been spent on healthcare *plus* the value of QALYs and other resources lost because of delays or new errors caused by safeguards. Decisions to commit resources to improve safety should be undertaken thoughtfully, because successive improvements in safety generally impose progressively higher costs for each increment of improvement gained. Consider the simplified model in Figure 9.1 showing the costs (or value) of both prevention and

---

[11] Given the systems causes of most errors, 'deliver an error' would be more accurate, but sounds strange as we are accustomed to blaming someone.

[12] From the point of view of society as a whole, amounts paid in compensation do not count, as they are simply a transfer from one party to another, though of course these payments matter very much to those who pay or receive them.

Figure 9.1 Cost of prevention and adverse events

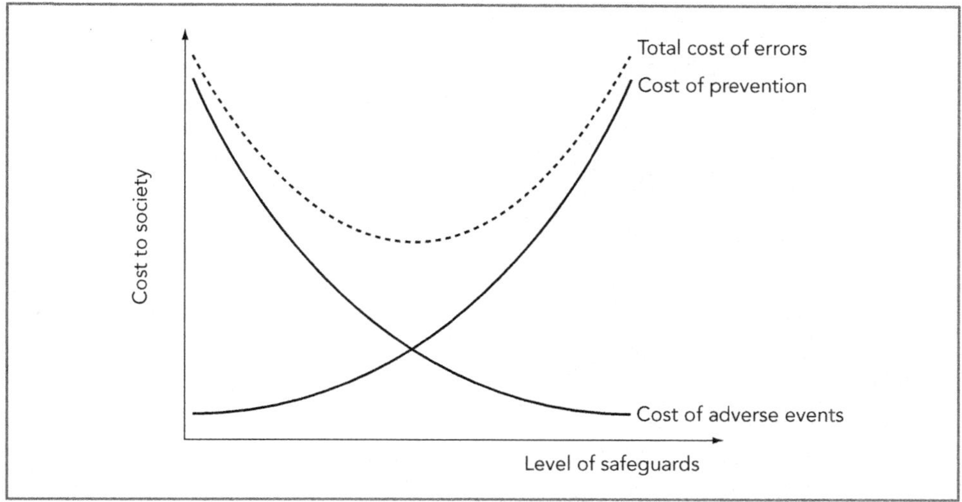

adverse events at various levels of safety precaution. (Only the costs of preventable adverse events, due to errors, are included in the figure.)

So how much safety is enough? If we consider only preventable adverse events and ignore the cost of improving safety, then perfect safety should be the goal. Once we consider the costs of prevention, though, we can see that we want to minimise the *sum* of the costs of adverse events and prevention. This sum is the dotted line in Figure 9.1 and it is U-shaped; we have enough safety at the bottom of the U. Improving safety beyond that point imposes marginal (extra) costs (from new safety precautions) that are larger than the marginal benefits (savings from newly avoided preventable adverse events).

A note about the shape of the curves in Figure 9.1: as drawn, the figure implies that safety improvements are adopted in order of cost effectiveness. Starting at the left, the steep slope of the dotted line indicates that total cost decreases rapidly as we first begin to improve safety, because initial safety improvements are relatively cheap (prevention cost increases very little) and quite effective (preventable adverse event cost drops significantly). The dotted line flattens out as we move towards the bottom of the U because later safety improvements cost a little more, and produce smaller benefits. Past the optimal level of safety (bottom of the U) the curve turns up; total costs increase because extra safety improvements are now quite costly yet produce only small benefits (little reduction in adverse events). This trade-off gets continually worse as we increase safety further past the optimum.

Arguably, healthcare safety will need to increase dramatically before we will be anywhere near the optimal safety level at the bottom of the U. But even in our current situation, we need to remember that every action comes at the expense of not doing something else. In the rush to improve patient safety, we need to remember that putting more effort into safety will likely force hospitals to put less effort into something else, at least in the short run.

Pause for reflection

How much safety is enough? Should health services aim for 'perfect' safety? Where could patient safety initiatives feasibly stop?

Costs and benefits – Why economic evaluation?

If more safety means less of 'something else', it becomes essential to ask: Which something else? What must we give up to make healthcare safer? There is no one answer to this question. For example, different safety improvements may either:

- cost very little, and create huge healthcare savings by avoiding patient injuries that can be corrected, but at great cost (Berwick 1998)
- cost very little, and save lives, but produce little in direct healthcare savings
- cost a great deal, and produce only small reductions in risk
- delay care or create new risks (Patterson et al 2002)
- increase workload, reduce employee satisfaction and make future changes harder
- streamline work and make it more rewarding, increasing employee buy-in and making future changes easier.

In clinical terms, as Merry notes subsequently in Chapter 11, extra safety checks may delay care and reduce patient throughput, endangering patients in situations where timeliness is essential. Without a fair assessment of the costs and effects (both intended and unintended) of proposed changes, it can be difficult to set priorities and impossible to know whether the best choice has been made. Yet most of the research now planned or in progress ignores costs and looks only at effects. This must change if we are to make sensible choices. We can turn to established methods in economic evaluation and technology assessment to inform these decisions, because the need to compare costs and effects is not unique to error reduction.

> **Pause for reflection**
>
> What do we give up when we try to make care safer? Do unintended consequences reduce the benefits in terms of safety and quality?

Setting priorities

When costs are not considered before action is taken, higher than acceptable costs can be the result. Most health regions can adopt only a fraction of recommended improvements due to constrained finances and limited staff time to safely implement change. This creates a danger of not adopting improvements in order of their cost effectiveness, and real examples exist: the universal precautions (an occupational health and safety initiative recommended by the US Centers for Disease Control to prevent worksite transmission of HIV to healthcare workers) cost from \$100,000 to \$1.7 million per QALY.[13] These precautions have been widely implemented in the US and Canada, yet many vaccines with much lower costs per QALY remain underutilised (even by Canadian regional health authorities responsible for both hospitals and immunisation).

Because human preferences must be considered in setting priorities, it is not possible to set rigid rules for the 'correct' value of a QALY. Despite general support for the use of QALYs in setting priorities (Bryan et al 2002) allocation preferences are affected by circumstances and patient characteristics (Schwappach 2002). Most people value

---

[13] Original estimate of C\$8 million to C\$128 million in 1990 per case of HIV seroconversion prevented from Stock et al 1990; updated and converted to US\$6.5 million to US\$104 million in 2002 by the author (Warburton 2005); cost per QALY based on 60 lost QALYs per seroconversion.

fairness and are willing to sacrifice some QALY gains to achieve more equality in access (Schwappach 2003). Perhaps healthcare workers are seen as more deserving of protection since they risk exposure to disease in their role caring for others. Alternatively, healthcare employers may have been willing (as in the case of universal precautions mentioned earlier) to incur high costs for prevention because of the difficulty and high costs involved in compensating and replacing skilled employees infected with HIV at work. The argument that the high cost paid to protect healthcare workers reflects preferences would be more compelling, however, if there were evidence that the high costs had been known *before* universal precautions were implemented; a credible rival hypothesis is that many non-optimal choices result from lack of information. (If employers believed employees to be deserving of special treatment, it means they understood that universal precautions were expensive, but felt the benefits outweighed the costs; alternatively, they might have made the decision not realising how expensive it actually was. It can't be both ways.)

While preferences might mean that we would not adopt improvements in exact cost-effectiveness order, we still would not expect huge discrepancies. Hence, it is hard to argue against estimating costs per QALY before (rather than after) initiating costly safety improvements.

Adopting costly, ineffective safety improvements when inexpensive but effective ones are available would be a double waste of resources; more would be spent than necessary on safety, and less obtained (in benefits) than was possible. In the US and the UK, reducing errors is seen as central to improving quality while controlling costs (Barach & Small 2000). Yet this hope is unlikely to be realised unless research examines both the costs and the effects of specific changes intended to reduce errors.

Pause for reflection

What information do we need before we embark upon safety improvement activities? How and by whom should this information be obtained?

Producing the evidence

In terms of the evaluation of safety improvements, it is important to apply both formative and summative evaluation tools. Formative evaluation (designed to shape and improve changes on the fly as they proceed) is important to ensure that the change is implemented as well as possible. This will avoid applying summative (after-the-fact) evaluation to a poorly implemented improvement.

A prime example of a formative tool is Deming's Plan–Do–Study–Act (PDSA) rapid-cycle change model of continuous quality improvement (Langley et al 1996), also discussed by Boaden & Harvey in Chapter 10. The PDSA cycle (Institute for Healthcare Improvement 2006) as shown in Figure 9.2 is powerful because first attempts to improve a complex system are rarely perfect, and it is important to re-assess and redesign flexibly until the intended results are achieved locally (or shown not to result even when the change is implemented as well as possible). The PDSA cycle holds out this promise. The cycle begins with three questions:

1. What are we trying to accomplish?
2. How will we know that a change is an improvement?
3. What changes can we make that will result in an improvement?

Quality improvement based on this model begins with discussion of these questions, leading to design of an improvement (*plan*). As the improvement is implemented (*do*), it is monitored (*study*) to determine effectiveness. Finally, it may be modified (*act*) as necessary based on experience and evidence. The cycle repeats itself to create continuous quality improvement.

Figure 9.2 The Plan–Do–Study–Act (PDSA) cycle

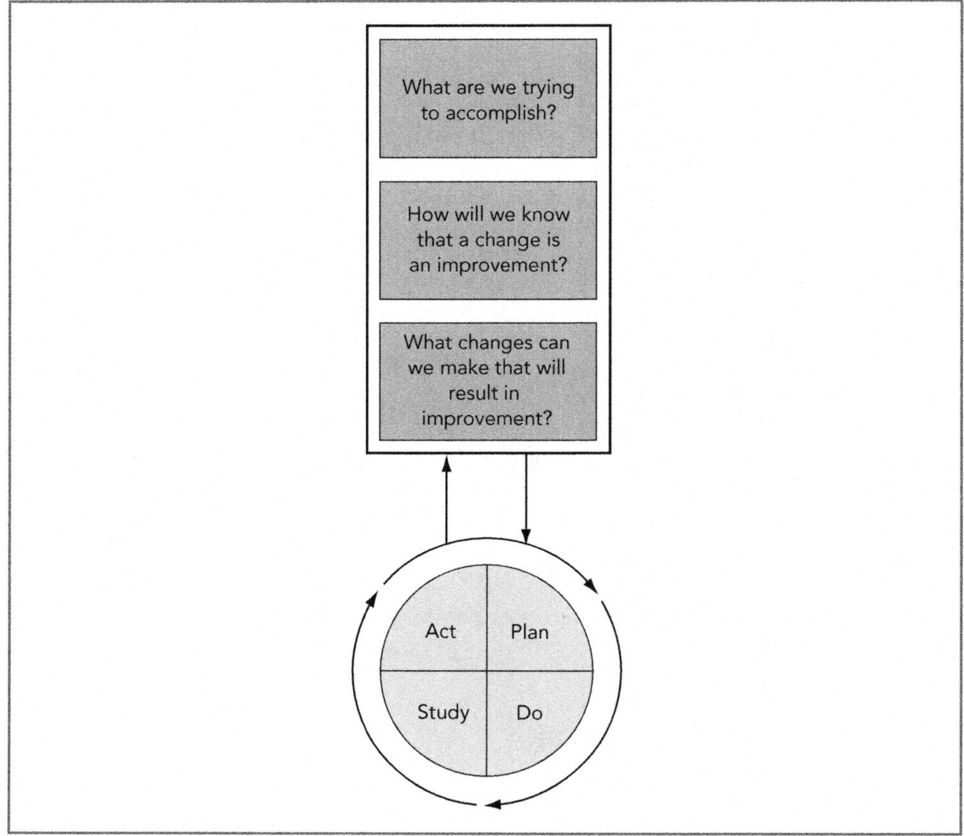

Even where PDSA cycles provide evidence that improvement projects have been successful, priorities for how and when to spread those improvements beyond the pilot sites requires evidence on costs and effects. To establish this stronger evidence, and ensure that the most cost-effective changes are implemented across the system, more rigorous summative evaluation methods are needed. An example is the Economic Evaluation Loop (EEL) (Warburton 2005). This model assesses the costs and benefits of a change, then tests plausible alternatives with a sensitivity analysis. Careful sensitivity analysis can reveal whether or not further information is needed before the results are sufficiently robust to be used in priority setting.

The EEL (shown in Figure 9.3) outlines a process that will ensure scarce research efforts are directed to the areas where new information has greatest value.

Box 9.1 sets out the three essential steps of the EEL process.

This new assessment loop can be used for small and large projects at the clinical, organisational and policy levels. It is consistent with and follows the excellent precedent set by the Technology Assessment Iterative Loop (TAIL) (Tugwell et al 1986, 1995) in recognising that the job of assessment must continue throughout the useful life of a technology because costs, effects and uses evolve. In the first cycle, the emphasis is on 'quick and dirty' assessment (Steps 1 and 2) to target future primary research (Step 3). As new data collection is completed, later cycles incorporate increasingly reliable evidence, and confidence in base-case results increases. Periodic reassessment is required to ensure that results remain reliable.

Figure 9.3 The Economic Evaluation Loop

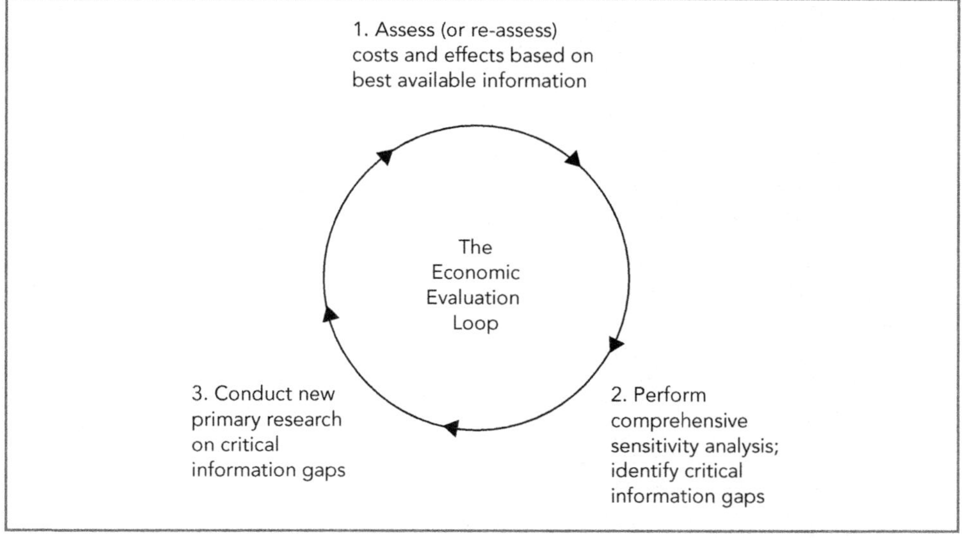

Box 9.1 Implications for practice – Steps in the EEL process

Step 1: An initial estimate is made of base-case (expected) costs and benefits (in QALYs) for all alternative strategies. This initial synthesis combines existing research, from whatever source, and may include modelling.

Step 2: The potential impact of uncertainty is explored in a comprehensive sensitivity analysis, again including synthesis of evidence from literature. All plausible alternative assumptions, and alternative values for key variables, are tested to determine what impact they have on results. Any plausible alternative values or assumptions that alter base-case conclusions are identified as critical information gaps; no firm conclusion can be reached until better information is obtained in these areas.

Step 3: New primary research is conducted to fill critical information gaps. The cycle begins again as these results are used to improve the estimates in Step 1, and to refine the sensitivity analysis in Step 2. Conclusions are deemed reliable only when no critical information gaps remain, and the sensitivity analysis reveals consistent conclusions under all plausible assumptions.

Where to start, without the evidence?

The preceding sections outline the evidence needed to gain the maximum benefit from improvements in healthcare. Unfortunately this evidence has not yet been generated. So where should improvement start? Because we now understand that healthcare is a high-risk industry and a complex system dependent for its safe operation on human

> **Box 9.2** Implications for practice – Creating the environment for improving safety and quality in healthcare
>
> Research already undertaken into quality improvement and patient safety and discussed throughout this book has shown that to operate safely, a complex high-risk industry needs:
>
> - a 'learning culture'
> - strong leadership on safety (both top-down and bottom-up)
> - a clear focus on the goal of changing procedures to make safety easy, and danger/harm hard
> - appropriate multidisciplinary teams
> - effective communication within and between teams and divisions.
>
> Leaders can be divided into two types: top-down and bottom-up. Top-down leaders (corporate or lay managers, administrators and policymakers) need to:
>
> - have a genuine understanding of patient safety issues
> - lead by example to foster a learning culture that takes a systems view of mistakes rather than a personal (blame–shame–name) view
> - provide adequate resources (improvement generally costs more at first, though it may save or make the use of existing resources more efficient, if successful)
> - continually demand (and support the development of) better data on safety
> - support the use of appropriate methods for improvement and evaluation.
>
> Bottom-up leaders (staff and point-of-care managers) need to:
>
> - regain (or maintain) hope of improvement and regain (or maintain) control of quality improvement in practical terms (make suggestions, learn PDSA, and apply)
> - be unafraid to make mistakes in improvement, but be afraid to make the same one twice!
> - celebrate 'good catches', and propose improvements to prevent it from happening again.
>
> Specific techniques that need to be in any organisation's safety toolbox include:
>
> - sort out the appropriate roles of boards, administrators, and staff in improving safety (Reinertsen 2003)
> - improve incident reporting systems of near misses as well as critical incidents
> - train staff in methods such as the PDSA improvement cycle; root cause analysis (RCA) (Hirsch & Wallace 2003) (RCA is an in-depth analysis when a complex system has failed and the cause is not clear); failure mode effects analysis (FMEA) (DeRosier et al 2002) (FMEA is a method of analysing the riskiness of a process); and safety huddles (routine, short staff meetings focused on safety hazards and fixes)
> - apply PDSA whenever an improvement is planned
> - apply RCA to analyse both critical incidents and near misses where causation is unclear; and use FMEA to assess the riskiness of planned process changes before they are implemented
> - use a trigger tool (Rozich et al 2003) to detect unreported adverse events (which may then require investigation using RCA)
> - manage shifts and shift transitions to minimise the danger of on-the-job fatigue (Dawson & McCulloch 2005).

beings, useful evidence to start improvement can come from outside healthcare. As noted earlier, useful insights have come from research in fields including complex systems, human factors engineering, reliable communication, and organisational culture and change, as well as from applications of that research in high-risk industries such as aviation and nuclear power. The single best source of good ideas presently is Don Berwick's Institute for Healthcare Improvement (IHI) (see Berding, Resources). More information on the following short list of necessary first steps and promising avenues for progress set out in Box 9.2 can be found at the IHI website (see www.ihi.org).

These success factors make clear that improved safety and quality is a shared responsibility of clinicians, support staff, managers, and funders at all levels. Administrators play a significant role in creating an environment that supports improvement and finds resources. Clinical staff must engage with improvement efforts and lead change on the ground. Beyond the health service organisation itself, boards, funders and policymakers can foster supportive environments and influence safety improvements through their policy decisions and recommendations (of the type that Jorm et al outline in Chapter 12).

In keeping with the intent to apply improvements in order of cost effectiveness, it is important to begin improvements in areas likely to provide the greatest benefits in proportion to resources spent, even where costs and benefits cannot be known precisely. This is called going after the low-hanging fruit first.

Box 9.3 Implications for practice – Examples of low-hanging fruit

These include:

- known high-risk activities, drugs or devices, such as:
  - care transitions (hand-offs or handovers) many problems result from poor attention to medication reconciliation and medical orders when patients are admitted, transferred or discharged, and at shift changes
  - high-risk medications – the top three are insulin, anticoagulants and sedatives
  - high-risk devices such as infusion pumps.

The Institute for Health Improvement and other organisations offer collaboratives and campaigns to support organisations as they take action in promising areas of improvement (see Berding, Resources). For an organisation deciding where to start, it is important not to go it alone.

It may seem paradoxical for this chapter to argue for the importance of implementing changes in order of cost effectiveness, and for the need to apply the EEL to changes so as to continually generate rigorous evidence on the costs and benefits of improvements, while recommending a laundry list of improvements whose cost effectiveness has not been demonstrated. The key to reconciling the apparent paradox is simple: implement, but evaluate. The way forward in patient safety is to ensure that as improvements proceed, knowledge of costs and benefits increases so that, over time, the most cost-effective changes can be identified and placed at top priority.

Pause for reflection

What low-hanging fruit exists in your organisation?

From patient safety to better overall quality of care

Much has been learned about patient safety, although there is still a long way to go. Nonetheless, we can be optimistic about the future because patient safety is the lever for improving quality generally. It is the 'foot in the door' for broad, sustained improvements in quality of care. Why might this be so, and why should we be optimistic? It is so because, as noted earlier, no one in healthcare can be complacent about patient safety. The issue is here to stay and new approaches are being tried. This is cause for optimism in terms of overall quality, because while excellent patient safety is necessary for high-quality care, it isn't sufficient.

The distinction between safety and quality is important. Safety is more qualitative than quantitative because it requires a cultural shift and a change in the distribution of quality. Think of quality in healthcare (overall, or in one organisation or site of care) as being distributed from low to high, something like Figure 9.4. Quality improvement is more quantitative because it involves incremental improvements in quality, and progresses by taking rigorous measures of patient outcomes and comparing them over time (see Boaden & Harvey, Chapter 10).

Figure 9.4 Distribution of quality of care

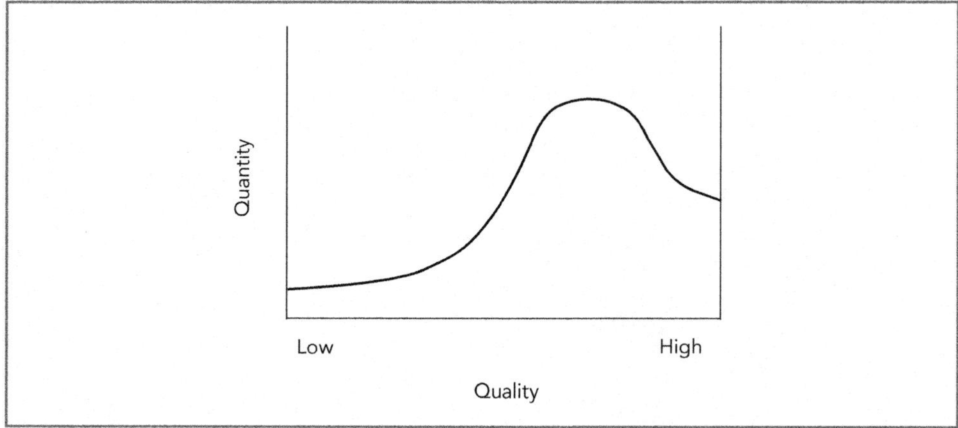

Patient safety is higher at the high-quality end, but some harm occurs to patients in all parts of the quality distribution. Preventable harm is presumably rare with high-quality care, though harm can still occur in ways that are (at our current stage of knowledge) not predictable, and hence not preventable. Preventable harm is presumably most common with low-quality care yet we hope few organisations or locations consistently provide low-quality care. Most care is routine, delivered at medium or average quality, and this is probably where most harm occurs to patients as well (simply because so much more care is delivered in this part of the quality distribution).

The goal of the patient safety movement is to reduce preventable harm to patients. In light of Figure 9.4, this goal can be seen to have two different components: to truncate or remove the low-quality end of the quality distribution, and to reduce harm in the middle part of the distribution. In general, the key method of improving patient safety is to improve processes of care in order to make safety easier (and risky care more difficult) than at present. However, the overall goal of improving quality is somewhat different. In this case the goal is to shift the entire quality distribution to the right. The ideal quality distribution being sought is more like Figure 9.5. This involves not only reducing harm, but also improving care to ensure that patients obtain the maximum health benefit possible.

Figure 9.5 Ideal distribution of quality of care

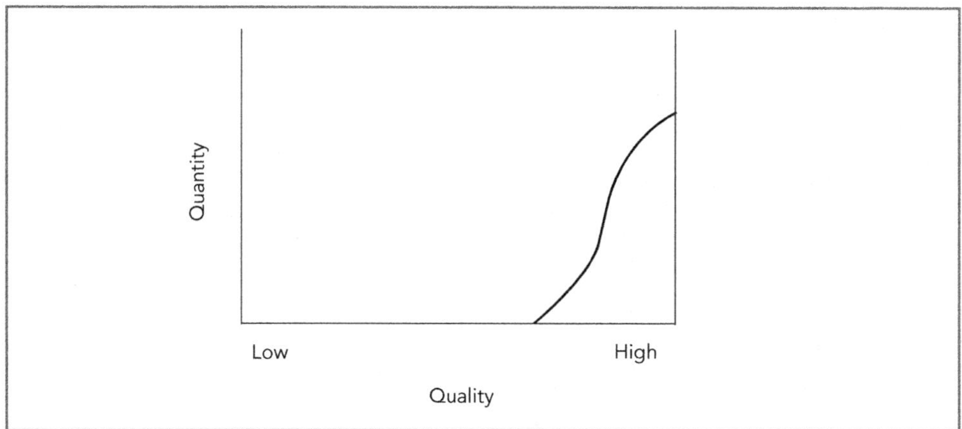

Why be optimistic that these two different tasks (improving safety and improving quality) are related? Because the actions needed to improve safety are fundamentally the same as those needed to improve quality, even though the initial goals are not the same. Pathways, for instance, as outlined by Boaden & Harvey in Chapter 10, can help ameliorate the poorest-quality care (for example where major delays or missed steps occur) and improve routine care (for example by bundling services that need to be done sequentially yet quickly for effective care). (See Berg, Schellekens & Bergen, Chapter 8.) The design and use of pathways requires a cultural shift from applying the clinical expertise of individual clinicians to individual patients to designing standardised evidence-based protocols for routine care for populations of patients undergoing similar treatment. Focusing on variation and flow, as Boaden & Harvey propose, and standardising processes to reduce the former and streamline the latter, as Berg, Skellekens & Bergen propose, can be formatively evaluated through PDSA cycles. Summative evaluation (comparing overall performance before and after pathway use via the EEL) would be appropriate only after sufficient experience shows that benefit is being gained.

Box 9.4 Implications for practice – Prioritising quality and safety initiatives

Steps in prioritising initiatives:

1. Focus on the goal; implement safety improvements in order of cost effectiveness (or likely cost effectiveness, if evidence is lacking).
2. Recognise the importance of leadership and cultural change.
3. Support staff to acquire and master essential tools such as improved incident reporting (including near misses); PDSA improvement cycles; trigger tools; RCA and FMEA.
4. Target improvement to known high-risk activities, drugs or devices such as care transitions, high-risk medications and high-risk devices. Employ both formative evaluation (to implement each change well) and summative evaluation (using the EEL as a framework) to guide the cost-effective spread of improvement based on experience. Collect data and generate evidence on costs and effects of changes.

Conclusion

Basing safety improvement recommendations on existing research evidence will not promote cost-effective reductions in patient harm, because few of the most promising improvements have been rigorously evaluated. However, waiting for complete evidence is not reasonable either; we have enough information to begin. The key to sustained improvements in safety, and perhaps in quality more generally, is to begin with plausible changes that seem likely to be cost effective; use PDSA improvement methods to implement changes as well as possible; and then apply the EEL to produce rigorous evidence on costs and effects. This more rigorously produced evidence can then guide the cost-effective spread of improvements to other settings, to help healthcare achieve its full safety and quality potential.

References

Barach P, Small S D 2000 Reporting and preventing medical mishaps: lessons from nonmedical near miss reporting systems. BMJ (Clinical research ed.) 320(7237):759–763

Berwick D M 2001 Is it wise to promote 'perfection' as a goal? Institute for Healthcare Improvement, Continuous Improvement, no 4

Berwick D M 1998 As good as it should get: making health care better in the new millennium. National Coalition for Health Care, Washington DC

Bryan S, Roberts T, Heginbotham C et al 2002 QALY-maximisation and public preferences: results from a general population survey. Health economics 11(8):679–693

Dawson D, McCulloch K 2005 Managing fatigue: It's about sleep. Sleep Medicine Reviews 9:365–380

DeRosier J, Stalhandske E, Bagian J P et al 2002 Using health care Failure Mode and Effect Analysis: the VA National Centre for Patient Safety's prospective risk analysis system. The Joint Commission journal on quality improvement 28(5):248–267, 209

Gillies A, Howard J 2005 An international comparison of information in adverse events. International journal of health care quality assurance incorporating Leadership in health services 18(4–5):343–352

Hirsch K A, Wallace P 2003 Conducting a Cost Effective Root Cause Analysis, Medical Risk Management Associates. Online. Available: http://www.rootcauseanalyst.com/costeffective.php 15 Nov 2007

Institute for Healthcare Improvement 2006 The Plan-Do-Study-Act Improvement Cycle. Online. Available: http://www.ihi.org 15 Nov 2007

Langley G, Nolan K, Nolan T et al 1996 The improvement guide: a practical approach to enhancing organizational performance. 1st edn Jossey-Bass Publishers, San Francisco

Patterson E S, Cook R I, Render M L 2002 Improving patient safety by identifying side effects from introducing bar coding in medication administration. Journal of the American Medical Informatics Association 9(5):540–553

Reinertsen J L 2003 Boards, administrators, medical staffs and quality: Sorting out the roles. Trustee September 1–11

Rozich J D, Haraden C R, Resar R K 2003 Adverse drug event trigger tool: a practical methodology for measuring medication related harm. Qual. Saf Health Care 12(3):194–200

Sackett D L, Richardson W S, Rosenberg W M C et al 1997 Evidence-based medicine: how to practice and teach EBM. Churchill Livingstone, New York

Schwappach D L 2003 Does it matter who you are or what you gain? An experimental study of preferences for resource allocation, Health economics 12(4):255–267

Schwappach D L 2002 Resource allocation, social values and the QALY: a review of the debate and empirical evidence. Health expectations: an international journal of public participation in health care and health policy 5(3):210–222

Stock S R, Gafni S R, Bloch R F 1990 Universal precautions to prevent HIV transmission to health care workers: an economic analysis. CMAJ 142:937–946

Tugwell P, Bennett K, Feeny D et al 1986 A framework for the evaluation of technology: the technology assessment iterative loop. In: Feeny D, Guyatt G, Tugwell P (eds) Health care technology: effectiveness, efficiency, and public policy. Institute for Research on Public Policy, Montreal, p 41–56

Tugwell P, Sitthi-Amorn C, O'Connor A et al 1995 Technology assessment. Old, new and needs-based. International Journal of Technology Assessment in Health Care 11(4):650–662

Warburton R N 2005 Patient safety – how much is enough? Health policy 71(2):223–232

Warburton R N 2003 What do we gain from the sixth coronary heart disease drug? BMJ (Clinical research ed.) 327(7426):1237–1238

Chapter 10

Organising for quality improvement and patient safety

Ruth Boaden & Gill Harvey

Introduction

Quality improvement efforts are focused on processes, regardless of whether they are clinical or managerial. However, clinical and managerial systems of process management and improvement are often treated as discrete, parallel activities within an organisation. This runs the risk of misaligned objectives, duplication of effort and a lack of focus on the things that really matter in terms of improving patient safety and quality outcomes.

The challenge for healthcare organisations is to continue to improve both clinical and managerial processes, while also recognising their interaction. To do this, it is important to understand the roots of both clinical and managerial improvement so that common themes and interactions can be identified.

In this chapter we outline the history and development of quality improvement from both a clinical and managerial perspective, including the influence of industrial approaches to improvement. A number of common challenges are set out that organisations need to address to achieve a whole systems approach to improvement. Specifically, the chapter discusses:

- the concepts of quality
- quality improvement in healthcare organisations
- the challenges for organisations.

Concepts of quality

Clinical concepts of quality

The development of healthcare quality is associated with the profession of medicine as a craft, with quality based almost solely on the skill of the 'craftspeople'. As outlined by Leggat in Chapter 2, this craft-based approach to professional practice vested the control of quality with individual clinicians more at an implicit level, within the overall scope of their professional practice. Consequently, the competence of individual practitioners is a major contributor to the delivery of high-quality care, something that has traditionally been regulated through controlling entry into the profession and upholding standards of professional education.

The influence of the craft-based model is apparent in some of the early approaches to quality evaluation in medical practice. For example, in outcome-related morbidity and mortality studies, clinical case conferences and the early introduction of medical audit, the emphasis was on closed discussions about quality and standards, typically through applying peer review methods (Harvey 1996). As quality became a more prominent feature in healthcare policy, so too more formal requirements for doctors to engage in quality and audit emerged, for example through the mandatory introduction of medical audit in the UK in the late 1980s (Department of Health 1989). For some doctors, these changes were seen as a threat to the traditional craft-based organisation of medical work, resulting in resistance to medical audit and distinctions being drawn between audit as an internal, peer review activity and audit as an external, regulatory mechanism (Shaw 1980).

Throughout these developments, a number of prominent clinicians have challenged traditional ways of thinking and pioneered developments in medical quality evaluation and improvement. As early as 1916, Ernest Codman, a US surgeon, used and published the 'ends results' system of auditing surgical care (Codman 1916). In the 1960s and 1970s, Avedis Donabedian went further, presenting quality as a multidimensional concept, influenced not just by the technical quality of care, but also by features of the interpersonal relationship between doctor and patient and by the physical amenities of care (Donabedian 1966). He is perhaps best known for his structure–process–outcome model of quality.

More recently, influential figures such as Don Berwick have led the way in calling for a move beyond medical audit towards more improvement-based approaches to quality (Berwick 1992) largely because of perceived failures to act on the results of audit to achieve meaningful change. In refocusing efforts towards the action phase of audit, the medical profession needs to look beyond its immediate sphere of knowledge and experience defining and measuring standards and criteria, towards more general theories of organisational change and industrially based approaches to quality improvement. As such, the narrow evaluation of practitioner performance needs to be widened to a more patient/client-focused view of quality, with clinicians taking on a so called new set of 'clinical skills', including skills in teamworking, process analysis, guideline development and collaborative working with patients, managers and other professional colleagues (Berwick et al 1992).

Other professional groups in healthcare have been less influenced by the craft-based model of practice, largely as a result of their position in the professional hierarchy relative to medicine. The nursing profession, for example, had their own pioneer of quality and standards in the early work of Florence Nightingale. However, early developments in nursing quality evaluation were largely focused on methods of external monitoring, through the development and application of quality indicators and measurement instruments (Harvey 1996). Such developments were superseded by more practitioner-based methods that typically involved local teams of practitioners working together to identify and work on topics for improvement. These approaches had more in common with industrially based approaches such as quality circles, although sometimes failed to become integrated within overall organisational systems for quality management (Morrell et al 1997). More recent clinically focused initiatives such as practice development in nursing that aim to transform the context and culture of care (McCormack et al 2004) may have the same effect.

Approaches to clinical quality improvement

More recently, developments emanating from the evidence-based medicine movement and from public inquiries into major healthcare failures have introduced a number of new concepts to the field of clinical quality, which may have the potential to create better integration with organisational quality. The evidence-based practice agenda, with its focus on synthesising existing research through systematic review methods, has contributed to the development of clinical guidelines, described as 'systematically developed statements to assist practitioner and patient decisions about appropriate healthcare for specific clinical circumstances' (Institute of Medicine 1992, cited in Duff et al 1996:888). A key defining attribute of clinical guidelines is that they should be based on available research evidence (Duff et al 1996) and the focus on distilling evidence of clinical and cost effectiveness into recommendations for clinical practice is an attempt to standardise care, within the operations management methods outlined by Leggat in Chapter 2. However, despite the extent of investment in guideline development, evidence to date suggests that their impact on actual practice and patient outcomes is variable (Grimshaw et al 2004), highlighting the challenges and complexities involved in translating evidence into practice.

Care pathways are another tool that has been applied in healthcare in an attempt to standardise processes of care delivery (see Claridge & Cook, Chapter 4). Pathways have been used in different ways, for example as a way of translating national guidelines into local practice or as a way of mapping ideal processes for specific care groups. Typically they are presented as structured, multidisciplinary plans of care designed to support the implementation of clinical guidelines and protocols, providing guidance about each stage of the management of a patient with a particular condition, including details of both process and outcome. They aim to improve continuity and coordination of care and enable more effective resource planning, as well as providing comparative data on many aspects of quality of care. Claims made are that they reduce variation and improve outcomes (Middleton et al 2001).

Clinical governance, defined as the 'action, the system or the manner of governing clinical affairs' (Lugon & Secker-Walker 1999:1), developed as an overall strategy within a policy on quality in the UK's National Health Service (NHS) (Department of Health 1989). After a high-profile failure of care in a hospital providing paediatric cardiac surgery services that highlighted organisational shortcomings (Kennedy 2001), statutory changes were introduced to impose a legal duty of quality on the chief executives and boards of NHS organisations, for the first time creating a corporate responsibility for the quality of clinical care. The significance of this is apparent in cases where poor clinical quality is observed and the boards of healthcare organisations are held to account for this, as opposed to individual clinicians or clinical teams, as illustrated by the case study in Box 10.1 later in the chapter.

In summary, developments in clinical quality have been professionally led and reflect the different traditions and ways of working within the profession. As a consequence, a range of healthcare definitions and 'dimensions of quality' have developed (see Table 10.1). Over time, there has been a move away from uniprofessional, clinical quality initiatives towards more multiprofessional, patient-centred models that are integrated within wider organisational structures and processes. This, in turn, has led to increasing awareness and application of some of the industrially based approaches and techniques that are described in the next section.

Table 10.1 Definitions of healthcare quality

Donabedian (1987)	Maxwell (1984)	Langley et al (1996)	Institute of Medicine (2001)
• Manner in which practitioner manages the personal interaction with the patient • Patient's own contribution to care • Amenities of the settings where care is provided • Facility in access to care • Social distribution of access • Social distribution of health improvements attributable to care	• Access to services • Relevance to need • Effectiveness • Equity • Social acceptability • Efficiency and economy	• Performance • Features • Time • Reliability • Durability • Uniformity • Consistency • Serviceability • Aesthetics • Personal interaction • Flexibility • Harmlessness • Perceived quality • Usability	• Safety • Effectiveness • Patient centredness • Timeliness • Efficiency • Equity

'Industrial' concepts of quality

The concept of 'quality' in industry can again be argued to have developed from early models of production management (see Leggat, Chapter 2) but was formalised through Shewhart's work on statistical process control (SPC) in the 1920s (Shewhart 1931) with the result that 'the management of quality acquired a scientific and statistical foundation' (Kolesar 1993:319). Many of the concepts of SPC are now being applied in healthcare with evidence that 'SPC is a versatile tool which can help diverse stakeholders to manage changes in healthcare and improve patients' health' (Thor et al 2007:387).

The concepts of quality then were developed by a number of key figures ('gurus'). Four in particular stand out:

1. *W Edwards Deming* developed a 14-point approach (Deming 1986), his management philosophy for improving quality and changing organisational culture. He was responsible for developing the concept of the PDCA (Plan–Do–Check–Action) cycle (more often referred to in healthcare as the Plan–Do–Study–Action (PDSA) cycle) (Langley et al 1996) (see Warburton, Chapter 9).

2. *Joseph Juran* (Juran 1951) focused on the managerial aspects of implementing quality and argued that by reducing statistical variation and therefore improving quality, productivity and competitive position is improved. He promoted a trilogy of quality planning, quality control and quality improvement and maintained that providing customer satisfaction must be the chief operating goal.

3. *Philip Crosby*'s philosophy is summarised as: improving quality reduces costs and raises profit; he defined quality as 'conformance to requirements' (Crosby 1979:15). He too had 14 steps to quality and his ideas were very appealing to both

manufacturing and service organisations. Best known for the concepts of 'do it right first time' and 'zero defects', he believed that management had to set the tone for quality within an organisation.

4. *Armand Feigenbaum* (Feigenbaum 1961) defined quality as a way of managing (rather than a series of technical projects) and the responsibility of everyone. His major contribution was the categorisation of quality costs into three: appraisal, prevention and failure, and his insistence that management and leadership are essential for quality improvement. His work has been described as relevant to healthcare (Berwick 1989).

Until the 1980s most of the emphasis on quality improvement, and most of the empirical utilisation of the associated techniques, was within the manufacturing industry. However, the field of 'service quality' developed initially from a marketing focus (Groonroos 1984) but relatively little attention is paid explicitly to the 'service' aspects of healthcare quality. This is despite the fact that many of the philosophies that underpin industrial quality improvement and the techniques that are associated with it are increasingly being applied in the healthcare sector in both the US and Europe.

During the same period there was also an increasing emphasis on overall organisational approaches to quality improvement, such as total quality management (TQM): a 'set of powerful interventions wrapped in a highly attractive package' (Hackman & Wageman 1995:339). Its attractiveness may have been its apparent simplicity; it offers 'a unified set of principles which can guide managers through the numerous choices [open to them] or might even make choosing unnecessary' (Huczynski 1993:289). Similar claims have been made for other packages of improvement such as business process re-engineering (BPR) (McNulty & Ferlie 2002).

Other techniques that are also described as approaches to quality improvement include six sigma, an improvement approach initially developed by Motorola in 1987. A sigma score represents the amount of variation in a process, and the term 'six sigma' refers to a process that has at least six standard deviations (6σ) between the process mean and the nearest specification limit, that is, a defect rate of 3.4 parts per million. Many argue that six sigma is both a set of improvement tools and an overall philosophy, with the tools 'strikingly similar to prior quality management approaches', although the way in which six sigma is implemented is claimed to 'represent a new organisation structural approach to improvement' (Schroeder et al 2007). The evidence for applying six sigma in healthcare is limited (Sehwail & DeYong 2003) and often methodologically weak with studies based on the assumption that six sigma can be applied in healthcare, rather than whether it is appropriate.

The concepts from lean thinking based on the Toyota Production System (Womack & Jones 1996) have become popular recently in healthcare. Although there are now reviews of its implementation in the public sector (Radnor et al 2006), including health (Kollberg et al 2007), there is as yet little systematic evaluation of its impact.

Pause for reflection

Attempts to improve quality are often instigated because they are the latest 'fashion' or reputed to have a significant impact. Is this an appropriate way to improve quality? What factors need to be taken into account before adopting an approach already tried elsewhere?

Quality improvement in healthcare organisations

In many countries healthcare provision is part of the public sector, and this raises new challenges for quality improvement. Compared with the private sector, public healthcare can be characterised by:

- the range and diversity of stakeholders
- its complex ownership and resourcing arrangements
- the professional autonomy of many of its staff (Pollitt 1993).

Many believe that healthcare systems are 'uniquely complex' (Benneyan et al 2004) but argue that this does not mean that quality improvement approaches are irrelevant (Silvester et al 2004). Indeed, the extent to which knowledge, theories and models from the private sector can be transferred to public sector healthcare organisations is described in the meta-analyses reported by Golembiewski et al (1982) and Robertson & Seneviratne (1995) who show that public and private sector interventions had similar patterns of results, whether positive or negative.

Some argue that everyone in healthcare agrees that quality should be improved – they just differ in their views on how it can be achieved. Øvretveit (1997:221), for instance, believes that 'quality has become a battleground on which professions compete for ownership and definition of quality'. The development of quality improvement as something that involves more than the clinical professions has therefore led to 'the quality movement being equated with a change in power or a bid for power by managers within [European] healthcare systems' (Øvretveit 1997:221). There is some indication now that clinicians are prepared to acknowledge the common issues: 'in matters of quality improvement, healthcare can indeed learn from industry – and perhaps, equally important, industry can also learn from healthcare. The fundamental principles of quality improvement apply to both' (Berwick et al 1990/2002:xiv, 2002 edition).

Non-clinical processes drew early attention when quality improvement was first formalised within healthcare and this has continued, although as Sorensen & Iedema argue in Chapter 1, a focus on clinical processes is vital if healthcare is to improve. Early work on quality improvement showed that healthcare organisations may need a broader definition of quality, and we now know that these must include the whole patient experience – not just clinical outcomes and organisational costs. Systems of measurement and improvement need to focus on outcomes and process, as well as the interaction between the two. The emphasis on process can go too far, as happened with TQM (Shapiro 1996:178) – 'has process taken over purpose?' However, outcomes are not only the result of clinical processes, but may be influenced by organisational processes too.

What about safety?

The issue of errors and patient safety is also important (see Sorensen & Iedema, Chapter 1; Warburton, Chapter 9; and Merry, Chapter 11). The link between quality and safety is not always clear although more recent definitions of quality (refer back to Table 10.1) include 'safety' as one of its key dimensions. Many assert that it is a prerequisite for quality: 'achieving a high level of safety is an essential first step in improving the quality of care overall' (Institute of Medicine & Committee on Quality Healthcare in America 2001:46). A review of patient safety research (Cooper et al 2001:2) concluded that there is 'substantial ambiguity in the definition of patient safety ... the boundary between safety and quality of care is indistinct'. While most interviewees in this study viewed safety as a part of quality, they recognised that there was a tendency to utilise the most fashionable term: 'patient safety has become the issue "du jour" and so almost everything gets redefined in that' (Cooper et al 2001:8). There is a strong argument for regarding patient safety as one aspect of quality improvement and ensuring that learning from other types of quality improvement are also applied when safety is the focus, rather than reinventing the wheel (Walshe & Boaden 2006).

The challenges for organisations

Any organisation wanting to improve quality of care and align its organisational and clinical processes needs to recognise the common underlying principles of approaches to improvement that include (Bendell et al 1995):

- quality is an effect caused by the processes within the organisation that are complex but understandable (Hackman & Wageman 1995)
- focus on the customer (Deming 1986) and their needs
- most human beings engaged in work are intrinsically motivated to try hard and do well
- teamwork is an important ingredient (Ishikawa 1985 – who pioneered the quality circle concept)
- statistical methods should be simple (this is linked with careful data collection and can yield powerful insights into the causes of problems within processes) (Berwick et al 1992)
- the need for appropriate tools and techniques
- management commitment and awareness is essential (Deming 1986).

The common challenges for organisations, including for healthcare organisations, can therefore be summarised as:

- understanding what 'quality' means in the organisation
- focusing on processes – because it is these which determine quality
- identifying customer needs and meeting them
- recognising the role of the people in the organisation, their motivation and how they work together
- using appropriate methods to collect and analyse data
- providing effective leadership and management to support quality improvement.

Each of these challenges is discussed briefly in turn.

Understand what quality means

This is often where the conflict between clinical and managerial priorities is most apparent, especially when performance metrics are associated with tangible aspects of process quality, such as waiting times, rather than patient experience or clinical outcomes. Most commentators agree that quality is a multidimensional concept, encompassing factors such as the effectiveness of care, accessibility, equity and appropriateness of services offered, efficiency of delivery and so on (again, see Table 10.1). At a strategic level, many organisations use a so-called 'balanced scorecard' approach to performance measurement to ensure that overall performance is judged against a set of key indicators (financial, internal process, customer and learning and growth measures), thus enabling a more complete picture of quality to be obtained

(Boaden 2006). However, in practice there is a danger that some sets of performance metrics get prioritised above others, particularly where external inspection and ranking of organisational performance takes place, as is the case, for example, with many national, government-led performance management systems. In these situations what gets measured by external inspection can become the main definer of quality within the organisation, as the example in Box 10.1 illustrates. In this example, the organisation became focused on one set of performance measures at the expense of other important dimensions of quality.

> **Box 10.1** Case study – Balancing clinical and organisational priorities: A case of focusing on performance targets at the expense of quality of care
>
> In the UK National Health Service (NHS), as in many other healthcare systems across the world, explicit performance monitoring and management by central government is now commonplace. NHS organisations are subject to an annual performance rating, determined by a composite measure of a number of key performance indicators, including financial and waiting time targets, alongside broader measures of performance such as staff and patient survey data.
>
> One hospital providing acute services was subject to a special investigation by the external regulator for healthcare standards in England and Wales (the Healthcare Commission) following two outbreaks of clostridium difficile infection, each of which resulted in 19 patient deaths. The investigation report (Healthcare Commission 2006) highlighted the failure of senior managers to prioritise infection control, as illustrated by their decision not to set up isolation facilities for infected patients, despite the advice of infection control specialists. This decision was attributed to the management's concern at the cost of establishing an isolation ward and the knock-on effect this would have on achieving their key performance targets. The investigation team were particularly critical at the time of the second outbreak of infection, that the organisation's leaders failed to learn from the first outbreak and remained focused on other targets at the expense of managing clinical risk. This is reflected in the following remarks made in the official report of the investigation.
>
> *'Following the first major outbreak, the trust's leaders chose to implement some changes but none that might compromise their strategic objectives. They failed to bring the second outbreak quickly under control because they were too focused on the reconfiguration of services and the meeting of the Government's targets, and insufficiently focused on the management of clinical risk. It took the involvement of the Department of Health and national publicity to change their perspective ... The failure of the trust to implement the lessons from the first outbreak, combined with a dysfunctional system for governance which did not incorporate the assessment of risk into its decision making, nor make the board aware of the significance of the outbreaks, meant that it took longer than it should to control the second outbreak. There was a serious failing at the highest levels of the trust to give priority to the management of the second major outbreak. The trust followed neither the advice of its own infection control team nor that of the Health Protection Agency. We are clear that this failing is on the part of the trust and its incorrect interpretation of national priorities. It is our conclusion that the approach taken by the trust compromised the control of infection and hence the safety of patients. This was a significant failing, and we would re-iterate to NHS boards that the safety of patients is not to be compromised under any circumstances.'* (Healthcare Commission 2006:9)

Focus on processes

Taking a process view, it is argued, is one of the key characteristics of organisations that are successful in improvement, along with adopting evidence-based practice, learning collaboratively and being ready and able to change (Plsek 1999). It is not sufficient, however, to focus on anything less than the total process (system) of patient care, when doing so could lead to too much focus on one element at the expense of others. This 'systems thinking' can be described as exploration of 'the properties which exist once the parts [of the system] have been combined into a whole' (Iles & Sutherland 2001:17) and is in some ways simply a combination of processes. Systems thinking has been proposed as a means of understanding medical systems (Nolan 1998) based on the following principles that:

- a system needs a purpose to aid people in managing interdependencies
- the structure of a system significantly determines the performance of the system
- changes in the structure of a system have the potential for generating unintended consequences
- the structure of a system dictates the benefits that accrue to various people working in the system
- the size and scope of a system influence the potential for improvement
- the need for cooperation is a logical extension of interdependencies within systems
- systems must be managed
- improvements in systems must be led.

This process view is therefore not only about changing organisations but also examining and improving the interaction between elements of the organisation, including the individuals who work within them. It can also be seen in the clinical emphasis on systematisation and standardisation, such as pathways and the use of clinical guidelines. Box 10.2 gives an example.

Identify 'customer' needs and meet them

All 'industrial' approaches to quality improvement involve identifying the customer, who may be internal or external to the organisation, and, subsequently, their needs. The purpose of the process has to be clear before improvement can take place. It is in this area that the issue of professionalism and the increasing role of the patient have an impact; while much rhetoric about healthcare systems states that they are patient driven, this does not appear to be the case in practice. Whether the 'customer' can be defined as the patient is open to question but it is clear that to date patient involvement in quality improvement has been limited, and has been noted in regard to the lack of attention to the presence of the patient in processes (Shortell et al 1995a).

Recognise the role of the people in the organisation, their motivation and how they work together

Most perspectives on improvement focus on the motivation and beliefs of individuals in the organisation, which contribute to defining the culture as well as the behaviour that results from them. In one study a participative, flexible, risk-taking culture was strongly associated with the implementation of quality improvement (Shortell et al 1995b). However approaches to culture in the literature are ambiguous. On the one

Box 10.2 Case study – Aligning organisational and clinical processes: Improving cancer services through cross-organisational networks

Cancer services is one area where significant attempts have been made to align clinical and organisational processes, for example, through applying principles of system redesign and the development of patient pathways. One particular methodology that has been used to achieve this is the improvement collaborative approach developed by the Institute of Healthcare Improvement in the US, sometimes referred to as the 'breakthrough' model (Kilo 1998). The breakthrough improvement collaborative methodology derives from continuous quality improvement theories, combined with more general organisational theories of initiating, implementing, monitoring and evaluating change. The improvement collaborative methodology has been adopted by a number of different countries including the US, the UK, Scotland, Sweden, France and Australia, all of whom have applied it to set up national system redesign initiatives for cancer services. In the UK, for example, the National Health Service (NHS) established a Cancer Services Collaborative in 1999. Planned improvements were set out in the NHS Cancer Plan (Department of Health 2000) and an ambitious target was set to reduce the mortality rate from cancer in the under 75 age group by at least 20% by 2010 (against the 1995–2007 deadline).

Starting in 1999, the initiative progressed in three distinct phases, gradually rolling out the improvement methodology across a total of 34 cancer networks. Within each network, the infrastructure for the initiative included a clinical and managerial service improvement lead person, as well as service improvement facilitators whose role was to work with multidisciplinary teams to enable them to review services and introduce service redesign. By March 2003, it was reported that half of the 1600 specialist cancer teams in the UK had been involved in the collaborative. A total of 28,000 changes had been tested (using the PDSA cycle), resulting in at least 2800 improvements for cancer patients across the UK, including improved patient experiences, shorter waiting times and more choice about treatment (NHS Modernisation Agency 2003).

The main evaluation in relation to cancer service collaboratives (Robert et al 2003) shows that, in terms of the impact of the collaborative, the views of staff were positive, especially in relation to changes in attitudes towards improvement, staff empowerment and the provision of time and training opportunities. However, experiences were seen to be highly context specific, with notable variations across and within program sites.

In attempting to explain the variation in findings, the researchers highlight a number of process issues (defined as the key levers for change) that appeared to influence the outcome of the collaborative at a project team level. They also highlight: the importance of these levers for change, alongside a receptive organisational context; the need to review measurement and reporting mechanisms and requirements within the collaborative methodology; a need to build in more preparatory work; and the development of greater local ownership of the collaborative.

Overall, the findings from research highlight that improvement collaboratives are complex, multifaceted interventions: there does not seem to be a single 'right' way of implementing a collaborative; and experiences and outcomes vary considerably both across and within organisations. Of particular importance seems to be an ability to get the right balance between top-down initiation and leadership of the collaborative and bottom-up ownership and commitment to the collaborative process.

hand, some authors describe a 'quality culture' as one 'whereby everyone in the organisation shares a commitment to continuous improvement aimed at customer satisfaction' (Wilkinson & Brown 2003:184). Others believe that culture cannot be 'managed' (Schein 1985) despite many policy innovations intended to achieve exactly this.

However, the 'people' implications are broader than organisational culture, relating to individual employment arrangements, and need to take into account both individuals and systems and the way they interact (see Stanton, Chapter 3). In particular, professional motivation is important in improving quality, and organisations would do well to review the lessons already learnt 'the hard way' by many others in different sectors who have attempted to improve process and outcome quality.

Use appropriate methods to collect and analyse data

This involves identifying the key characteristics of the process in terms of variation and flow raised in Chapter 4 by Claridge and Cook:

- *Variation* within a process is inherent, and it is argued that understanding and analysing the variation are keys to success in improvement (Snee 1990). This is especially true in healthcare (Haraden & Resar 2004) in terms of clinical (patient), flow and professional variability. Patient variability is 'random' and cannot be eliminated or reduced, but must be managed, whereas non-random variability should be eliminated. It is argued that 'it is variation ... that causes most of the flow problems in our hospital systems' (Institute for Healthcare Improvement 2003:6). Consideration of variation leads to a clear requirement for data about the process that can then be used to measure the key aspects of its performance, one of which will be variation.
- *Flow* and managing the flow of patients through a process is similarly important, and can to some extent draw on approaches widely used in manufacturing (Brideau 2004). Understanding and evaluating flow requires more detailed understanding of demand and capacity than has often been the case in healthcare organisations (Horton 2004). Many performance metrics for healthcare systems have focused on flow through the use of proxy measures such as waiting times. Zimmerman (2004) proposes that studying and improving flow leads to a need to consider alignment – within the whole healthcare system, within pre-hospital care, and of goals within the system, especially those of both managers and clinicians. This will inevitably lead to whole-systems approaches to improvement.

Provide effective leadership and management to support quality improvement

The involvement of top management, use of teamwork and the ability to foster innovation were shown to be important in quality improvement (Parker et al 1999). In fact, quality improvement can be seen to be dependent on leaders, both in relation to clarifying the overall mission and strategy and creating a commitment to change (Berwick et al 1990/2002). Leaders have a key role to play in planning for quality, creating the right cultural conditions and setting organisational structures that empower staff to become actively involved in improvement (Juran 1989). These views are supported by research undertaken by Stanton et al reported in Chapter 3.

Conclusion

The contingency approach to improvement and organisational change argues that there is no one 'best way' of changing organisations: 'different organizations face different situations and therefore must vary their change strategies accordingly' (Burnes

> **Box 10.3** Implications for practice – Organising for quality
>
> Attempts to improve quality often fail to address clearly how quality is defined before starting to change organisations and processes. *It is important to explore what is meant by 'quality' before attempting to improve it* – but care must also be taken to ensure that this step does not take too long.
>
> It is clear that whatever approach is taken to improve quality, *the identification of the process is a vital first step.* This chapter shows clearly that processes will have both clinical and organisational elements and should not be separated but integrated. Clinical processes in particular must take account of the organisational resources necessary for them to function effectively. However organisational processes must also recognise the clinical decisions that are necessary as patients go through the process.
>
> *It must not be assumed that an individual patient is the only 'customer'* where healthcare is provided within the public sector; this is an over-simplistic approach. Other important 'customers' include those who commission healthcare, as well as the wider public and perhaps those with political interests.
>
> Quality will only improve where the behaviour of individuals within the system changes and this has to date often been ignored or underplayed in quality improvement efforts. *Understanding what motivates the individuals within the healthcare system, especially those with a clinical professional background, is vital.*
>
> *Data about performance and quality is needed* – it should be appropriate and enable improvement action. Improvement based on gut feelings about what is wrong is not likely to be effective or sustainable.
>
> *Organisations and whole health systems need to be effectively led and staff empowered to improve quality.* Quality will not improve throughout the system when the actions or words of those at the top do not support quality improvement. The relationship between quality and cost is something about which great care should be taken since cost reduction is often interpreted as implying deterioration in quality.

1996:11). This undoubtedly applies to quality improvement and although the underlying principles may be true for all organisations, selecting which elements of quality improvement approaches to use requires a level of understanding that is not always apparent. 'If you understand the theory behind the tools and realities of your own situation, you will then have a better chance of understanding the appropriate techniques and of knowing how to tailor them to the unique needs and opportunities facing your company' (Shapiro 1996:xiv).

Given the variety of perspectives on quality improvement, especially those from an organisation/process perspective and those developed by professionals, there are challenges for all to address if improvement efforts are to achieve their maximum potential. At a general level, quality improvement needs to be demystified: 'much of it is common sense, accessible to all and not the preserve of a few. The tendency for each new quality improvement theory to generate its own jargon and esoteric knowledge must be resisted' (Locock 2003:56). Healthcare professionals need to recognise their role and responsibility to the wider system, including in healthcare, particularly 'the need to balance clinical autonomy with transparent accountability, to support the systematization of clinical work' (Degeling et al 2003:649). Equally, managers need to recognise the limits of their authority in improvement, for instance, 'There is no evidence at all to support the view that managers … alone could produce an intervention strategy that would generate active participation from clinicians in processes of innovation adoption' (Dopson & Fitzgerald 2005:216).

In the continually changing world of healthcare, quality will always be important. Managers and clinicians need to work together to address priority area for process improvement within a whole systems approach, underpinned by an organisational culture that promotes collaboration, information sharing and collective learning.

References

Bendell T, Penson R, Carr S 1995 The quality gurus – their approaches described and considered. Managing Service Quality 5(6):44–48

Benneyan J C, Lloyd R C, Plsek P E 2004 Statistical process control as a tool for research and healthcare improvement. In: Grol R B R, Moss F (eds) Quality Improvement Research. BMJ Books, London, p 184–202

Berwick D 1989 Continuous Improvement as an Ideal in Healthcare. New England Journal of Medicine 320:53–56

Berwick D 1992 Heal thyself or heal thy system: can doctors help to improve medical care? Quality in Healthcare 1(Supplement):S2–S8

Berwick D, Endhoven A, Bunker J P 1992 Quality Management in the NHS: the doctor's role. BMJ 304:235–239, 304–308

Berwick D, Godfrey A B, Roessner J 1990/2002 Curing Healthcare (paperback edition July 2002 ed). Jossey-Bass, San Francisco

Boaden R, 2006 The Quality Management Contribution to Patient Safety. In: Walshe K, Boaden R (eds) Patient Safety Research into Practice. McGraw Hill/Open University Press, Maidenhead

Brideau L P 2004 Flow: Why Does It Matter? Frontiers of Health Services Management 20 (4):247–50

Burnes B 1996 No such thing as … a 'one best way' to manage organizational change. Management Decision 34(10):11–18

Codman E A 1916 A Study in Hospital Efficiency: The first five years. Thomas Todd Co, Boston

Cooper J B, Sorensen A V, Anderson S M et al 2001 Current Research on Patient Safety in the United States. National Patient Safety Foundation, Chicago

Crosby P 1979 Quality is Free. McGraw Hill, New York

Degeling P, Maxwell S, Kennedy J et al 2003 Medicine, management, and modernisation: a 'danse macabre'? BMJ 326 (7390):649–652

Deming W E 1986 Out of the Crisis. Centre of Advanced Engineering Study, MIT, Cambridge

Department of Health 1989 Working for Patients: Medical Audit (Working Paper No.6). HMSO, London

Department of Health 2000 The NHS Cancer Plan. A plan for investment, a plan for reform. HMSO, London

Donabedian A 1966 Evaluating the quality of medical care. Milbank Memorial Fund Quarterly 44(3, Part 2):166–206

Donabedian A 1987 Commentary on some studies of the quality of care. Health Care Financing Review, Annual Supplement:75–85

Dopson S, Fitzgerald L (eds) 2005 Knowledge to Action? Oxford University Press, Oxford

Duff L A, Kitson A L, Seers K et al 1996 Clinical Guidelines: an introduction to their development and implementation. Journal of Advanced Nursing 23:887–895

Feigenbaum A 1961 Total Quality Control (1st edition). McGraw-Hill, New York

Golembiewski R, Proehl C, Sink D 1982 Estimating success of OD applications. Training and Development Journal 72:86–95

Grimshaw J M, Thomas R E, Maclennan G et al 2004 Effectiveness and efficiency of guidelines dissemination and implementation strategies. Health Technology Assessment 8(6)

Groonroos C 1984 Strategic Management and Marketing in the Service Sector. Chartwell-Bratt, London

Hackman J R, Wageman R 1995 Total quality management: Empirical, conceptual and practical issues. Administrative Science Quarterly 40(2):309–342

Haraden C, Resar R 2004 Patient Flow in Hospitals: Understanding and Controlling It Better. Frontiers of Health Services Management 20(4):3–15

Harvey G 1996 Quality in Healthcare: Traditions, influences and future directions. International Journal for Quality in Healthcare 8(4):341–350

Healthcare Commission 2006 Investigation into outbreaks of Clostridium difficile at Stoke Mandeville Hospital, Buckinghamshire Hospitals NHS Trust. Commission for Healthcare Audit and Inspection, London

Horton S 2004 Increasing Capacity While Improving the Bottom Line. Frontiers of Health Services Management 20(4):17–23

Huczynski A 1993 Management Gurus. Routledge, London

Iles V, Sutherland K 2001 Organisational Change: a review for healthcare managers, professionals and researchers. National Co-ordinating Centre for NHS Service Delivery and Organisation R&D, London

Institute for Healthcare Improvement 2003 Optimizing Patient Flow: Moving Patients Smoothly Through Acute Care Settings. Institute for Health Improvement, Boston

Institute of Medicine, Committee on Quality Healthcare in America 2001 Crossing the Quality Chasm. Institute of Medicine, Washington DC

Ishikawa K 1985 What is total quality control: The Japanese way. Prentice-Hall, Englewood Cliffs

Juran J (ed) 1951 The Quality Control Handbook (4th ed). Mc-Graw Hill, New York

Juran J 1989 Juran on Leadership for Quality. Free Press, New York

Kennedy I 2001 Learning from Bristol: the report of the public enquiry into children's heart surgery at the Bristol Royal Infirmary, 1984–1995. Command Paper cm 5207, London

Kilo C M 1998 A framework for collaborative improvement: Lessons learned from the Institute of Healthcare Improvement's Breakthrough Series. Quality Management in Healthcare 6(4):1–13

Kolesar P J 1993 The relevance of research on statistical process control to the total quality movement. Journal of Engineering and Technology Management 10(4):317–338

Kollberg B, Dahlgaard J, Brehmer P 2007 Measuring Lean Thinking Initiatives in Healthcare Services: issues and findings. International Journal of Productivity and Performance Management 56(1):7–24

Langley G J, Nolan K M, Nolan T W et al 1996 The Improvement Guide. Jossey-Bass, San Francisco

Locock L 2003 Healthcare redesign: meaning, origins and application. Quality and Safety in Healthcare 12(1):53–58

Lugon M, Secker-Walker J (eds) 1999 Clinical Governance: making it happen. Royal Society of Medicine Press, London

Maxwell R 1984 Quality Assesment in Health. BHJ 288:1470–1472

McCormack B, Manley K, Garbett R (eds) 2004 Practice Development in Nursing. Blackwell Publishing, Oxford

McNulty T, Ferlie E 2002 Reengineering Healthcare: the complexities of organisational transformation. Oxford University Press, Oxford

Middleton S, Barnett J, Reeves D 2001 What is an Integrated Care Pathway? What is...? 3(3):1–8

Morrell C, Harvey G, Kitson A L 1997 Practitioner based quality improvement: a review of the Royal College of Nursing's Dynamic Standards Setting System. Quality in Healthcare 6 (1):29–34

NHS Modernisation Agency 2003 Cancer Services Collaborative Improvement Partnership: A Quick Guide, Vol 2004

Nolan T W 1998 Understanding Medical Systems. Annals of Internal Medicine 128 (4):293–298

Øvretveit J 1997 A comparison of hospital quality programmes: lessons for other services. International Journal of Service Industry Management 8(3):220–235

Parker V A, Wubbenhorst W, Young G et al 1999 Implementing quality improvement in hospitals: the role of leadership and culture. Am J Med Qual 14(1):64–69

Plsek P 1999 Quality Improvement Methods in Clinical Medicine. Pediatrics 103(1):203–214

Pollitt C 1993 The struggle for quality: the case of the NHS. Policy and Politics 21(3):161–170

Radnor Z, Walley P, Stephens A et al 2006 Evaluation of the Lean Approach to Business Management and its Use in the Public Sector. Scottish Executive, Office of Chief Researcher, Edinburgh

Robert G, McLeod H, Ham C 2003 Modernising Cancer Services: an evaluation of phase I of the Cancer Services Collaborative, Research report number 43. University of Birmingham: Health Services Management Centre, Birmingham

Robertson P J, Seneviratne S J 1995 Outcomes of planned organisational change in the public sector: a meta analytic comparison to the private sector. Public Administration Review 552(6):547–558

Schein E H 1985 Organisational Culture and Leadership. Jossey-Bass, Oxford

Schroeder R G, Linderman K, Liedtke C et al 2007 Six Sigma: Definition and underlying theory. Journal of Operations Management, doi:10.1016/j.jom 2007.06.007

Sehwail L, DeYong C 2003 Six sigma in healthcare. International Journal of Healthcare Quality Assurance 16 (4):i–v

Shapiro E 1996 Fad Surfing in the Boardroom. Capstone Publishing, Oxford

Shaw C D 1980 Aspects of Audit. BMJ 280:1256–1258

Shewhart W A 1931 Economic control of quality of manufactured product. Van Nostrand, New York

Shortell S, Levin D, O'Brien J et al 1995a Assessing the evidence on CQI: is the glass half empty or half full? Journal of the Foundation of the American College of Healthcare Executives 40 (1):4–24

Shortell S M, O'Brien J L, Carman J M et al 1995b Assessing the Impact of Continuous Quality Improvement/Total Quality Management: Concept versus Implementation. Health Services Research 30 (2):377–401

Silvester K, Lendon R, Bevan H et al 2004 Reducing waiting times in the NHS: is lack of capacity the problem? Clinician in Management 12(3):105–111

Snee R D 1990 Statistical Thinking and Its Contribution to Total Quality. American Statistician 44(2):116–121

Thor J, Lundberg J, Ask J et al 2007 Application of statistical process control in healthcare improvement: systematic review. Qual Saf Healthcare 16:387–399

Walshe K, Boaden R (eds) 2006 Patient Safety: Research into Practice. Mc-Graw Hill/Open University Press, Maidenhead

Wilkinson A J, Brown A 2003 Managing Human Resources for Quality Management. In: Dale B G (ed) Managing Quality. Blackwell, Oxford, p 177–202

Womack J P, Jones D T 1996 Lean Thinking. Simon and Schuster, London

Zimmerman R S 2004 Hospital Capacity, Productivity and Patient Safety – It all flows together. Frontiers of Health Services Management 20(4):33–38

Chapter 11

Managing risks to patient safety in clinical units

Alan Merry

Introduction

Unintended harm to patients from failures in healthcare is now recognised as a public health problem of considerable importance (see Sorensen & Iedema, Chapter 1). There is more at stake than the possibility of direct harm to patients. There are a number of dimensions of quality in healthcare and risk that may manifest at different organisational layers within the system (see Figure 11.1).

A balance must be found between investing in safety and the need to provide as much healthcare to as many patients as possible. An undue emphasis on safety by individual practitioners may lead to delays in treatment, increase the burden of illness experienced by patients on waiting lists, and in some cases reduce the effectiveness of the delayed therapy (because the benefit of some treatments depends on the timeliness with which they are provided). Redundancy (in the form of extra checks, extra staff, reserve power supplies, reserve equipment and so on) is an important way of promoting safety, but may also be seen as reducing efficiency. It may be difficult to work out the optimal balance between these conflicting considerations.

There may also be conflicts between risks for staff and the organisation and risks for individual patients – sometimes staff may feel that their own safety is best served by inactivity (declining to take on a difficult surgical case for example) or excessive activity (over-investigation of a patient before anaesthesia for example) in situations where some pragmatic middle course would be in the patient's best interests.

Managing risks to patient safety in clinical units depends on interdisciplinary teamwork and on a cultural commitment to quality (which includes safety). In this chapter I will discuss critical aspects of effective risk management that include:

- understanding risk and the ways in which it can be measured
- appreciating the legal implications of risk

- understanding errors and violations and how these may occur in complex systems
- proactively identifying risks within one's own unit
- actively reducing risk to acceptable levels without unduly impeding service delivery
- responding effectively when patients are harmed by healthcare.

Figure 11.1 The dimensions of quality and organisational layers of healthcare

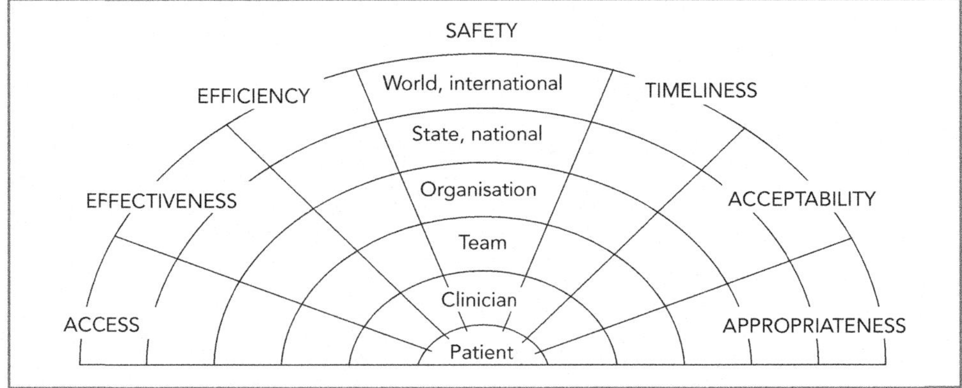

(Source: reproduced with permission from Runciman et al 2007)

Understanding risk

Many individuals find it difficult to evaluate the risk of infrequent events. People do not tend to use Bayesian logic when making decisions. Instead, they tend to be influenced by the nature of the hazard, their own personal experiences, social norms, and many other factors whose relevance may be more personal than logical. Marked fear of snakes or spiders is quite common, and generally out of proportion with any real hazard created by these animals. Furthermore, people who fear one do not necessarily worry about the other. Complacency about the substantial risks of smoking is common, but goes hand in hand with public expectations for the government to spend extraordinary amounts of money to further reduce the already infinitesimal risk of viral transmission through donated blood.

Expressing the risks of a particular procedure

From a clinical perspective, interest is typically in the risks of specific procedures. Published data tend to come from high-volume units, often from academic institutions, and often represent the best attainable results rather than the average. The actual risk of a procedure in the hands of one practitioner or one team may be quite difficult to establish because of the high numbers required to estimate the incidence of given adverse events with reasonable confidence limits. It is not often appreciated that (as a rule of thumb) a zero incidence of an event in x procedures could be associated with an upper 95% confidence limit of one event in $x \div 3$ procedures. Thus no adverse events in 10 procedures could be compatible with a true rate of 33%, and simply reflect a run of good luck. Conversely, one or two adverse events in a short series of procedures might be associated with surprisingly low true incidence. For example, two adverse events in 20 cases would give a point estimate of risk as 10% but with 95% confidence limits of 1% and 32%. Twenty events in 200 cases would give 10% (6%, 15%), and 200 in 2000 would give 10% (9%, 11%) – with all estimates rounded to the nearest integer.

Some ways of expressing the difference between two risks

Risk can be expressed in a number of ways. The most common expressions are 'relative risk' and 'absolute risk', the 'odds ratio', 'numbers needed to treat' (NNT) and 'numbers needed to harm' (NNH) set out in Table 11.1.

Table 11.1 Expressing risk in healthcare

Expression of risk	Discussion and example
The risk of an event	The rate at which the event occurs, e.g. 10 events per 1000 exposures would be a 10% risk rate.
The odds	The number of patients having the event compared with those not having it, i.e. using the above example, the odds ratio is 10:90, or 1:9.
Relative risk and odds ratio	The extent to which a treatment reduces the likelihood that an event will occur. For example, if a treatment reduces the occurrence of a particular event from 0.5% to 0.25%, the relative risk is 50%. The odds of the event without the intervention are 1:199 and with it 1:399. The *odds ratio* is therefore 1/399 ÷ 1/199. This is very nearly the same as the relative risk reduction. When the risks are higher, however, the difference between these two measures becomes greater. For example, reducing a risk of 50% to 25% also gives a relative risk of 50%, but the odds are 1:1 and 1:3 so the odds ratio in this case is 1/3 ÷ 1/1, that is 33%.
Absolute risk reduction	The difference between having a treatment and not having it. In our first example, the reduction in absolute risk is 0.25%, but in the second it is 25%. This expression perhaps describes the true benefit of each intervention or treatment more realistically than does relative risk.
Number needed to treat	The number of patients who need to be treated before a beneficial outcome occurs in one person. In the first example above, the NNT would be 400.
Number needed to harm	The number of patients who need to be treated before an episode of harm occurs in one person.

The importance of exposure

An attempt is often made to compare risks of a medical procedure with those of a common every day activity. For example, anaesthetists often say that the risk of an anaesthetic is comparable with that of driving a car in traffic. This sounds plausible because the lifetime possibility of dying from one or the other event may be similar. However, for most people exposure to traffic is much greater than exposure to anaesthesia. It is important, therefore, to relate risk to exposure. The risk of undergoing anaesthesia in a developed country has been estimated as 1000 deaths per 100 million hours of exposure, while that of being in traffic (in any capacity) is only 50 deaths per 100 million hours of exposure. Interestingly, in relation to time of exposure, flying in a commercial aircraft is more dangerous than being in traffic, with a risk of 100 deaths per 100 million hours of exposure. Note that the way in which exposure is defined can make a difference here: if distance travelled were used as the denominator, then flying would be safer than driving a car (Runciman et al 2007).

The importance of underlying risk

The value of an initiative to reduce risk is dependent on the underlying rate of the adverse event in question. For example, a treatment that could reduce the risk of coronary artery disease by 10% would have no value if given to children, because they hardly ever get coronary artery disease. It is possible to stratify adults according to their risks of coronary disease, and it makes sense to invest in those groups at highest risk. A 10% reduction in this risk would give an absolute risk reduction of 0.1% if the underlying rate of the disease was 1%, and of 2% if the underlying rate was 20%.

Refining the concept of harm

One point often missed about studies like the Harvard Medical Practice Study (Brennan et al 1991) is that many of the deaths identified in these studies occurred in very sick patients who did not have long to live anyway (Hayward & Hofer 2001), and therefore, although not acceptable, they are not quite comparable with most deaths caused by road traffic accidents.

In addition to mortality rates, it might help to define the burden of iatrogenic harm in order to measure the quality adjusted life years (QALYs) (Murray & Lopez 1996) lost in this way, although there are limitations to the value of these indicators as well (La Puma & Lawlor 1990).

The importance of balancing loss against gain

Another limitation is the uni-dimensional nature of the results of these studies. Very little attempt has been made to balance the burden of adverse events from admissions to acute care institutions with the reduction in the burden of disease associated with the same admissions. When quantifying risk, some measure of accomplishment is useful to place into context the data on harm.

Process in healthcare – in pursuit of six sigma quality

Many medical activities are relatively straightforward, and it should be possible to achieve reliability levels equivalent to those now expected as normal in certain industries. The concept of 'six sigma quality' involves expressing the reliability of a given process in terms of standard deviations from the mean of a normal distribution. In effect, six sigma quality implies 3.4 failures per million events (procedures undertaken, or products produced). This level of reliability is expected in many industrial and manufacturing processes today, but if all adverse events are considered (not just deaths), it is not often achieved in healthcare, if ever. For routine processes this is no longer acceptable. It is time to clearly identify aspects of healthcare that lend themselves to process management, and adopt an approach for these that is process oriented, standardised, and strictly compliant with clearly defined and monitored guidelines.

On the other hand, it must also be recognised that not all aspects of healthcare lend themselves to the methods of industry. In general, diagnosis tends to be more demanding and depends more on experience and judgment than procedural work. Patients do not usually present with diagnoses emblazoned on their foreheads. A systematic and standardised approach will no doubt improve the likelihood of a correct diagnosis, but not all patients present in accordance with the textbooks. Even after a correct diagnosis has been made, there are many conditions for which the question of what to do next remains controversial. It is not easy to allow for uncertainty of this type when measuring the quality of healthcare.

Many procedural activities also involve considerable variation from case to case, and extend skilled practitioners to the limits of their ability. Performing a triple heart valve replacement in a 78-year-old patient is a very different proposition from replacing a single valve in a 40-year-old, for example. As another example, in major trauma each patient presents a unique combination of problems and requires sustained and creative effort from a large number of people working in unison. An activity of this sort is more like trying to win the World Cup in Rugby than like managing an industrial process.

Casemix and risk scores

Units that regularly undertake more complex and acute cases are likely to have more adverse events than those that concentrate on the routine and the straightforward. Some measure of differences in casemix is needed to take this variation into account. Various scoring systems have been adopted for this purpose – the EuroSCORE for cardiac surgery being one example (Nashef et al 2002) and the Goldman Index of cardiac risk for patients undergoing non-cardiac surgical procedures being another (Goldman et al 1977). Scores of this type are generated using regression analysis of information collected in large databases, and then validated by testing in other populations. They tend to become dated quite quickly as methods of managing medical conditions advance, and may not be reliable if applied to patient populations different from the ones in which they were developed.

Measuring performance over time

It is important to know not only whether a team or individual's rate of adverse events is comparable with benchmark statistics, but also whether it is stable. Most time series of biological data exhibit variation, which can be of two types. *Common cause variation* may be thought of as 'noise'. Thus a unit might have an infection rate that fluctuates by ± 2% around a mean of 5%. Fluctuation of this type usually reflects random variation from day to day, and the underlying rate may be stable from one year to the next. On the other hand, something may change. Some failure in process or alteration in resistance of microbes might lead to a jump to (say) 7% ± 2%, or some initiative to improve sterile procedures or the timely administration of antibiotics might lead to a fall to 3% ± 2%. The challenge is to detect *special cause variation* of this type in a reliable way. This is particularly important in relation to monitoring the effect of interventions to promote safety. Not only may such interventions fail to achieve their aim, they may even make matters worse (through so called 'revenge effects' (Tenner 1997)).

Simply comparing rates at two time periods may be misleading, in the absence of information about the long-term stability of the process in question. There are a number of better ways to distinguish special cause from common cause variation over time. Cumulative sum (cusum) charts (Bolsin & Colson 2000) and control charts (Carey 2002a, 2002b) are two examples. The data for these charts may or may not be adjusted for risk. One method of using risk-adjusted data to monitor the ongoing performance of an individual or a unit is the variable life-adjusted display (VLAD) chart. It is sometimes used in cardiac surgery, where it is possible to calculate an expected survival rate using scoring systems and each patient's known risk factors. Outcomes (death or survival) can be plotted against numbers of cases operated on. If a particular patient has an expected survival probability of 0.9 (or 90%) and survives, the plot is moved one unit along the X-axis and 0.1 along the Y-axis in a positive direction. If such a patient dies, the plot is moved one unit along the X-axis and 0.9 units along the Y-axis in a negative direction. At the end of 10 cases, if as expected one dies and nine survive, the plot will have moved 10 points along the X-axis and will be at zero on the Y-axis. Statistical limits can be set to identify points at which it becomes likely that one is dealing with special cause variation rather than common cause. VLAD charts have much to offer in relation to procedural work where high levels of standardisation are possible, and where clearly definable adverse outcomes (such as death) are relatively common. A Microsoft Excel spreadsheet for creating VLAD charts on the basis of the logistic EuroSCORE can be downloaded from The Clinical Operational Research Unit at University College, London.[14]

Defining acceptable standards

A point often missed in relation to any of these methods is that results are inevitably defined as acceptable in relation to the norms for a particular group. It is important to understand certain implications of this approach. In any one clinical unit it is a statistical inevitability that one practitioner will get the best results and another will get the worst. If one had 10 surgeons, evaluated results and fired the worse performer in the name of quality improvement, one would simply have reduced the group to nine, with a different surgeon in the bottom place. In the same way, demands that all practitioners should be better than average are statistical nonsense. Some adequately performing clinicians must, by definition, be operating below the average, and there is no possible way of changing this fact.

> **Pause for reflection**
>
> Some healthcare professionals are 'insiders' and in the privileged position of knowing the results of their colleagues. Would such a person elect to undergo cardiac surgery from the member of the unit who has the worst outcome data? Would the decision to choose the surgeon with the best results be (a) rational and (b) ethical?

This discussion is not trite, because no patient, if asked, would say he or she wanted to be operated on by a surgeon whose results were 'below average', let alone the worst surgeon in a group. However, in a clinical unit, all surgeons have to contribute to the work.

Yet another difficulty is that the clinical situations that lend themselves to an analysis of this type are very much in the minority. Is it equitable that many cardiac surgeons today are required to have their results publicly scrutinised while their colleagues in general medicine, psychiatry and geriatrics are not? Actually, even their anaesthetic colleagues tend to be left out of this process, notwithstanding evidence that the anaesthetist may contribute to outcome after cardiac surgery (Merry et al 1992). It could be argued that there is merit in applying sound methods or monitoring performance where possible, and in working towards improving the situation where it is not. Alternatively it could be argued that the inequitable application of harsh standards to isolated groups is likely to do little more than promote gaming. For example, risk scores are known to be inaccurate at the extremes, so in practice patient selection will probably influence the results of a VLAD chart even though this should not happen in theory.

Two more points are relevant to this debate. Statistics apply to groups rather than individuals. A risk of 10% means that 10 of the next 100 patients are likely to die, but for each patient the result will be unpredictable, and will be either life or death (not

---

[14] http://www.ucl.ac.uk/operational-research/downloads/VLADdownload2

10% death). Morbidity is also important – in the example of cardiac surgery the risk of stroke is significant, may differ from the risk of death, and may be more feared by patients, but strokes are seldom incorporated into risk scores or monitored with VLAD charts. Also the management of patients goes beyond procedural results, and includes decision making in the first place, and then the whole amalgam of interpersonal skills, compassion and professionalism that might be very important to individual patients. Thus it can be seen again that the use of a uni-dimensional measurement such as a mortality rate is inadequate as a means of measuring performance in an endeavour as complex as healthcare.

Where databases are large, and many individuals contribute to the data, a normative approach based on reasonable outcome measures is fairly satisfactory, but its limitations should not be forgotten. In most cases the difference in outcome between the best and worst clinician in a unit should be small. Any difference will become statistically significant if very large numbers of data are available for analysis, but ideally the difference between individuals within one unit should not be clinically important. In fact the point is not whether one is the best or worst performing individual available to a patient, but whether one's performance is good enough. The same thing can be said of units (see Box 11.1)

Box 11.1 The Bristol Enquiry (Kennedy 2001)

At the paediatric cardiac unit of the Bristol Royal Infirmary 29 children died and four were left brain damaged following open heart surgery between 1984 and 1995. This was twice the expected mortality rate. A major inquiry was undertaken, and 198 recommendations were made, which led to many reforms in medical practice in the UK, including the establishment of more rigorous requirements for monitoring the results of surgery.

It can be seen that there may be clinical units in which the important question is not which surgeon is the best on the team, but rather whether the team as a whole is functioning to a standard that is acceptable at all.

The importance of the team

Many of the difficulties associated with monitoring performance become less marked if the emphasis is placed on the team rather than on the individuals within it. This approach still depends on making sure that all individuals are performing adequately, but it is more likely to be associated with standardisation, the universal adoption of evidence-based approaches, teamwork and supportiveness, and better outcomes for all patients.

Given the large numbers of units across the world, there is no reason why one's own unit should not aspire to being better than average. If all units worked hard to achieve that goal, the average standard overall would improve (even if the number below average remained obdurately at 50%!).

Legal implications of risk in healthcare

Increasingly, risk management is being driven by legislative requirements. Some of the legal pressures are proactive – explicit demands for accreditation for example. Others are reactive – litigation in response to patient harm for example. In most countries today legal considerations weigh heavily when decisions have to be made about how much of a limited resource should be invested into risk management.

Accreditation

Accreditation is a formal process for demonstrating that an organisation complies with certain standards. The degree to which accreditation of healthcare is compulsory varies from country to country and so does the process by which it is achieved. In the US the Joint Commission on Accreditation of Healthcare Organizations (JCAHO) provides accreditation required to obtain reimbursement from Medicare and Medicaid (healthcare funding for the elderly and poor respectively). In Australia and New Zealand there is a trend towards greater emphasis on accreditation. For example, the Australian Commission on Safety and Quality in Healthcare developed a national standard for credentialling and defining the scope of clinical practice in 2004, and this has formed the basis for initiatives by state governments such as introducing a policy for the credentialling of senior doctors appointed to public health services in Victoria.[15]

Compliance with standards can be assessed by considering structure, process or outcome (Donabedian 2003). In theory, if it were possible to measure relevant outcomes adequately, there would be little need to measure anything else, but in practice this may be much more difficult than establishing that the required buildings, equipment and personnel are in place (i.e. that the structure of the organisation is adequate) and that the right protocols, clinical pathways and other process tools have been established and are in use.

Tort

In many countries there has been a substantial increase in the cost of litigation related to healthcare during the second half of the last century, and in the UK, US and Australia the costs of the tort system now amount to 1% of expenditure on healthcare (Runciman et al 2007). In New Zealand a no-fault system of accident compensation was established following the 1967 Sir Owen Wodehouse report, and it is essentially unknown for doctors to be sued for negligence (Merry & McCall Smith 2001). Today the Accident Compensation Corporation is responsible for promoting safety within the healthcare system proactively and for compensating patients after they have been harmed. The tort system tends to be slow, inefficient and somewhat capricious in the degree to which it achieves any worthwhile outcomes for patients, healthcare professionals or the system as a whole. From first principles the New Zealand approach appears to be more effective, and it is popular with New Zealanders. Individual practitioners are still held to account through the investigations of the Health and Disability Commissioner and through disciplinary actions by the Medical Council, but on the whole, organisations are less at risk from the repercussions of harming patients than they would be if lawsuits were still possible. It is hard to obtain data on the relative effectiveness of these different systems in promoting safety, but it is at least possible that the loss of the tort system from New Zealand has removed one incentive for hospital administrators to invest in safety initiatives.

Criminal law

It ought to go without saying that the role of criminal law in healthcare is to deal with seriously culpable behaviour (Merry & McCall Smith 2001). Unfortunately, in New Zealand in the 1990s, and more recently in the UK, there has been a tendency to respond to tragic accidents that have resulted in the deaths of patients by charging healthcare

---

[15] www.health.vic.gov.au/credentialling

176

professionals with manslaughter. In many cases the level of negligence involved has been minimal (Ferner & McDowell 2006) and only a minority of the charges have been successfully prosecuted, but the impact on all concerned has been very substantial. This topic has been discussed in greater depth elsewhere (Merry 2007).

Whose risk should we manage?

One of the difficulties with legal responses that focus on punishing individual practitioners, and even with those in which the primary aim is to provide compensation for patients, is that they do little to promote safety at an organisational level. In fact, the motivation for many so-called safety initiatives is the protection of administrators, clinical leaders and individual practitioners. This is particularly true of some policies instituted in the name of safety or quality (see Box 11.2).

Box 11.2 Policies to protect administrators

Recently in New Zealand a consultant practitioner was found in breach of the Code of Patient Rights because he did not obtain consent from a patient for a trainee doctor to be present (simply as an observer) during a bedside consultation. In reaching this judgment it was considered relevant that the hospital had a policy that specified the need to obtain informed consent for all teaching activities. It was therefore held that the hospital administrators had discharged their responsibilities and that the blame lay fairly with the practitioner for failing to follow the policy.

A meeting was subsequently held to discuss the wider implications of obtaining informed consent in a major teaching hospital in New Zealand (not necessarily the same one). It became apparent that there are many circumstances in which it is very difficult to obtain informed consent simply in order for a trainee (a medical or nursing student, or a junior doctor) to be present as an observer. For example, anaesthetised patients in the operating room, babies in a paediatric unit, unconscious patients admitted to an emergency department, and patients on ventilators in intensive care units are all in a different position from that of an alert and competent patient who can easily be asked if it is acceptable for a student to be present. It is perhaps not impossible to obtain consent from some other appropriate person in each of these situations, but it may be difficult and very time consuming to do so, and there are wider implications of proxy consent that might also need to be considered.

Given that staff are required by the hospital to teach students and juniors it was accepted, even by senior managers present at the meeting, that the policy about informed consent for this activity was effectively impossible to implement as it stood, and served primarily to protect management rather than to promote proper practice. It was decided to implement a new policy that would include a blanket approach to obtaining informed consent for basic educational activities at the time of admission. Even this would be only partially satisfactory, and there may still be situations in which staff might find it difficult to marry the requirements to teach future generations of health professionals with the need to obtain meaningful consent to do so, but at least some of these difficulties have now been made more explicit.

Legislating for safety

The well-known series of disasters in British hospitals involving the inadvertent injection of the anti-cancer drug vincristine into the spinal fluid instead of the blood stream is illustrative of the failure of a harsh legal response to improve safety (Merry in press). Criminal charges against junior doctors involved in these tragic mistakes have not been effective in promoting safer practice. Instead, the elements have been left in place for the same mistake to happen again and again (over 14 times so far) in different institutions and with different casts of players. This is not surprising, because junior doctors have very little if any ability to improve the system.

James Reason (2004) made the following comment about these disasters.

> When a similar set of conditions repeatedly provokes the same kind of error in different people, it is clear that we are dealing with an error prone situation rather than with error prone, careless, or incompetent individuals.

> (Reason 2004:ii29)

This implies that the key to managing risk of this sort lies in moving the focus from the individual to the process of care. This depends on engaging those who are able to influence these processes. One of the interesting aspects of the equally well-known events at Bristol Royal Infirmary in relation to paediatric cardiac surgery (see Box 11.1) was the fact that a senior administrator was among those held accountable for the failures in this service. This was facilitated by his being a registered medical practitioner. In many systems hospitals are administered by generic, lay managers and it is not always obvious how these people could be held to account for failures to ensure the safety of their organisation. It does seem irrational to insist on rigorous requirements for registering doctors and nurses in the name of patient safety, but not for those who, through the financial processes of healthcare, also have a great influence on the system in which these doctors and nurses have to provide safe care for their patients.

If the ultimate aim is to protect patients, legislative processes must be developed that place this responsibility onto the shoulders of all concerned with the provision of healthcare. This will require systems of governance that include within the responsibilities of clinicians a duty to ensure fiscal prudence, and in the responsibilities of administrators a duty to ensure patient safety.

Understanding error and violation

Many adverse events (not all) are attributable to error. To be effective, clinical risk management must be predicated on a basic understanding of the nature of human error. Surprisingly, some of the adverse events are actually attributable to violations, and these also need to be understood. Regular educational activities on the nature of errors and violations are essential if a culture of safety is to be nurtured. Space precludes more than a brief synopsis of the key points of this very large subject, and readers are referred to other sources for more information (see Reason 1990, 1997, Merry & McCall Smith 2001, Runciman et al 2007).

Complex systems

Perrow (1999) has characterised processes on two dimensions. The first is the degree to which outcomes are coupled to actions. In a tightly coupled system, the link between actions and outcomes is direct. Many interactions in healthcare are tightly coupled – giving the wrong drug to a patient can produce instant adverse effects. Poor hand hygiene on the part of staff will result in an increase in nosocomial infection, not necessarily in every patient, but certainly overall. The second dimension is the interaction scale. Interactions can be linear or complex. Any collection of two or more interacting components can be thought of as a system. A system can be considered complex when the possible interactions exceed the number at which it is possible to predict its long-term behaviour. Healthcare is a complex system. Perrow argues that in complex systems accidents are inevitable, and therefore 'normal'. It follows that such systems are intrinsically unsafe. Considerable investment and constant vigilance will be required to achieve safety if the coupling of a system is tight and consequences of failure potentially severe.

Healthcare is a particularly hazardous complex system. It differs from many other complex systems (such as aviation) in its diversity, in the vulnerability of the patients within it, and in the degree of uncertainty that characterises many of the problems faced by practitioners (Runciman et al 2007).

Errors

An error can be formally defined as is 'the unintentional use of a wrong plan to achieve an aim, or failure to carry out a planned action as intended' (Runciman et al 2003:975). More simply, an error occurs 'when someone is trying to do the right thing, but actually does the wrong thing' (Runciman et al 2007:112). The fundamental point is that errors are unintentional (note that this essential element has not been captured by all published definitions of error). Identifying a failure as an error does not depend on outcome – errors may have no effect on outcome, or may even lead to a better outcome than anticipated (for example, one might forget to give a prophylactic antibiotic to a patient, who unbeknown to anyone is actually allergic to this drug, and thereby avoid an anaphylatic reaction). Equally, adverse events can occur in the absence of any identifiable error. The outcome of an error is largely dependent on chance.

Pause for reflection

Can an adverse event really occur without any error (or violation)? For example, if one attempts to repair an acute aortic aneurysm and the patient dies despite no obvious mistakes or deficiencies in management, does this not imply either:

- errors (or at least imperfections) occurred that were not identified or perhaps even understood given the present 'state of the art'
- it was a mistake to undertake the case in the first place.

These views are only meaningful with the benefit of hindsight: assuming there was a reasonable chance of success at the time of the decision, there would have been no way of knowing in advance that the outcome would be unsatisfactory. Similarly, future gains in knowledge and technique lie in the future – one can only characterise actions as errors in relation to what was known and possible at the time. This of course can create difficulties in perception when old cases are brought before the courts: the tendency is to judge past events by present-day standards.

The classification of errors

There are many different ways of classifying errors, but the central point is that errors are classifiable, rather than random: they occur in particular ways and under recognisable circumstances, so it is possible to understand the factors that predispose to error.

This implies that it is possible to address so called 'latent factors' (previously known as 'latent errors') in the system that make errors more likely (Reason 1990). James Reason's 'Swiss cheese' model of accident causation is very well known (Reason 2000). It depicts the defences in the system as slices of Swiss cheese, with the holes representing latent vulnerabilities in their effectiveness. Accidents seldom occur from a single error – usually it is necessary for several of these latent factors to manifest at the same time – depicted as the holes lining up.

One classification widely used in the context of healthcare is based on the thought processes involved in the generation of the error. Skill-based errors (slips and lapses) involve failures in actions during learned behaviours with no conscious engagement of the mind (classically, a person who has just given up taking milk in tea might accidentally add milk to a cup without thinking). Mistakes involve failures in decision making. Technical errors are a little different, and in effect represent a mismatch between the (variable) challenge provided by patients and the (variable) skills of practitioners (see Box 11.3) (Runciman et al 2007).

Box 11.3 Golf – a prime example of technical errors

All golfers make errors (which are not slips or lapses, nor are they mistakes – although golfers may make both of these types of error as well) otherwise the ball would end up in the hole at least on every shot within reach of the green. These errors can be thought of in terms of *tolerance* – skilled golfers tend to play within tighter tolerances than beginners. However some courses are harder than others, so tolerances vary not only with the skill of the person, but also with the challenge he or she faces.

In the same way, success at undertaking an epidural injection (for example) is a factor of the skill of the practitioner and also of the difficulty presented by the unique anatomy of each patient. The more skilled the practitioner the greater the likelihood of success, indicating some imperfection on the part of his or her less-skilled colleagues that can be thought of as technical error.

Violations

The important difference between violations and errors is that violations are intentional, although this does not imply that there is any intention to harm patients. Stated simply, a violation is 'an act which knowingly incurs a risk'. More formally: 'a violation is a deliberate – but not necessarily reprehensible – deviation from safe operating procedures, standards or rules'.

Many violations occur in healthcare, largely because people are struggling with an imperfect system, and following the rules can often be difficult within the overall constraints of heavy workloads and inadequate resources. Occasionally it is appropriate to break a rule (in a real emergency an anaesthetist might forgo a complete check of the anaesthetic machine before using it to administer oxygen for example). There are in fact too many rules in many healthcare institutions; the problem with an excess of rules (or policies) that are widely perceived to be trivial, unhelpful or unworkable is that people do break them (indeed they may not even be aware of many of the policies, and may often break them unintentionally) and breaking any rule is the first step on the slippery road to a culture of denial of the value of rules.

Violations are not all equally culpable. Exceeding the speed limit by one kilometre per hour is obviously a different moral proposition from exceeding it by 20. On the other hand, there are two major reasons for taking violations very seriously:

1. violations predispose to error and tend to make the consequences of error worse when errors occur (speeding is a good example of this)
2. unlike errors, violations are intentional, so (in theory at least) they should be totally avoidable.

Much emphasis is placed on the idea of promoting a culture of safety in healthcare. An absolutely central element of such a safety culture is a commitment to avoiding unnecessary risk, and a respect for 'safe operating procedures, standards or rules'.

Pause for reflection

One type of violation, the 'optimising' violation, is characterised by a desire for self-gratification, and is very common in healthcare. It is often driven by doctors' desire to be the 'best' and to be known as 'outstanding' – often defined in relation to being fast, clever, exceptionally technically able, and so on. In fact safety is not about being the best – it is about doing the right thing, which is often routine and boring, and sometimes slows down the process. This means that the safety conscious person often runs the risk of being seen as 'slow' or 'unhelpful' when compared with those who appear more accommodating and who perhaps take shortcuts to 'get the job done'.

Deliberate harm

Deliberate harm to patients is very rare in healthcare, notwithstanding the high profile of Harold Shipman, the English general practitioner who murdered over 200 of his patients (Richards 2006). James Reason calls this 'sabotage' (Reason 1990). It does occur and should not be tolerated but has received far too much emphasis in relation to patient safety. The vast majority of adverse events in hospitals occur because good doctors and nurses who intend to help their patients fail in this endeavour, and not because of anyone who got up in the morning with the intention of hurting people.

Categories of human activity

Effective risk management can be facilitated by an appreciation of the different types of activities that occupy health workers, because the risks are different in each. These categories of activity are:

- routine operations
- maintenance activities
- dealing with abnormal conditions (sometimes in emergencies)
- creative activities (sometimes in emergencies).

Routine and maintenance activities are very common in healthcare. Indeed, promoting a routine approach to common problems is a cornerstone of high-quality and safe practice. The most common errors in these activities are slips and lapses. These are not easily avoided, but the design of equipment, processes and facilities can make them less likely. For example, the use of forcing functions can eliminate specific errors (pin indexing systems on gas cylinders used to avoid inadvertent misconnections when using anaesthesia machines are one example of this). Alarms and checklists may also be helpful.

The risk of a mistake is increased, in comparison with that of skill-based errors, when dealing with abnormal conditions. The first response to an abnormal condition usually involves identifying and applying a rule, and this is likely to go wrong if the person concerned has not seen the particular condition before. Creative activities are relatively uncommon in healthcare (in contrast with engineering for example), but dealing with an abnormal condition that has not been seen before may require a creative response. The problem with creative thinking is that it takes time, which may not be available in an emergency. It follows that an important technique for clinical risk management is to increase the number of conditions for which rules have been specified. Traditional medical training, case conferences, mortality and morbidity meetings and many other educational techniques are all predicated on trying to increase the number of relevant conditions likely to be correctly identified by staff working in a particular unit, and to increase awareness of standard rule-based responses to these. Another technique for improving the likelihood of success in responding to an abnormal condition involves the use of appropriate algorithms[16] (Runciman & Merry 2005).

Proactively identifying risk in a clinical unit

The starting point in reducing risk is to identify the factors likely to create risk in one's own unit.

Expertise, standardisation and evidence-based medicine

The importance of expertise cannot be overemphasised. A system of credentialling clinical staff to ensure that training and experience is appropriate for the work done in the unit is essential. The peer-reviewed literature relevant to the clinical problems dealt with in the unit should be reviewed regularly, and key publications should be presented and discussed at continuing education meetings. Policies should be developed to standardise the management of patients along evidence-based lines so far as possible. Where evidence is equivocal or lacking, agreement should be reached among senior clinicians in the unit on one reasonable method of dealing with particular clinical problems, based on first principles and experience, and this method should be adopted as the standard for the unit.

Incident reporting

Incident reporting has gained considerable traction in healthcare over the past decade and many institutions have set up systems for incident reporting. In many cases these systems have been implemented on a hospital-wide or even state-wide basis. The key for risk management in one's own unit is to ensure that staff are proactive in reporting relevant incidents, including near misses, and that these reports are reviewed locally as well as centrally.

The objective of incident reporting is to improve patient safety. This means that it is more important for information that might reduce risk to be shared with those who can act upon it than it is to count events or punish clinicians for mistakes or wrongdoing.

Regular meetings should be held to review incidents. These can be based on forms that have been completed by members of staff, but it is worth also encouraging

---

[16] An algorithm is a systematised approach to solving a problem.

spontaneous verbal reports of things that have gone wrong, nearly gone wrong or simply concerned members of staff. These meetings should be run on a confidential no-blame basis. In many jurisdictions this can be formalised by registration of the meetings and the incident reporting process as quality assurance programs. Blame-oriented processes can run in parallel to confidential incident reporting, and the provision for confidentiality in this way does not impede access to information in any other way, such as through a patient's notes, interviewing staff for the express purpose of investigating a complaint, and so on.

It is important to 'close the loop'. This implies that some action must follow the confidential meetings. Minutes that are limited to the issues, and points for action, are a reasonable way of facilitating this. Someone, such as the clinical director of the unit, must be responsible for implementing the recommendations that arise from the meetings.

Recording and responding to events

It is important to measure the rate of specified outcomes in order to track performance over time and to compare the performance of one's own unit with that of comparable institutions and with results published in the literature. This is a different exercise from incident reporting, with different objectives, and the two should not be confused.

Key performance indicators or clinical indicators may be used to monitor selected processes. For example, it may be relevant to track the percentage of patients who have been assessed by an anaesthetist before surgery. On the other hand, if this is the standard of care in one's own unit, and compliance is 100% (or very nearly 100%), there would be no point in monitoring this indicator.

Serious adverse events should certainly be tracked, and the rates of these reviewed regularly. For many units, mortality rate is an important indicator of quality, but for others death is too infrequent to provide meaningful information about clinical performance. However, there may be other outcomes that are more common and worth monitoring to provide early warning of problems in the management of patients – nosocomial infections being an obvious example.

Sentinel events are serious adverse events that should not be allowed to happen. A number of events have been specified as 'sentinel' in various jurisdictions, and the reporting of these is required by law. However it may be appropriate to designate certain events as 'sentinel' for the purposes of a particular unit. It may not be necessary to pre-specify these – in many cases it is obvious to all concerned when a serious adverse event occurs that is out of the ordinary and demands special attention.

Root cause analysis (RCA) is a formalised process to identify the underlying causes of an adverse event, in order to prevent it from happening again. The term means different things to different people, but the approach developed by the Veteran's Administration in the US is particularly thorough, and has been described in detail elsewhere (Runciman et al 2007). It is usual for the process for RCA to be set up at an institutional level, and this is appropriate for several reasons, not the least of which is the considerable resource required. However, there may be times when a RCA should be initiated locally, at the level of a clinical unit, in response to an event that is serious and unexpected, or to a series of events identified by incident reporting (for example) that collectively demand action.

Other processes may be appropriate instead of, or in parallel to, unit-based actions to deal with adverse events. For example, deaths related to surgery should generally be reported to a coroner, and coronial inquiries may be very helpful in identifying actions to improve safety within a unit.

It is important to review the results of these activities regularly and to take action if they indicate a problem. In doing this, the use of appropriate statistical techniques to differentiate special cause from common cause variation is essential (see above).

Complaints

Complaints are an important means of identifying risks in healthcare, and should be actively encouraged. It is reasonable for patients who have had a bad experience in a clinical unit (or their families) to complain. Complaints may also be received from visitors, and from other people who have had some interaction with the unit. Poor communication often underlies complaints and open disclosure of adverse events may reduce their likelihood.

All clinical units should have formal processes for dealing with complaints, which should be aligned with the processes of the overall institution, and should include support for all parties. It is inevitable that some complaints will end up going beyond these processes but the aim should be to resolve complaints locally and promptly if possible. Part of this response should be to identify factors that could be improved in the future, and to record and implement these. Many patients who complain say that they do so to prevent future incidents (and also to get an explanation, to obtain compensation and to promote accountability). It follows that this part of the response is important not only for managing future risk, but also for resolving the present complaint.

Actively reducing risk in a clinical unit

Identifying risk is half way to reducing it, but measurement alone will not improve patient safety: action is needed, and this implies the investment of time and money.

Safe staff – the importance of the team

Effective risk management requires commitment and cooperation from all disciplines involved directly and indirectly with the care of patients – doctors, nurses, pharmacists, laboratory staff, managers and even orderlies and cleaning staff (see Box 11.4).

> **Box 11.4** Case study – An orderly's dedication to safety
>
> This author spent four days in a major pubic hospital after suffering a comminuted fracture of his tibia and fibula. The fracture was very low, and required difficult surgery that involved inserting a rod into the tibia and a number of screws to secure the position of the fragments. On the day of discharge an orderly was entrusted with taking him by wheelchair from the ward to a waiting car, and with assisting him in moving from the wheelchair to the car.
>
> The orderly discharged his duty with a care and diligence that reflected great pride in his work. When thanked, he summarised the situation perfectly saying, 'There wouldn't be a lot of point in all that skilled surgery if you were allowed to trip over while getting into your car and managed to break your leg again, would there?'
>
> When asked, he said he had been in the job for over 20 years, knew the hospital and its medical and nursing staff very well indeed, and was proud to be part of an organisation dedicated to patient care.

This commitment must be present at all levels of the system, from politicians and senior government officials right down to the clerk who coordinates the appointments for outpatient clinics. Safety requires all those who work in healthcare to understand that the focus of all activities should ultimately be the patients (refer back to Figure 11.1). This includes everyone from financial officers to the staff who prepare meals in the hospital kitchen. In short, safety in healthcare is a function of teamwork, the team is very large, and the patient's outcome depends on the weakest link in the team.

An unfortunate trend in healthcare in recent years has been towards greater mobility in staff, the use of contractors rather than employees for functions such as cleaning and catering, and the increased use of agency staff and locums for clinical services. Two important safety measures have been lost in this change from long-term employees:

1. the opportunity for individuals to develop thorough knowledge of their clinical unit, the people who work in it, the types of patients who present to it, the location of the equipment, the other disciplines who interact with it and all the myriad factors essential for the successful management of patients
2. the opportunity to develop strong team identities: people who believe themselves to be part of an identifiable and well-performing team will often go beyond the strict boundaries of their paid employment to promote the goals of the team (in this case high-quality patient care).

The things that go wrong in hospitals are not random. As explained above, errors and violations can be classified, their causes understood, and their occurrence often predicted. Thus a nurse who has been in a clinical unit for many years will have seen many adverse events, and will often recognise the signs of the next one in the making. He or she will be able to intercept the mistake about to be made by the house officer, the new staff nurse, or even the new catering contractor (errors in providing meals to patients being a prime source of adverse events in hospitals).

Investing in safety

The concept of risk as a homogenous organisation-wide phenomenon, likely to be solved by major initiatives to improve the culture and change the entire system, is only partially correct. Many risks manifest uniquely at a local level, and the risks faced in a psychiatry ward are different from those faced in the operating room. It follows that many solutions are also local, and those who work in clinical units often know what the key risks are and quite often have innovative or simple, sensible ideas about how to address them. These ideas need to be acted upon, and the resources need to be provided to facilitate safe practices that are specific to specific clinical situations. Obviously good ideas should also be shared, but often this is as much a matter of communication between different institutions as between units within the same institution, and the medical and nursing peer reviewed literature is often the most effective vehicle for this.

A major challenge to improving the safety of healthcare processes lies in having to justify the cost of this investment, in a sector that finds it difficult to meet the financial demands of providing service even at current levels of risk. It may be very difficult to quantify the benefits for any specific intervention to reduce risk. Ironically, misuse of the concept of evidence-based medicine may itself be a barrier to appropriate investment in safety.

Sackett has made it clear that evidence-based medicine is 'the conscientious, explicit and judicious use of current best evidence in making decisions about the care of individual patients' (Sackett et al 1996:71). For some clinical questions, the randomised controlled trial (RCT) is the best source of evidence, but there are many questions for which other forms of evidence are more appropriate (Merry et al 2000). Furthermore, the lack of evidence to support an intervention is not the same as evidence that it has no value; error prevention is a young field, and one in which the commercial incentives to fund large randomised trials are less than they are in relation to the development of new drugs (for example), so evidence is not yet particularly abundant. RCTs are not always feasible in relation to safety interventions, because randomisation and/or blinding may be impossible or because adverse events, although occasionally catastrophic, are actually quite infrequent. For example, the inadvertent administration of intrathecal vincristine alluded to above has occurred at a frequency that is totally unacceptable from a clinical perspective but too low for use of this outcome as an endpoint in an RCT.

Leape et al (2002) have put the matter this way in relation to anaesthesia.

> ... the anesthesia community has measured its progress over time, accumulating a 'time series' track record whose signal is virtually incontrovertible. To say that convincing evidence of progress and effect is lacking because randomised trials of all safe anesthesia practices have not been conducted would be Luddite.

> (Leape et al 2002:506)

RCTs are best suited to evaluating the efficacy of individual interventions or therapies, whereas patient safety is primarily a function of how well the system of care is performing – evaluating safety is more like evaluating the effectiveness of a treatment in actual practice. For example, the efficacy of prophylactic anticoagulation to prevent venous thromboembolism can be demonstrated in an RCT, but the impact of anticoagulation in clinical practice also depends on patients receiving the appropriate drug, on time, at the right dose, every time, and if these elements fail it is actually possible for the outcome to be worse than if no attempt is made to use anticoagulation at all. The safe provision of anticoagulation is in fact a function of the system, and depends on the application of human factors theory, process engineering, and systems theory. This involves the iterative institution of small changes guided by repeated evaluations through a cycle of continuous quality improvement (See Warburton, Chapter 10). This is not a process that can easily be studied by RCTs. It may be possible to follow outcomes using sequential statistical tools (such as control charts) provided one is dealing with a frequent end point. For infrequent but disastrous adverse events, not even these methods are viable. Often, one simply has to resort to first principles, which in the case of safety includes such things as standardisation, simplification, and using checklists. Many of these initiatives can be justified on the basis of common sense and evidence from industry. As Leape et al (2002) say

> [F]or policymakers to wait for incontrovertible proof of effectiveness before recommending a practice would be a prescription for inaction and an abdication of responsibility. The prudent alternative is to make reasonable judgments based on the best available evidence combined with successful experiences in health care. While some errors in these judgments are inevitable, we believe they will be far outweighed by the improvement in patient safety that will result.

> (Leape et al 2002:507)

Establishing a safety culture

In order for a team of long-term staff to reduce risk rather than entrench it, they must habitually display behaviour appropriate for this objective. This behaviour can be conceptualised as reflecting certain attributes (see Figure 11.2). There is no doubt that health professionals need knowledge and skill, and often a great deal of both.

In Figure 11.2 the attributes of individuals (there may often be more than two people in a clinical unit) and of the clinical unit to which they belong are each depicted as three sides of a safety triangle. The culture of a clinical unit (or any other

Figure 11.2 The safety triangle

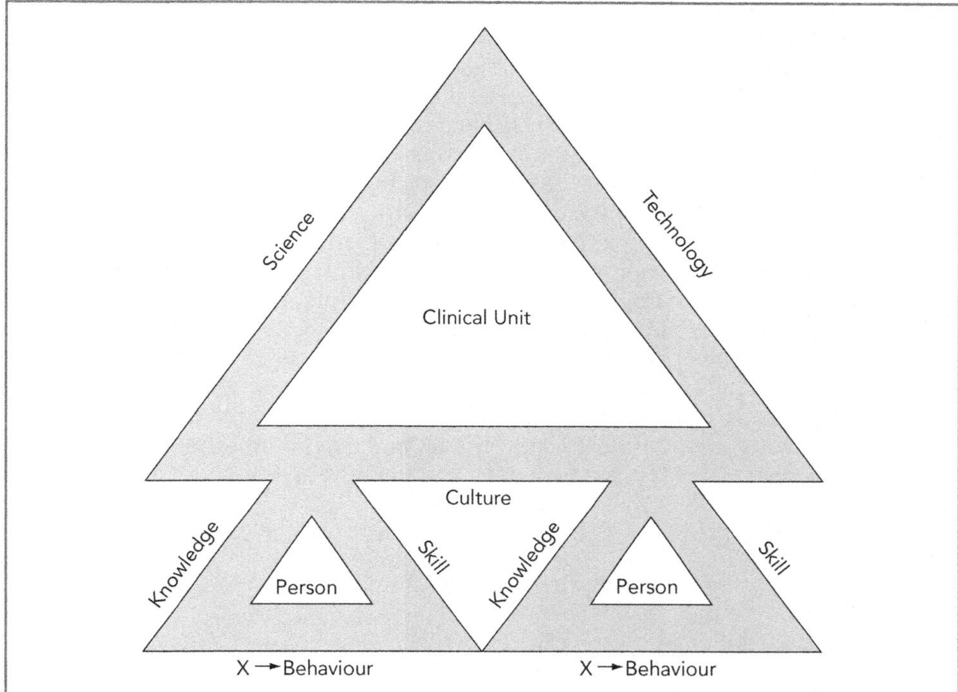

organisation) reflects the collective attributes of the people who make it up (modified from Runciman et al 2007). The contribution of Dr Richard Morris to this concept is acknowledged.

There is an additional factor that can be recognised as important, but is harder to define. An exercise sometimes used in teaching clinicians is to ask them to identify the features of the doctor or nurse in their own unit who they would like to have caring for their own family. There is no doubt that there is a factor over and above knowledge and skill, that relates to a complex mix of attributes that people in the know take into account when making such a choice. This mix has been called the X-factor (Runciman et al 2007); it is not easily defined, but it is recognisable, and manifests in the individual's behaviour.

In a similar way there are a number of attributes one might identify as desirable in clinical units (or indeed any organisation in healthcare). These include the empirical and scientific knowledge on which it operates (its 'science'), its technology, and its culture (see Figure 11.2). The knowledge of its people adds up to its 'science' and their skills are largely dependent on its technology. Science and technology are applied within a culture. In the end, the culture of a clinical unit is no more than the collective manifestation of the individual behaviour of the people within it. The behaviour of each individual is influenced by the behaviour of the others within the unit, so a new entrant to the community may well be drawn into a strongly established culture, implying that a desirable culture, once established, tends to be self-propagating (and so does an undesirable one).

How then can a culture of safety be achieved? Obviously the more the focus of those responsible for the unit is on safety, the better. However, a personal focus on safety by every individual, demonstrated by safe behaviour, is an essential contribution to such a culture. If a culture places greater value on throughput and is tolerant of carelessness, individuals will be more likely to disregard safety. Thus every individual's behaviour is modified by the prevailing culture, but, in a cyclical way, this behaviour creates and reinforces that very culture. Thus the discussion returns to the point that the culture of any group is a product of the collective attitudes and behaviour of the individuals within it. If the culture of a system is to change, then the behaviour of the individuals within it must change. It follows that the responsibility for the safety of any unit lies with every individual.

Of course clinical units do not exist in a vacuum, and aligning the culture and risk management activities of the clinical unit with those of organisational management can be a major challenge, particularly when the former are strongly grounded in clinical work and the latter are predominantly from lay backgrounds. Perhaps the most important step towards this goal is regular communication, both formal and informal. The more people talk to each other the more likely they are to understand the other's view of the organisation's objectives and risks. It is important to articulate these formally. A small set of carefully chosen practical indicators of performance in relation to goals and risks can then be monitored. It is essential that relevant clinical data is fed back to organisational management, and that organisational management demonstrates responsiveness to those data, and the information they represent.

> **Pause for reflection**
>
> In a safety-oriented culture, the motto should be: 'If you don't know it's safe, it isn't safe.'
>
> The responsibility for alerting the team to any concern over safety lies with each individual within the team. This does not always mean that the team will change course – it does mean that critical information on which to make a safe decision is more likely to be shared.

Responding to an adverse event

For the foreseeable future adverse events will occur however effectively risk is managed within clinical units. A very important part of a risk management program is to ensure that the immediate response to these events is appropriate (see Box 11.5 overleaf).

The most important thing is to recognise that a serious adverse event warrants focused and detailed attention, and that arrangements need to be made to ensure that the staff involved in the event are able to deal with the aftermath. This may imply cancelling other work, or finding other staff to take over. It is also important that senior staff not directly involved with the incident become involved in the response, to provide support for those who were involved and may be distressed and (understandably) lacking in objectivity. A more detailed account of this important topic is available elsewhere (Runciman et al 2007).

Conclusion

Managing risk to patients is an essential activity in healthcare, and should involve all levels of every organisation. The steps taken at the level of the clinical unit are particularly important, and need to be proactive, planned, coordinated and grounded in the science of human factors, cognitive psychology and safe systems design.

Many of the risks faced by patients are specific to particular clinical units, and no one is better placed to identify these, and respond to them, than those who work at the front line of clinical medicine. Culture is important, and is largely determined at the level of whole institutions, but the contribution to each individual in developing and maintaining a safety-oriented culture cannot be overestimated. Reducing risk requires the investment of time and money, and the justification for this along traditional business lines may be difficult – but the investment still needs to be made.

Risk management is very much a team affair (see Box 11.6). Risk is determined by the weakest link in any chain. Every member of the clinical unit should be engaged in

---

Box 11.5 The immediate response to an adverse event

1. Secure the situation by:
   - making sure the patient is safe
   - making sure no one else is likely to be harmed.
2. Record the event and the actions taken to deal with it.
3. Communicate with the patient and/or family.
4. Support:
   - the patient and/or family
   - the staff involved in the event.
5. Inform:
   - the hospital risk managers, unit directors etc (and complete an incident report)
   - liability insurers as appropriate.
6. Plan:
   - ongoing care of the patient if necessary
   - follow-up meetings with the family and patient
   - appropriate investigations (e.g. root cause analysis).

Box 11.6 Implications for practice – Accounting for clinical risk and patient safety

- Staff at the level of the clinical unit have a major role in any organisation in managing risks to patients.
- The risks that matter in each particular unit should be identified and proactive steps taken to mitigate these.
- The clinical data provided to organisational management from a clinical unit should be carefully chosen to reflect these key risks and progress managing them.
- The distinction between errors and violations should be understood within clinical units, and every effort made to identify and reduce factors contributing to both.
- The response to adverse events that do occur should be given high priority to ensure that both patients (and their families) and staff are properly and promptly cared for and supported.
- Complaints present an opportunity to improve the quality of care provided by a clinical unit, and should be handled proactively, fairly and constructively.
- A culture of safety begins with a personal commitment to safety by every individual within an organisation.

this activity. The development of stable groups of long-term staff who identify strongly with their clinical units is therefore the cornerstone of safety.

References

Bolsin S & Colson M 2000 The use of the Cusum technique in the assessment of trainee competence in new procedures. International Journal for Quality in Health Care. 12(5):433–8

Brennan T A, Leape L L et al 1991 Incidence of adverse events and negligence in hospitalized patients – results of the Harvard Medical Practice Study I. New England Journal of Medicine 324(6):370–376

Carey R G 2002a Constructing powerful control charts. Journal of Ambulatory Care Management 25(4):64–70

Carey R G 2002b How do you know that your care is improving? Part I: basic concepts in statistical thinking. Journal of Ambulatory Care Management 25(1):80–87

Donabedian A 2003 An Introduction to Quality Assurance in Health Care. Oxford University Press, New York

Ferner R E, McDowell S E 2006 Doctors charged with manslaughter in the course of medical practice, 1795–2005: a literature review. Journal of the Royal Society of Medicine 99(6):309–314

Goldman L, Caldera D et al 1977 Multifactorial index of cardiac risk in noncardiac surgical procedures. New England Journal of Medicine 297:845–850

Hayward R A, Hofer T P 2001 Estimating hospital deaths due to medical errors: preventability is in the eye of the reviewer. JAMA 286(4):415–420

Kennedy I 2001 Learning from Bristol: The Report of the Public Inquiry into Children's Heart Surgery at the Bristol Royal Infirmary 1984–1995. Online available: www.bristol-inquiry. org.uk/final_report

La Puma J, Lawlor E F 1990 Quality-adjusted life-years: ethical emplications for physicians and policy makers. Journal of the American Medical Association 263(21):2917–21

Leape L L, Berwick D M et al 2002 What practices will most improve safety? Evidence-based medicine meets patient safety. Journal of the American Medical Association 288(4):501–507

Merry A F 2007 When are errors a crime? – Lessons from New Zealand. The Criminal Justice System and Health Care. Erin C, Ost S (eds). Oxford University Press, Oxford

Merry A F, Davies J M et al 2000 Qualitative research in health care. British Journal of Anaesthesia 84(5):552–555

Merry A F, McCall Smith A 2001 Errors, Medicine and the Law. Cambridge University Press, Cambridge

Merry A F, Ramage M C et al 1992 First-time coronary artery bypass grafting: the anaesthetist as a risk factor. British Journal of Anaesthesia 68:6–12

Murray C J L, Lopez A D (eds) 1996 The global burden of disease and injury series, volume 1: a comprehensive assessment of mortality and disability from diseases, injuries, and risk factors in 1990 and projected to 2020. Cambridge, MA:, Harvard School of Public Health on behalf of the World Health Organization and the World Bank, Harvard University Press

Nashef S A, Roques F et al 2002 Validation of European system for cardiac operative risk evaluation (EuroSCORE) in North American cardiac surgery. European Journal of Cardiothoracic Surgery 22(1):101–105

Perrow C 1999 Normal Accidents: Living with high-technologies. Princeton University Press, Princeton New Jersey

Reason J 1990 Human Error. New York, Cambridge University Press

Reason J 1997 Managing the Risks of Organizational Accidents. Aldershot, Ashgate

Reason J 2000 Human error: models and management. British Medical Journal 320:768–770

Reason J 2004 Beyond the organisational accident: the need for 'error wisdom' on the frontline. Quality and Safety in Health Care. 13(Suppl 2):ii28–ii33. Online. Available: http://qhc.bmj-journals.com/cgi/content/full/13/suppl_2/ii 28 Jul 2006

Richards T 2006 Chairwoman of Shipman inquiry protests at lack of action. British Medical Journal 332(7550):1111

Runciman W B, Merry A et al 2007 Safety and Ethics in Healthcare: A Guide to Getting it Right. Ashgate, Aldershot

Runciman W B, Merry A F 2005 Crises in clinical care: an approach to management. Quality and Safety in Health Care 14(3):156–63

Runciman W B, Merry A F et al 2003 Error, blame, and the law in health care – an antipodean perspective. Annals of Internal Medicine 138(12):974–9

Sackett D L, Rosenberg W M et al 1996 Evidence based medicine: what it is and what it isn't. British Medical Journal 312(7023):71–72

Tenner E 1997 Why Things Bite Back – Technology and the Revenge of Unintended Consequences. Vintage Books, New York

Chapter 12

The changing dynamic of policy and practice in Australian healthcare

Christine Jorm, Margaret Banks & Sara Twohill

Introduction

Managing clinical work to achieve the best possible quality of care requires systems to be established and information to be shared. Policy is a mechanism through which these ends can be realised, and while often defined in a formal sense as a blueprint of intentions, health policy can also be described informally as the 'courses of action that affect that set of institutions, organisations, services and funding arrangements' in the healthcare system (Palmer & Short 2000:2). Recent policy in Australia has been directed to health system reform, but 'good policy intentions' are often hampered by complex funding and governance arrangements, specifically, in the case of Australia, by the politics of federalism where both state and federal levels of government share responsibility for health services. The duplication and division that shared responsibility brings impedes reform (Willis et al 2005), and the funding provided by the Commonwealth to state public hospitals via the Australian Healthcare Agreements (negotiated between both levels of government) provides the Commonwealth with opportunities to influence the shape and direction of reform. There is no easy 'solution' to the federal–state issue, although redesign efforts are occurring at multiple levels in the system to better link funding models with incentives for improved outcomes (Swerissen & Duckett 2002). The difficulty remains in determining which outcomes are chosen, how they are measured and the incentives and sanctions offered.

Health reform is made more complex by a range of other structural factors, including a substantial private sector that accounted for 41% of hospital beds in 2003–04, and an increasing emphasis on the responsibility of individuals for their own healthcare needs. There are the pressures from the professions, specifically the medical profession about their changing place in the system, and from consumers about the level and standard of service provided. Together with the life and death nature of healthcare decisions, these complexities in the system all impact to make health a fraught policy arena and, within this contested environment, the concern that health policy may do harm (Spitz & Abramson 2005) is a significant challenge for policymakers. Examining health policy from the recent past can illuminate important modern practices and provide clues for the future. In this chapter we examine two 'small' policy directives and conclude that small policy directives struggle to guide and control care, just as large policy initiatives do.

Health Policy 1990

For the purpose of our discussion, two 1990 policy circulars from New South Wales are reproduced and appended to this chapter: Circular 90/29 (Appendix 1) issued in April 1990 and Circular 90/122 (Appendix 2) issued in December 1990. Both are representative of policy issued by Australian state and territory health departments at that time. They are examples of 'control and command' statements that presume the organisationally shared understanding of authority, direction and discipline that is a hallmark of classical management theory. These policies were issued to the public health system in the form of a paper-based notification intended to guide the actions of health practitioners and managers.

Circular 90/29 is brief and deals with two separate issues: first, the commencement of labelling of blood units with a warning of possible infectious transmission; and second, the possibility of directed donations of blood from first-degree relatives causing graft versus host disease, and a central office directive that these blood donations be irradiated in future. These issues are separate but related. The discovery of the transmission of HIV (and other infections such as hepatitis C) via blood transfusion resulted in an increased demand for directed donation. This relationship is not made explicit in the document and multiple ambiguities are encoded into this circular: Which infections might be in the blood and undetected by screening? What data would help doctors and patients decide about the relative risks and benefit of transfusion if the blood could be infected? Are directed donations to be discouraged or encouraged? How are arrangements made for blood irradiation? Who is the label for? Is it to 'protect' the blood bank? The label warns, but doesn't inform, nor does the circular.

Circular 90/122 is even briefer. Published later in 1990 it has acquired a letterhead and logo, increasing the appearance of legitimacy. It refers to a new procedure for billing for inter-hospital air transports. A previous fixed charge is to be replaced by full cost recovery. This is to be met within existing budgets. No reasons are given for the directive. It appears to be an attempt to reduce the demand for, and therefore the cost of air transport by introducing a user-pays mechanism. It is ambiguous in terms of the potential size of full cost recovery charges, and the implications for regional areas could be significant, but there is no suggestion of special budget consideration. There is no information about how clinical appropriateness of air transport might be assessed.

The circulars detail the authors' contact details and file references available within central office. While the files may have contained information on the circular development, including the issues that precipitated the development of the policy statement (and possibly the evidence base and development methodology), this information does not appear on the circular. Policy statements at this time rarely referenced published literature or evidence, and it was infrequent that evidence informed their development. The methodology used to develop such a circular varied and included brief stakeholder consultation through to central composition by a single author.

Policy papers in 1990 needed to be printed, generally off site, and mailed to recipients in health services from the central health department in accordance with a pre-determined distribution list. Inclusion, or indeed exclusion, from the distribution list was determined by the policy officer. Their level of understanding of the operations of health services varied, therefore distribution could exclude groups vital to the policy's implementation. For Circular 90/29 the print run was 136 copies and these were distributed to directors

194

within the health department (25 copies), public health units (21 copies), health services (29 copies), health professional associations and related organisations, which would have included the 12 medical colleges (19 copies), public hospitals (27 copies) and private hospitals and day procedure centres (15 copies). Further distribution was reliant on these organisations having effective dissemination mechanisms.

The size and fragmentation of the private hospital sector, which at that time consisted of over 33% of available hospital beds (National Health Strategy Working Group 1991), meant this sector was unlikely to consistently receive new policy directives. Copies could be accessed directly from the health department if it was known they existed. The system did not have a reliable mechanism for dissemination of circulars to the 18,000 doctors registered in NSW in 1990 (Australian Institute of Health and Welfare 2001) nor to the approximately 30% of these doctors practising in a specialty area where they were likely to order and administer blood.

When viewed, the documents look ancient (a manual typewriter has been used) although they are comparatively recent. We ask what might these directives look like if they were developed now?

Health policy today

Outlined in Box 12.1 are the elements that would be expected to be taken into account when health policy is being formulated today.

Box 12.1 Case study – Health policy today

A policy directive developed today would be expected to contain the following elements:

- definition of the problem in terms of service provision for clinical stakeholders e.g. 'health services have had n instances of this issue, which has had x effects on patient outcome (e.g. four deaths) and resulted in the following resource requirements'
- detailed reference to the current evidence
- a methodology – the process of consultation and development for the policy would be described e.g. a reference group consisting of participants/representatives of a number of specified groups and the outcome of their deliberations
- consideration of risks of implementation
- specification of expectations around implementation, resourcing and standardisation, e.g.
  - state-based standardisation of a process and protocol
  - quarterly reporting against specified indicators
  - to be funded either within existing budget, via seeding funding or new recurrent program funding
- identification of whose responsibility implementation was – if it was sufficiently high level it would be included in managers' and practitioners' performance contracts (e.g. that of the blood bank director for a health area)
- links to multiple other relevant policy documents
- often inclusion of implementation tools, mechanisms for monitoring, and at times evaluation requirements, e.g. the safety and quality manager's tool kit, use of the state-wide incident monitoring system.

The boxed elements reflect a number of significant developments in Australian health policy in the 17 years since the 1990 documents were created. We highlight four:

1. explicit use of best available evidence
2. significant participation by stakeholders
3. improved accessibility of information
4. introduction of accountability mechanisms.

Each element seems both compelling and essential, indeed a clear improvement over earlier policy processes. Yet when we explore them, their circumstances are complex, their value is contested and the quantity and quality of evidence supporting the benefits of the changes is variable. We discuss each element in turn, examining the current versions of exemplar policy circulars before moving on to the fourth element, accountability mechanisms.

Elements in health policy development and implementation

Explicit use of best available evidence

Policy statements in 1990 rarely if ever referenced published literature or evidence and indeed evidence infrequently informed circular development. Circular 90/29 existed as policy until it was superseded by Circular 92 issued in 2002 – well behind the systems and technology that addressed safety and quality assurance issues (although more likely in a clinical domain).

The term evidence-based medicine emerged less than 20 years ago and is no longer the province of clinical practice alone, with public health practice and policymaking increasingly looking to evidence to support effective health policy development and implementation (Sheldon 2005, Shortell et al 2007). As the healthcare sector becomes inherently more complex, expensive and demanding of greater attention to safety and quality, there is pressure to apply evidence to practice. Yet numerous barriers to its application exist (Canadian Heath Services Research Foundation 2007) and evidence informs policy to a lesser degree than might be expected. As an example, when issuing advice in areas where evidence is available, the World Health Organization rarely uses systematic reviews to inform this advice, relying on expert consensus (Oxman et al 2007).

The influential role that research should play within health policy is hard to dispute. Research has the potential to strengthen and improve healthcare systems when used as the basis for policy decisions. Nonetheless, policymakers presently view research and the evidence base that it produces as limited and problematic. There is a real need for systematic, rigorous and global methods for identifying, interpreting and applying evidence (Dobrow et al 2006). While research in the areas of dissemination and implementation of research into clinical practice is increasing in frequency, there is still a paucity of research into the effectiveness of interventions intended to improve the delivery of care. For instance, despite the sizeable investments made in patient safety, there is little evidence to support links between organisational factors in healthcare, medical errors and patient safety (Hoff et al 2004). Quality improvement strategies also lack a strong evidence base (Shojania & Grimshaw 2005) and there is a deficiency in quality scientific evidence produced through appropriate clinical trials (Tunis et al 2007), for instance for the appropriate use of medications.

Two major arguments have been advanced for this research policy gap: the differing nature of policy and research, and communication challenges in the relationship between researchers and policymakers. We briefly discuss each in turn.

The differing nature of policy and research – compromise versus clarity

If policymaking is to establish agreement between competing claims, this can only be done via compromise (Booth 1988). This agreement may be general and ambiguous, enabling the resulting policy to be flexible in scope and thus more likely to being open to interpretations (as was our exemplar 1990 blood policy). Policy derived from this methodology is adaptable to varied aims and interests and therefore more likely to be accepted.

On the flipside, research is precise in its attempt to provide clarity to inform policy decisions. It does this by taking a number of variables and examining them in a controlled and systematic manner but 'rarely provides the breadth of vision policymakers require' (Booth 1988:230). Obtaining an increased understanding of an issue may increase the difficulty and challenge in arriving at an agreed policy decision (especially where experience and opinion are major influences upon health policy development) (Bowen et al 2005). Hence policy and research derive from very different streams of thinking and methodological frameworks. The fluid and ever-evolving environment in which policy is created is a challenge for researchers. The appropriate entry points for evidence-based research into a policy process are rarely controlled, and they are not the same in all instances. Evidence rarely enters into the genesis of a policy proposal because there is a lack of empirical evidence outlining the best methods for effective knowledge transfer into the policy domain (Almeida & Bascolo 2006). There are also apparent or real inadequacies in the timeliness, quality and relevance of research (Innvaer et al 2002). Thus the current utilisation of research in both policy and practice is subtle and indirect.

Relationship between researchers and policymakers – communication challenges

Another theory contends that a lack of communication between researchers and policymakers is the major reason for the policy research gap (Meyer et al 2006). The 'two communities' theory maintains that research and policy players are two factions unable to realise the perspectives and realities of one another's sphere (Innvaer et al 2002). Moreover, with communication lines weak, any endeavour to 'pair up' these spheres remains a significant challenge in part because of an absence of personal contact between key players within these domains and because of their mistrust (Meyer et al 2006). Other critics simply advocate the use of '[policy] user-friendly formats' (Laupacis & Straus 2007) for research reviews. By this is meant that research should be brief and focused on validity, applicability and implementation.

A further concern stems from the recently developed pejorative phrase 'policy-based evidence making' (House of Commons Science and Technology Committee 2006: para 89) referring to government use or commissioning of research that supports an already-determined policy approach. Doctors in the UK, for example, disbelieve that the National Institute of Clinical Evidence (NICE), the organisation responsible for developing national guidelines, acts independently; 85% of UK doctors state that they would ignore NICE guidance if they thought it 'was wrong' – presumably based on the perception that tainted or biased evidence was used (McLoughlin & Leatherman 2003). Consequently, Culyer & Lomas (2006) advocate for transparent deliberative processes allowing policymakers to develop 'evidence-informed' decisions. While this might seem an ideal solution, NICE is considered an exemplar of deliberative processes (Culyer & Lomas 2006) but it is still not always considered credible (Milewa 2006).

In summary, while it is easy to suggest that closing the current gap between research and policy is essential for effective health policy development, there are barriers. Research and policy are two very different entities that struggle to align. A number of reasons may account for this difference: there is an overall paucity of policy relevant research; research is often considered to fail policymakers in its appropriateness and timeliness; and there is a lack of mechanisms to appropriately review, disseminate and implement research.

Significant participation by stakeholders

In Australia in 1990 few substantial stakeholder structures existed and the roles and expectations for stakeholders in the policymaking process were ill defined: the current peak national consumer body, the Consumers Health Forum of Australia, had only been founded in 1987; the Commonwealth Department of Health established the Australian General Practice Network and the National Rural Health Alliance in late 1992.

In the absence of defined structures, policymakers met with individuals or representatives of very small groups. Engaging in a process of multiple negotiations with stakeholders was thus impractical, time consuming and expensive. Not surprisingly, the policymaker assumed a position of authority, justified from the perspective that policy legitimacy derived from its enactment by a professional bureaucracy accountable to an elected government (Nagel 2006). The published documents reflect this sense of the policymaker 'knowing best'. Stakeholders were often brought into the process late, such as at 'final draft' stage, and Harvey (1991:14) commented that to establish an efficient and effective healthcare system 'the three rules are: (1) find out what works; (2) choose what to do – after considering what value is obtained for each additional dollar spent;(3) make sure it happens'. This simple process formulation did not reflect the need for stakeholder engagement or its value.

In the case of the 1990 circular concerning transfusion practice, it is not known who might have been involved in the development of this directive. Such a directive now would involve haematologists, the blood bank, the Therapeutic Goods Administration (TGA), medical managers, medical colleges, associations and foundations, accreditation bodies, nurses, doctors and consumers. Extensive discussion would be expected with consumers about directed donations (including issues of patient and family choice and rights) and about how to appropriately involve patients in the discussion about newly recognised risks of blood transfusions. Educational material for patients would be developed during the process.

Modern policy practice sees stakeholder consultation as part of the enactment of policy (see Box 12.2). The multiple expectations of the stakeholder process include education, influence, lobbying and listening. Policy is communicative work. Via these communications, policymakers can have three aims: to manage stakeholders, to seek opportunities for creative problem solving, or to build legitimacy for the process of change (Nagel 2006). These aims are not always compatible, and there is little evidence to support which is more effective or important (Nagel 2006). Sometimes the very substance of the policy is devised by communicative work with stakeholders – the deliberative democracy perspective (see Mooney, Chapter 13). Such an approach allows for flux and transformation and accepts that organisation (here content and agreement) may emerge from chaos (Morgan 1997). However, if the substance of policy is determined by the process, the definition of success and measurement or evaluation of success factors becomes difficult.

> **Box 12.2** Case study – Current practice in stakeholder consultation
>
> A detailed documentation of the stakeholder process now forms a regular part of policy development. A good example is the recently released national Australian Palliative Care Needs Assessment Guidelines (Girgis et al 2006), which have as appendices a list of the 58 organisations and groups involved in the review, and details of the individuals that represented these groups at a national consensus meeting. However the investment of time and resources required can be substantial, and may not always seem appropriate for the issue. For instance, one recent improvement initiative in a single London sexual health clinic had representatives of approximately 65 stakeholder groups involved in the oversight group (Greenhalgh 2007). This caused process and practical difficulties including obtaining sufficiently large venues. The Australian Commission's review of national safety and quality accreditation had involved 125 meetings (from one-on-one to focus group), reviewed over 140 written submissions, published four discussion papers and presented at multiple conferences to develop an alternative accreditation model. However, this is a potential policy reform that will affect the whole healthcare system and this investment in stakeholder consultation is critical to its success.

Enhanced stakeholder engagement remains problematic. Harvey (1991:14) goes on to naively say that 'if the agreed objective is to achieve the greatest health benefit to the community, an equitable distribution of health services and programs will be possible'. Rather, stakeholders will campaign for their own definitions of an equitable distribution. A Victorian study suggests that the major influence on health policy comes from a relatively small network of powerful individuals (Lewis 2006). Public interest groups and social movements have limited bargaining power: 'People join such groups as part of active citizenship. Their commitment to these social movements – for example to the environment … or disability rights is usually additional to their … work in paid employment' (Willis 2002:182). If stakeholder tools are protests and lobbying, they can only bargain with government when they have an organisation able to represent their interests.

Stakeholders also include private interest groups such as the Australian Medical Association (AMA) and the medical colleges who 'act as conservative self-serving lobby groups and as forces for reform' (Willis 2002:183). 'Private groups have expertise that the government must take into account for political reasons. They are able to make informed critical comment on government policy' (Willis 2002:184–185). As Dzur (2002:178) notes, the professions are 'crucial dimensions of the intermediary realm between individual and state. They are political entities, not just when they form interest groups, but because in the intermediary realm of civil society, professions possess the power to distract, encourage, limit and inform public recognition of and deliberation over social problems'. Attempts to engage clinical stakeholders may appear adequate on paper, but often fail in practice if only those with the time and interest to attend meetings are consulted. There is a need to ensure stakeholders are representative members of a community (Bound 2006) and this is especially so where policy is co-created.

Improved accessibility of information

The modern versions of the one-page 1990 policy directives would now take longer to develop due to the need to incorporate evidence and stakeholder input. However they would be immediately available, once 'signed off', to anybody in the health system with access to the intranet, including frontline staff (see Box 12.3). Accessibility also brings implicit accountability for actions contained in the policy and the potential for ad hoc implementation, although this may not be an issue if an implementation plan accompanies a policy directive.

Box 12.3 Implications for practice – Disseminating policy

The internet is not as profound a means of communication as might appear. Alert systems for what is new and important are not well developed. Departmental websites are complex and information rich, but require a high level of skill to navigate. Sophisticated search engines are rarely available. Few staff have the knowledge of structures that would determine the potential location. As an example, a search on the NSW Health internet site for a guideline that was said to accompany a circular entitled 'Management of fresh blood components' was made using the terms 'transfusion guidelines', 'blood guidelines' and 'management of fresh blood components' and produced no items. A search simply using the term 'blood' produced 365 documents.

For some staff the content of policy directives may become like the 'small print' on a banking document – what could be described as 'white policy noise', something not for one to read or act on, yet whose existence provides a veiled threat. The potential is for a culture to develop defined by loss of control – 'they keep making rules'. Clinicians may feel unable to influence, or even read or find the volume of policy material that is relevant to their work. Clinicians receive around one policy circular per week in NSW (personal communication). Further, the complexity of more highly developed policies may limit implementation, as the message is no longer simple, and a large volume of material will dissuade people from reading it in detail unless they 'have to'. Those who 'have to' read such policies are managers, and some organisational power undoubtedly comes from managers understanding the rules and regulations which 'they' apply variably. Yet there are those who don't 'have to' read them for whom the policy may have direct impact, or should inform their work. Policy is not well able to penetrate beyond the professional bureaucracy to practitioners; doctors in particular often don't see themselves as accountable for implementation of policy, including safety and quality strategies (Shekelle 2002).

The term 'system' is often used to describe health services organisation, and doctors objectify, reify and distance themselves from 'the system' (Jorm et al 2006). Vilification of management is the norm. The problems of a teaching hospital in Sydney were recently attributed by doctors to the (local) management's 'obsession with filling out useless forms and mindless application of protocol' (Benson & Wallace 2007:10). The call was to '(f)ire all the middle management in hospitals who have created this environment and contribute nothing and you will have plenty of hospital funding' (Benson & Wallace 2007:10).

According to Lipsky (1980) public policy is not best understood as made by government or by high-level bureaucrats but created by the daily actions of 'street-level' workers. These street-level workers are the professionals actually involved in service delivery and they make policy in three ways: by possession of information (e.g. indicators), by policymaking by discretion (the choices professionals have about the extent to which they follow policy) and by cumulative action (e.g. mass refusal). This means that messages, information and influence pass from top to bottom *and* bottom to top.

Policy directives in 2007

Policy directives in 2007 are quite different from those in 1990 (see Box 12.4). Those relating to blood and payment of ambulance transport are freely available on health department intranet sites and the internet. Each circular still contains a distribution list, which is still the subset of staff who 'have to' receive, read and take responsibility for others acting on the directive. However, the mechanism for reaching managers and clinicians is still inconsistent and relies on people at multiple decision points within the health department and corporate structures of private services being aware of the policy and recognising its applicability to their service. Further, many medical staff don't functionally report to a manager as many are part-time contractors.

Box 12.4 Case study – Policy directives in 2007

The ambulance transport charges document has been regularly updated, most recently in 2004 and still deals exclusively with transport charges. The charges are now detailed; the document is three pages long, and the costs for a transfer capped at just under $4000, but there is still no reference to the broader context of the clinical and social aspects of patient transfers.

The blood directive has also been updated multiple (10) times and 2002/92 is now a circular entitled 'Management of Fresh Blood Components'. It has increased in size to two pages with a cover sheet detailing status. It was published on 27 January 2005 and is due for review in 2010. It has four major headings. The first is the 'Purpose of this circular'. This is stated to be: '… For use by clinicians, hospital transfusions staff and health service managers … involved in the collection, storage and transfusion of fresh blood and blood components. It sets out the mandatory requirements for … transfusion therapy'. The circular references an accompanying guideline that includes the mandatory requirements and additional information on better practice. Justification is also given for both the circular and the guidelines; these are: avoiding transfusion reactions and appropriate use of a 'precious resource'. After 'Purpose', the subsequent headings are 'Obligations of a clinician', 'Obligations of the hospital transfusion service' and 'Obligations under clinical governance'.

The complex committee structure (that includes many stakeholders) for the governance of blood and blood products in NSW is also available on the NSW Health internet site (see www.health.nsw.gov.au/public-health/clinical_policy/blood/nswarrangements/index.html), but is not included or referenced in either the circular or the guidelines. The 'Guidelines' are a 21-page document referenced with both legislative requirements and evidence. The guidelines do include mention of the subjects of the 1990 memo: information on directed blood donation and a mention of a reporting route for graft versus host disease. However while the need to obtain patient consent and explain the risks and benefits of transfusion forms part of the guideline (Appendix on Clinical Care) no details of the risks are provided. There is no tool to discuss risks with patients, yet such a tool is surely necessary for compliance. Internationally the adoption of decision aids to support patient choice has been tardy, despite evidence of the value of such aids (O'Connor et al 2007). The circular specifically details three items that represent only a small part of the total guidelines: transfusion verification procedure, the procedure for collecting and labelling specimens and the statement that small facilities must not store RH negative blood. It is not clear why these three items have been selected to feature in the circular.

The introduction of accountability mechanisms

Here we discuss the introduction of accountability mechanisms, and consider the effect that the safety and quality movement has had on the dynamic development of policy and of practice. We also consider the place of clinical governance as an organisational framework for accountability and improvement, and, last, we discuss the place of regulatory policy.

The effect of the safety and quality movement on the dynamic of policy and practice

Safety and quality introduce special policy issues to health. These are often emotive, used by both politicians and healthcare professionals to achieve their policy aims as stakeholders, and, at times, to resist change. Healthcare is also the subject of intense media coverage, and in the UK the ratio of negative to positive stories in the print media has increased (Alia et al 2001).

It is customary to ascribe the origins of the quality and safety movement to the Harvard Medical Practice study (Brennan et al 1991), the Quality in Australian Healthcare Study (Wilson et al 1995) and the Institute of Medicine report 'To Err is Human' (Kohn et al 1999). However, public trust in Australia wavered after a series of high-profile public inquiries into failures in safety and quality of care, namely those concerning:

- The King Edward Memorial Hospital, Perth (Australian Council for Safety and Quality in Healthcare 2002)
- The Camden and Campbelltown hospitals, Sydney (Pain & Lord 2006)
- The Bundaberg Hospital, Queensland (Forster 2005).

The processes, quality and balance of inquiries can vary. Often they take on the characteristics of a witch-hunt (Beckett 2002) as release of information leads to wider, damaging consequences where the innocent can be punished and an atmosphere of hysteria leads to false accusations. But public inquiries can also bring public catharsis (Walshe & Higgins 2002) and substantially alter public opinion (Brunton 2005), especially if they produce appealing and plausible interpretations of events to repair damaged social institutions (Brown 2003), if they become a lever for change (Walshe & Higgins 2002) or through regulatory reform (Quick 2006). Against this backdrop the safety and quality movement uniquely drives policy (Liang 2004) providing reasons to increase regulation (Mello et al 2005) and accountability, the latter often via clinical governance mechanisms.

Clinical governance

The term clinical governance, introduced in 1998 (Donaldson & Gray 1998), describes an organisational accountability framework for improvement, to safeguard high standards and for excellence to flourish in clinical care. Many specific items have subsequently been added to this framework or 'umbrella'. The NHS clinical governance support team (http://www.cgsupport.nhs.uk/about_cg/) states: 'Underneath this umbrella are several key components and themes, all of which, when effective, combine to make up good clinical governance ... each [element is] of equal value and importance ... interdependent and mutually reinforcing.' While the components in published lists vary, elements can be separated into the disciplinary devices of inspection and moralising devices designed to enhance collaboration (Iedema et al 2005). Inspectorial devices include: data generation and analysis; performance monitoring and management; accreditation; guideline and protocol production and implementation; and the close integration of clinical work data with financial data. Moralising devices include: open disclosure, no blame, a just culture, a safety culture, leadership, teams, collaboratives, consumer involvement and patient centredness.

The current blood circular introduces the notion of 'obligations *under* clinical governance'. Clinical governance is a powerful policy framework able to comprehensively envelop all aspects of clinical care and work practices to engage frontline staff to control, direct and theoretically improve care. The multiplicity of devices under the umbrella of clinical governance assists policymakers in developing 'dispersed and devolved systems of policy implementation, where mechanistic and "top-down" command-and-control processes are ineffectual' (Flynn 2002:160). Clinical governance in the UK has been described as quite a fundamental shift in the relationship between the state and the healthcare professions (Flynn 2002). Employees are given responsibility for quality and *self*-surveillance, but performance is also monitored by managers via targets, incentives and sanctions. In Australia different structure and funding arrangements make clinical governance less visible than in the UK.

Regulatory policy

Embedding best practice is difficult (Greenhalgh et al 2005). Medical leaders alone have been unable to improve the quality of care (Dixon et al 2007) and mandating best practice via policy is seen as an alternative. In the 1990s policy directives were not accompanied by tools to implement or monitor uptake, and neither health services nor the health department had mechanisms in place to measure and evaluate policy uptake or effectiveness. Local health service managers were left to determine how policy was implemented, which, not surprisingly, resulted in a variety of processes and procedures across the entire system. Detailing policy specifications to overcome this variation has not been sufficiently successful, giving way to further attempts to enforce healthcare policy by regulation.

A further regulatory strategy commenced in the 1990s when contracts with services began to include performance targets for patient outcomes. These were later associated with sanctions, penalties and incentives. An extension of this strategy is contracting with individuals to achieve key performance indicators (KPIs), that is, requiring managers to meet clinical quality and efficiency targets. Types of accountability include financial accountability introduced in the 1970s (The 'Cogwheel' Reports 1967/1972/1974), and the introduction of pay-for-performance (P4P) schemes that link clinical and financial accountabilities. Nagel (2006:4) suggests that 'the trend in public management is focused on outcome-based policy where public sector managers are held accountable for results and afforded more discretion as to the means of their achievement'. This approach, implemented widely in the US (see for instance the AHRQ resources at www.ahrq.gov/qual/pay4per.htm), is seen by McLoughlin & Leatherman (2003) as imperative to achieve improvements in care in the UK. Paying general practitioners in the UK to ensure basic management of chronic disease, for instance, has proven effective (Dixon et al 2007), albeit unexpectedly expensive. Queensland is trying a more limited approach via the development of clinical networks based on the Queensland Health Clinical Practice Improvement Centre (CPIC) (Ward 2006) that use clinical practice improvement payments to provide a financial incentive for good-quality care linked to performance against defined targets that requires networks to collect and report data.

Further, patient safety has been used to justify a push for so called 'responsive regulation' to replace self-regulation (Healey & Braithwaite 2006). Mello et al (2005:375) in turn call for 'rational regulation' arguing that '(p)atient safety today exemplifies that eclectic mix of regulation that can occur when a new problem is exposed to the general public'. Australian regulation is undoubtedly eclectic. The mix of accreditation, licensing and the requirements of private insurers and government departments is a duplicative, expensive and unreliable way of ensuring the safety and quality of healthcare. Other regulatory experiments in Australia include the Quality Systems Assessment (QSA) program that aims to provide evidence of assurance of compliance with policies, standards and guidelines and assessment of the level of development of a patient safety system, clinical quality improvement, improvement at a local, facility and systems level and the identification of future risks to patient safety (see www.cec. health.nsw.gov.au/moreinfo/more_QSA.html).

Individual inquiries into health services also bring increased regulation. The Health and Quality Complaints Commission (HQCC) was established in Queensland following the Forster Report (2005) into Bundaberg Hospital. This oversight body aims to guide health service providers about what is expected in the areas of monitoring and improving the quality of health services. Following its inception, the HQCC has released statutory standards under section 20 of the Act establishing a legal duty that '(a) provider must establish, maintain and implement reasonable processes to improve the quality of health services provided by or for the provider, including processes: (a) to monitor the quality of health services and (b) to protect the health and well being of users of health services'.

Conclusion

A view often expressed in health circles is that despite the rhetoric of reform little has changed. We do not share this view and our examination of policy instruments over the past 17 years indicates just how far the system has come. Policy developed now reflects myriad developments in healthcare improvement that are in turn reflected in the dynamics of policy development and implementation. Policy directives in healthcare in 2007 are very different in format and in the nature of their development from those of 1990.

Modernising policymaking has been irregular across Australia and across the health sector, but it has occurred. Stakeholders are more visible, are consulted in greater numbers and more often. Engaging stakeholders early in the policy process is now commonplace. Distributing policy is electronic and immediate. This alone does not necessarily translate into greater penetration of policy, but the increasing accompaniment of policy initiatives by guidelines, tools and extensive education and training suggest that implementation is being taken seriously and is being more effective. Evidence may never quite have the place in policymaking that some desire; there are good reasons why it sits apart, but efforts are under way to maximise its use in policymaking.

Accountability mechanisms have taken on a broader framing in health policy in response to quality and safety concerns. Clinical governance is a somewhat vague umbrella of elements that constrain and direct practice, reinforced by an increasing tendency to regulation. The hybrid of clinical governance aims to codify clinical standards and to evaluate performance while giving the semblance of delegated autonomy, but in reality professional expertise becomes subject to increased managerial control (Flynn 2002). There is nothing protective about the umbrella of clinical governance. It will not protect the status quo but it will have a profound effect on practice. Indeed, the proliferation of accountability mechanisms may mean that there is a risk that monitoring can become an end in itself (Michael 2005).

Clearly, in this context the key questions for modern health policy are: What is the best mix of policy levers to improve health system performance? (Dixon et al 2007); and What will health policy look like in the future? Hopefully there will be less ambiguity. While ambiguity serves to protect the writers and implementers of policy against failure, it must be reduced. The best way to reduce it is by using policy pilots. 'Although pilots or policy trials may be costly in time and resources and may carry political risks, they should be balanced against greater risk of embedding preventable flaws into a new policy' (Government Chief Social Researcher's Office 2003:2). Policy pilots give more prominence to the whole process of evaluation that can then continue into long-term outcomes evaluation. Policy pilots do have significant resource implications, but 'getting it wrong' also has costs, and those that pay in healthcare are the patients who ultimately suffer from unsafe and poor-quality care. Policy developers must build motivation to participate via communicative work at all levels during development and add to it via training. Health policy must be allowed to do its job – to better manage clinical work.

References

Alia N, Lo T et al 2001 Bad press for doctors: 21 year survey of three national newspapers. BMJ 323(7316):782–783

Almeida C, Bascolo E 2006 Use of research results in policy decision-making, formulation, and implementation: a review of the literature. Ca Saude Publica, Rio de Janeiro 22: sup: S7–S33

Australian Council for Safety and Quality in Healthcare 2002 Lessons from the Inquiry into Obstetrics and Gynaecological Services at King Edward Memorial Hospital 1990–2000. Canberra, Australian Council for Safety and Quality in Healthcare

Australian Institute of Health and Welfare (2001) Health and Community Services Labourforce 1991(AIHW cat no HWL 19). Australian Institute of Health and Welfare, Canberra

Beckett C 2002 The Witch-Hunt Metaphor (And Accusations against Residential Care Workers). British Journal of Social Work 32:621–628

Benson K, Wallace N 2007 No commitment to care: staff bemoan lack of care. The Sydney Morning Herald. Sydney

Booth T 1988 Developing Policy Research. Avebury Aldershot, Hants, England; Brookfield, VT

Bound H 2006 Assumptions within Policy: A Case Study of Information Communications and Technology Policy. Australian Journal of Public Administration 65(4):107–118

Bowen S, Zwi A et al 2005 What evidence informs governmental population health policy? Lessons from early childhood intervention policy in Australia. NSW Public Health Bulletin 16:11–12

Brennan T A, Leape L L et al 1991 Incidence of adverse events and negligence in hospitalized patients. Results of the Harvard Medical Practice Study I. New England Journal of Medicine 324(6):370–6

Brown A 2003 Authoritative Sensemaking in a Public Enquiry Report. Organization Studies 25(1):95–112

Brunton W 2005 The place of public inquiries in shaping New Zealand's national mental health policy 1858–1996. Australia and New Zealand Health Policy 2(24): doi10.1186/1743-8462-2-24

Canadian Health Services Research Foundation 2007 Received Wisdoms: How health systems are using evidence to inform decision-making. Vancouver, Canadian Health Services Research Foundation

Culyer A, Lomas J 2006 Deliberative processes and evidence informed decision making in healthcare: do they work and how might we know? Evidence and Policy 2(3):357–371

Dixon J, Chantler C et al 2007 Competition on Outcomes and Physician Leadership Are Not Enough to Reform Health Care. JAMA 298(12):1445–1447

Dobrow M, Goel V et al 2006 The impact of context on evidence utilisation: A framework for expert groups developing health policy recommendations. Social Science and Medicine 63:1811–1824

Donaldson L, Gray J 1998 Clinical Governance: a quality duty for health organisations. Quality in Health Care 7(suppl):S37–S44

Dzur A 2002 Democratizing the Hospital: Deliberative-Democratic Bioethics. Journal of Health Politics, Policy and Law 27(2):177–211

Flynn R 2002 Clinical governance and governmentality. Health, Risk and Society 4(2):155–173

Forster P 2005 Queensland Health Systems Review – Final Report. Brisbane, Qld Government

Girgis A, Johnson C et al 2006 Palliative Care Needs Assessment Guidelines. Department of Health and Ageing, Canberra

Government Chief Researcher's Office 2003 Trying it out: the role of 'pilots' in policy-making. Cabinet Office Strategy Unit, London

Greenhalgh T 2007 Evidence as complex innovation. public lecture for National Institute of Clinical Studies, 20 Jul 2007, sydney

Greenhalgh T 2007 Evidence as complex innovation. Public lecture for National Institude of Clinical Studies, 20 Jul 2007, Sydney

Greenhalgh T, Robert G et al 2005 Diffusion of Innovations in Health Service Organisations. A systematic literature review. Blackwell, Oxford

Harvey R 1991 Making it Better. Strategies for improving the effectiveness and quality of health services in Australia. Background Paper No 8. Australian Government, Canberra

Healey J, Braithwaite J 2006 Designing safer health care through responsive regulation. Medical Journal of Australia 184(10):S56–S59

Hoff T, Jameson L et al 2004 A review of the literature examining linkages between organizational factors, medical errors, and patient safety. Medical Care Research & Review 61(1):3–37

House of Commons Science and Technology Committee 2006 House of Commons Science and Technology Committee: Scientific Advice, Risk and Evidence Based Policy Making. The Stationery Office, London

Iedema R, Braithwaite J et al 2005 Clinical governance: complexities and promises. In: Stanton P, Willis E, Young S Health Care Reform and Industrial Change in Australia: Lessons, Challenges and Implications. Palgrave MacMillan, Basingstoke pp 253–278

Innvaer S, Vist G et al 2002 Health policy-makers' perceptions of their use of evidence: a systematic review. Journal of Health Services Research and Policy 7(4):239–244

Jorm C, Travaglia J et al 2006 Why don't doctors engage with the system? In: Iedema R (ed) Hospital Communication: Tracing complexities in contemporary healthcare organisations. Palgrave, Basingstoke, pp 222–243

Kohn L, Corrigan J et al 1999 To Err is Human: Building a Safer Health System. National Academy Press, Washington DC

Laupacis A, Straus S 2007 Relevance and Rigor of Systematic Reviews. Annals of Internal Medicine 147:273–274

Lewis J 2006 Being around and knowing the players: Networks of influence in health policy. Social Science & Medicine 62:2125–2136

Liang B 2004 A Policy of System Safety. Harvard Health Policy Review 5(1):6–20

Lipsky M 1980 Street-Level Bureaucracy: dilemmas of the individual in public services. Russell Sage Foundation, New York

McLoughlin V, Leatherman S 2003 Quality or financing: what drives design of the health care system? Quality & Safety in Health Care 12(2):136–42

Medical Professionalism Project 2002 Medical professionalism in the new millennium: a physician charter. Ann Intern Med 136(3):243–246

Mello M, Kelly C et al 2005 Fostering Rational Regulation of Patient Safety. Journal of Health Politics, Policy and Law 30(3):375–426

Meyer J, Alteras T et al 2006 Toward more effective use of research in state policymaking, The Commonwealth Fund:1–26

Michael B 2005 Questioning Public Sector Accountability. Public Integrity 7(2):95–109

Milewa T 2006 Health technology adoption and the politics of governance in the UK. Social Science and Medicine 63:3102–3112

Morgan G 1997 Images of Organization. Sage, London

Nagel P 2006 Policy Games and Venue-Shopping: Working the Stakeholder Interface to Broker Policy Change in Rehabilitation Services. Australian Journal of Public Administration 65(4):3–16

National Health Strategy Working Group 1991 Hospital services in Australia: access and financing. National Health Strategy Issues Paper No. 2. Australian Government Publishing Service, Canberra

O'Connor A, Wennberg J et al 2007 Toward The 'Tipping Point': Decision Aids And Informed Patient Choice. Health Affairs 26(3):716–725

Oxman A, Lavis J et al 2007 The use of evidence in WHO recommendations. The Lancet 369(9576):1883–1889

Pain C, Lord R 2006 Lessons from Campbelltown and Camden Hospitals. ANZ J Surg 76(Suppl 1): A42–A44

Palmer G, Short S 2000 Health Care and Public Policy 3rd Edition. Macmillan Press, Australia

Quick O 2006 Outing Medical Errors: Questions of Trust and Responsibility. Medical Law Review 14:22–43

Shekelle P G 2002 Why don't physicians enthusiastically support quality improvement programmes? Quality & Safety in Health Care 11(1):6

Sheldon T 2005 Making evidence synthesis more useful for management and policy-making. Journal of Health Services & Research Policy 10(Suppl):1–5

Shojania K G, Grimshaw J M 2005 Evidence-Based Quality Improvement: The State of The Science. Health Affairs 24:138–151

Shortell S, Rundall T et al 2007 Improving Patient Care by Linking Evidence-Based Medicine and Evidence-Based Management. Journal of the American Medical Association 298:673–676

Spitz B, Abramson J 2005 When Health Policy Is the Problem: A Report from the Field. Journal of Health Politics, Policy and the Law 30(3):327–365

Swerissen H, Duckett S 2002 Health Policy and Financing. In: Gardner H, Barraclough S (eds) Health Policy in Australia. Oxford University Press, Victoria, pp 13–48

The 'Cogwheel' Reports (1967/1972/1974). Joint Working Party on the Organisation of Medical Work in Hospital. HMSO, London

Tunis S, Stryer D et al 2007 Practical Clinical Trials Increasing the Value of Clinical Research for Decision Making in Clinical and Health Policy. JAMA 290(12):1624–1632

Walshe K, Higgins J 2002 The use and impact of inquiries in the NHS. BMJ 325:895–900

Ward M 2006 Queensland Clinical Networks: Safety and Quality Aspects. Online. Available: www.healthnetworks.health.wa.gov.au/acnc/docs/presentations/070424_Prof_Mike_Ward.pdf 4 Oct 2007

Willis E 2002 Interest Groups and the Market Model. In: Gardner H, Barraclough S (eds) Health Policy in Australia. Oxford University Press, Melbourne, pp 179–200

Willis E, Stanton P et al 2005 Health Sector and Industrial Reform in Australia. In: Stanton P, Willis E, Young S (eds) Workplace Reform in the Healthcare Industry: The Australian Experience. Palgrave Macmillan, Hampshire, pp 13–19

Wilson R M, Runciman W et al 1995 The Quality in Australian Health Care Study. MJA 163:458–471

Appendix 1 NSW Health circular 90/29 issued 24 April 1990

```
                                    DEPARTMENT OF HEALTH, N.S.W.

                                    McKell Building
                                    Rawson Place
                                    HAYMARKET   2000

A.  25          H                   217-6666 extn.   5979

B.  21          I                   (Dr. Gerard Cudmore)

C.  29          J 27                File No:  C6408

D.              K                   Circular No:    90/29

E.              L 15

F.                                  Issued:     24TH APRIL 1990

G.  19  (Distributed in accordance with Circular List/s
         A, B, C, G, J, L)
```

<u>BLOOD TRANSFUSIONS: TRANSMISSION OF
INFECTIOUS AGENTS
AND DIRECTED DONATIONS</u>

The Red Cross Blood Transfusion Service has advised that all blood packs issued in the future will have the following additional information on their label:

WARNING: THIS PRODUCT MAY TRANSMIT INFECTIOUS AGENTS

All health professionals involved in the administration of blood products should be advised that this warning has been instituted.

The Red Cross Blood Transfusion Service has also advised of recent evidence that directed blood donations from first degree relatives (parent, sibling or child) may cause graft versus host disease when transfused, even though the recipient may <u>not</u> be immunocompromised.

Although this complication appears to be uncommon, all directed donations from first degree relatives should be irradiated prior to issue. A suitable irradiator is operating on a 24-hour basis at the Red Cross Blood Transfusion Service at 153 Clarence Street, Sydney, Telephone (02) 229 4444.

Directed donations from first degree relatives which are collected in non-metropolitan areas without irradiation facilities may be irradiated at the Clarence Street Blood Bank by arrangement.

Irradiated blood has a shortened shelf life and has a 5 day expiry from the date of irradiation.

B J AMOS
<u>Director General</u>

Appendix 2 NSW Health circular 90/122 (issued December 1990)

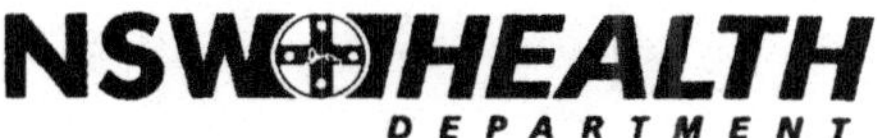

CIRCULAR

File No	C.8235/4
Circular No	90/122
Issued	17 DECEMBER 1990
Contact	John Neilson 391 9100 EXTN: 9164

INTER HOSPITAL HELICOPTER TRANSPORTS

Prior to 1 March, 1990, Area Health Services/hospitals were charged the Road Ambulance or Air Ambulance rates for helicopter transports, to a maximum of $1,800.

Effective from 1 March, 1990 the full cost of inter hospital helicopter transports including the cost of Medical Retrieval Services and any road ambulance component are charged to the Area Health Service/Hospital requesting such transport by helicopter as opposed to road and fixed wing. No charges are levied for primary response transports initiated by the Ambulance Service.

Billing of the charges are carried out by the Ambulance Service and payment to the Service is to be made within twenty one days of receipt of the account.

Funding of these transports is to be encompassed from existing budgets.

Mr R. Wraight,
A/g Director General

Distributed in accordance with circular list(s):

A 113	B 88	C117	D	E
F 38	G	H36	I	J107
K	L	M	N	P

73 Miller Street North Sydney NSW 2060
Locked Mail Bag 961 North Sydney NSW 2059
Telephone (02) 391 9000 Facsimile (02) 391 9101

Chapter 13

Involving communities in decision making

Gavin Mooney

Introduction

Ultimately, it is for patients that we seek to improve the management of clinical processes. In recent years, the place of patients and consumers of healthcare has shifted. The view of patients as passive receivers of healthcare is being replaced by one of communities as equal partners in decision making about healthcare priorities, contributing their opinions alongside those of bureaucrats and policymakers. Through 'deliberative democracy', this involvement takes a number of forms, such as citizens' juries in which the UK is leading the way (Bristol Primary Health and Social Care 2006, McIver 1998). As a process, deliberative democracy is being used in different ways and for different purposes. In this respect, the chapter discusses the issue of community governance and distinguishes different levels of community involvement: in decision making, principles setting and being consulted. It briefly outlines the historical context of community participation in health and the values and benefits of community participation in setting principles and priority setting.

The chapter examines the principles, purposes and advantages of bringing 'the community' more into decision making in healthcare, especially where the question arises of whose values are to be used. The principles on which deliberative democracy might be built are many but foremost are issues of democracy and social justice. The chapter goes on to address the question of what sorts of issues around decision making it is appropriate to bring community values to bear. Deliberative democracy holds out a number of advantages, including greater readiness to comply with policy and hence boost policy effectiveness and efficiency. At a much broader level, it can help to build a greater sense of community and enhance social cohesion.

While different processes exist for eliciting preferences from communities when decisions are being made, in this chapter citizens' juries are proposed as often the best way forward. Citizens' juries bring a random selection of citizens together, give them good information and a chance to quiz experts and thereafter discuss and reflect on certain questions about healthcare, against a background of resource constraints. An Australian example of a citizens' jury is presented and advanced as one that could be replicated to good purpose elsewhere. The way citizens' juries can be used to aid in setting priorities is outlined.

The chapter concludes by summarising the outcomes of community participation, the advantages it brings and how to manage the plurality of interests and grapple with balancing power in decision making. Finally, the impact of these outcomes is discussed as service objectives and priorities are reconsidered.

Background to community involvement

This section examines the principles, purposes and advantages in bringing 'the community' more into decision making in healthcare, especially regarding the question of the values to be used in healthcare planning and priority setting.

What constitutes community is clearly crucial to this discussion, and it is unfortunate that the concept is not agreed in the literature. The community is not 'all things to all people'; rather the existence of many different communities needs to be acknowledged. Boswell (1990:5) argues that the exploration of what is meant by community is 'hindered not by the complete absence of community ideas but by their pervasiveness. In fact, they are all around us but in immature, secondary or emasculated forms. This produces a widespread illusion that they are alive and well, and do not need intellectual effort'. Generally, communities are conceived of as geographically located. This represents the most common usage and the most long-standing usage historically. There are however various other possibilities. Prominent among these are social groupings that can be ethnically, religiously, sports or recreationally based.

In the context of economics, and possibly of other concerns, the issue that separates those who seek more emphasis on community and those of a more individualistic bent (most liberals and certainly neoliberals) is the nature and importance of choice. Bell (2004) argues that the former cast doubt 'on the view that choice is intrinsically valuable, that a certain moral principle or communal attachment is more valuable simply because it has been chosen following deliberation among alternatives by an individual subject'. Bell makes the further point that 'the valorization of greed in the Thatcher/Reagan era justified the extension of instrumental considerations governing relationships in the marketplace into spheres previously informed by a sense of uncalculated reciprocity and civil obligation', that is, what are in essence features of a strong community. Health and healthcare are included in these spheres, which were not previously, but now are often seen as able to be governed by the forces of the marketplace. There has been a move to 'commodify' healthcare in the past 20 years or so, with increasing tendencies to see it as a market good. This has been accompanied by a willingness to consider privatisation as the way to deliver healthcare well, where 'well' is seen in terms of market efficiency with equity disappearing from view. It would be an exaggeration to suggest that health has become a private good (it is not a good at all if that is defined as something that is capable of being traded); nonetheless the way that health is being seen in public policy places it more at the door of individual responsibility.

Individualism increasingly dominates even within public health services, for example in the measurement of health. Further, the language of the market and market-based managerialism is becoming more pervasive: public healthcare has 'providers', 'consumers' and 'business plans'. As the ethos of the MBA takes over, health services as social and community institutions succumb to quantification through performance indicators and worshipping at the altar of QEBM (quantified evidence-based medicine) (Mooney 2004). The notion of a community 'caring about' (Little 2000) its members and caring about community health is lost; not because it is absent, but because it is not measurable.

In this chapter, two important issues differentiate a community focus from the individualism of marketplace liberalism. The former allows for, indeed encourages, the inclusion of intangibles such as compassion and cultural diversity, and is more likely to encapsulate the value of process as well as outcomes. Conversely, the individualism of liberalism is concerned with consequences, that is, what is measurable at an individual level, and makes claims to be universal. Marketplace liberalism and certainly neoliberalism are concerned with freedom of choice, with the emphasis on individual choice. An added assumption is that individuals are willing, and able, to exercise consumer sovereignty, indeed that there is a moral goodness about individual choice. This strand can be further split into two parts: the first being about choice per se, and the notion, through choice, of 'revealed preferences', that is, that studying individuals' choices in the marketplace allows us to judge what their preferences and strengths of preferences are; and the second, the fact that this choice is *individual* choice.

To what extent, though, can choice be only individual when goods are held in common? As Taylor (1989) writes

> The crucial point ... is this: since the free individual can only maintain his identity within a society/culture of a certain kind, he has to be concerned about the shape of this society/culture as a whole. He cannot ... be concerned purely with his individual choices and the associations formed from such choices to the neglect of the matrix in which such choices can be open or closed, rich or meagre. It is important to him that certain activities and institutions flourish in society. It is even of importance to him what the moral tone of the whole society is ... because freedom and individual diversity can only flourish in a society where there is a general recognition of their worth.
>
> If realizing our freedom partly depends on the society and culture in which we live, then we exercise a fuller freedom if we can help determine the shape of this society and culture.
>
> Taylor (1989:47)

There is much to discuss in adopting a community perspective of choice and decision making. There are social aspects that a marketeer will choose to ignore or play down. The concepts of freedom are different, especially in the neoliberalism of the marketplace. Oddly, as Taylor hints, freedom is not consciously and overtly valued in the marketplace in the sense that it is not seen as being in need of protection. Rather it is taken for granted, as a given. The market delivers freedom. This is close to being a mantra: a fundamental belief, and as with most fundamental beliefs not open to question – not even subject to question. In a fully fledged market one individual freely exchanges with another individual and they only freely choose to do so if they both believe that they will thereby be better off. The case is proven!

The shaping of the economy follows from this two-person exchange, as the whole economy can be seen as simply a large number of such two-person exchanges all entered into freely. In recent years in the wake of inter alia Thatcher's famous statement that there is no such thing as a society, the economy and society have become – in neoliberal speech – synonymous, and the word citizen is obsolete as the consumer becomes all that individuals are seen to be. The shaping of society for those who still believe in such an entity can in turn be left to the market and individuals do not have to be concerned about it.

Emphasising community does three things. First, it shifts concern to the shaping of society and a belief that issues around health and healthcare cannot be left to individuals qua individuals. It is citizens as moulded by the society or the community who shape, and, importantly, are shaped by, the society or community. Here, community identity and individual identity are interlocked and interdependent. The distinction between citizen and consumer thus becomes critical. The distinction is well made by McPherson (1977) who claims that

> [o]ne can acquire and consume oneself, for one's own satisfaction or to show one's superiority to others … whereas the enjoyment and development of one's capacities is to be done for the most part in conjunction with others, in some relation of community. And it will not be doubted that the operation of participatory democracy would require a stronger sense of community than now prevails.

> (McPherson 1977:99)

Boswell (1990) makes a separate but related point regarding the distinction between citizens and consumers.

> The participatory democracy model has been sharply contrasted with the view which sees democracy primarily as an output mechanism, a begetter of wealth and economic growth. It has been said that this latter concept essentially views human beings as infinite consumers and accumulators … whereas under the participatory model we are to regard ourselves primarily as exerters and enjoyers of our capacities.

> (Boswell 1990:31)

Second, it is based on the assumption that community preferences will not equate with the summation of individuals' preferences. There are contexts in which individual votes cast in secret can be the way to reach decisions for the group or community, but having people debating and reflecting as a community on issues can come up with different answers and in some instances may be a preferable way of reaching decisions. Third, it brings out as important the idea of establishing what may be best described as the social good of healthcare. This might be simply in terms of 'outcomes' such as health, or perhaps through the 'capabilities' of Sen (1992); such capabilities being about freedoms to be or to act: in essence, freedoms to function.

Anderson (1993) argues at a general level that democratic institutions allow people to live in the sorts of social conditions where they have the autonomy to express and live their own values in ways with which they are happy. She is derisive of the idea of commodity fetishism where all that is valued by people is available in the marketplace. What is needed, she suggests, is to create institutions where people have voice directly and do not have to operate through so called experts. The same argument can be used more specifically for healthcare consumption and for health in general. Anderson's 'institutions of voice' are particularly important in healthcare if the healthcare system is seen as a social institution. There is very clearly a need for agency – the expert doctor assisting the ill-informed patient – at the level of the doctor–patient relationship. There is a tendency however for this issue to have a spillover effect when it comes to health services as systems. Doctors can become embroiled in discussions about the healthcare system as a system: whether it is adequately funded, what the priorities ought to be in terms of diseases or types of beds, lengths of waiting lists, and so on.

Such involvement is not necessarily problematic in itself, but it is too often conducted in terms that suggest doctors are experts at these levels. They are not.

Joan Robinson (1972) makes the point that

'[n]o-one who has lived in the capitalist world is deceived by the pretence that the market system ensures consumer's sovereignty'. She continues: 'The true moral to be drawn from capitalist experience is that production will never be responsive to consumer needs as long as the initiative lies with the producer... In a planned economy the best hope seems to be to develop a class of functionaries, playing the role of wholesale dealers, whose career and self-respect depend upon satisfying the consumer. They could keep in touch with demand through the shops; market research which in the capitalist world is directed to finding out how to bamboozle the housewife could be directed to discovering what she really needs; design and quality could be imposed upon manufacturing enterprises and the product mix settled by placing orders in such a way as to hold a balance between economies of scale and variety of tastes.

(Robinson 1972:274)

The parallels with healthcare are very real. Consumer sovereignty does not exist in healthcare and we can go further and argue that consumers do not want it to exist. It is not, as the standard health economics literature implies with agency, that the agent is there to assist the consumer to make decisions that he or she would make in the market if as well informed as the agent. This role cannot be played by the doctor. We need another type of 'functionary' as Robinson suggests (see above) 'whose career and self-respect depend upon satisfying' not the consumer but the patient. We have par excellence in healthcare a situation where 'production will never be responsive to consumer needs as long as the initiative lies with the producer'.

The healthcare sector needs to be responsive not to consumer needs per se but to community needs and preferences. The patient is often heavily dependent on the doctor to act in the role of his or her agent. There is information asymmetry between them. That is accepted by both sides. It is the main reason why we train doctors to such high levels and a reason why we ask them to abide by ethical codes of conduct. It would be grossly inefficient for patients to chase information themselves. Nonetheless, there is an unfortunate tendency to assume that the citizen suffers from information asymmetry in respect of decision making in healthcare and that he or she is willing to hand over decision making at this level to managers and senior doctors. In some instances they may, but they need to be asked, and when the doctors and managers are not willing, there need to be mechanisms available to allow citizens to be involved. This is where deliberative democracy comes into play.

Why bother with deliberative democracy?

There is a lengthy history of seeking to involve citizens or the community in health service decision making. In 1954, the World Health Organization (1954) argued for such a shift to embrace citizens' values in health service decision making. Such a move has been frequently endorsed since then (Vuori 1984), most recently by the Romanow Commission in Canada (Romanow 2002). Regardless, Australian governments have been slow to engage citizens in healthcare decision making.

To some extent the expectations of participation depend on the context in which it is set. At its most fundamental, there are two, perhaps three, overarching objectives in healthcare. The simplest is to make the health service 'better'; the second is to foster democracy and democratic governance; and, while furthering social cohesion and better social institutions is related to the second, it is given a separate heading here because of its potential importance. There are problems with 'doing better': What is meant by 'better' and how might such betterment be evaluated or measured? 'Better' is often interpreted as 'more efficient' (Abelson & Eyles 2002) and this objective is less likely to be achieved through technical efficiency than through allocative efficiency. The former is about doing better or doing more with the same resources. This is not something that citizens can be expected to get worked up about or to address with any degree of knowledge. It is a 'technical' matter. The public are likely to recognise that and to leave it to the technicians, that is, various healthcare professionals and managers.

Allocative efficiency is where the impact of community consultation is to be felt. It is about maximising benefit with the resources available – often described as 'doing the right thing'. Abelson & Eyles (2002) argue that 'public participation may potentially contribute to the effective performance of the health system by helping to create a fully informed citizenry, transparency and, ultimately, accountability, and in this way contribute to the achievement of efficiency goals'. By putting it in these terms Abelson & Eyles miss a key point. Allocative efficiency involves judgments about how best to use resources. This 'best' is value laden and switching from one group's values (say healthcare managers') to another's (say citizens') may well result in a different answer. There might be agreement between the managers and the citizens about the effectiveness of an intervention in, say, providing more care for the elderly living at home or about the effectiveness of another intervention for screening women younger than currently for Down syndrome, but how the two groups judge the relative value of the two effects may differ. This is a major part of what allocative efficiency is about; it is where citizens' values may lead to a different allocation of resources.

It becomes obvious that trying to evaluate and measure any impact on allocative efficiency using citizens' values is difficult. The role of the public official or bureaucrat in the absence of citizens' values should not be to use his or her own values but to try to reflect the values of the community served. Thus, provided that any consultative process manages to elicit genuine community values – and assessing that is hard – then if the process results in some recommendation to alter the allocation of resources from that which the managers would have recommended, there has to be an improvement in allocative efficiency. Thus, in pursuing allocative efficiency, it is clearly better to use direct community values than public officials' proxies for community values.

Fostering democracy and democratic governance is an accompanying issue. While perhaps instrumental, some writers (Kashefi & Mort 2004) argue for this as an outcome, consequence or benefit in its own right. Kashefi & Mort warn against some of the problems of settling for instrumentality. 'Incidental' consultations are deeply mistrusted and can be seen as 'social control disguised as democratic emancipation' or 'simply … ways of deflecting criticisms of mainstream (un)democratic practice' (Glasner 2001:44). These same authors express concern at 'the heavy reliance by health and social care agencies on the extractive, incidental outputs of the consultation industry'. Certainly, there are risks associated with public consultation. It can result in a cynical response in attempting to build democratic governance, and this author has experienced such cynicism in facilitating citizens' juries, albeit from a small minority of jurists. Most enthusiastically endorse the process and express positive feelings (even delight!) at being involved.

Despite the reservations of some observers (e.g. Abelson & Eyles 2002), the experience of this author (e.g. Mooney & Blackwell 2004, Mooney 2007) is that in asking people to put on their citizens' hats and think and act and judge and express preferences as citizens about some big broad issues such as: What values should underpin your health service? They revel in doing so. Abelson & Eyles' experience is clearly different; they feel more comfortable in getting citizens to pursue issues in which they have a self-interest. The differences are no doubt real. This author has encouraged citizens to be citizens of whatever jurisdiction was relevant, such as a citizen of the state of Western Australia and not of Perth or Geraldton or Kalgoorlie. Of course they bring their values to the table, but they seem able to be 'state' citizens rather than 'town' citizens, and most importantly, 'citizens' rather than 'consumers' or 'patients'.

Building democratic governance into health services will never be easy. If it is to happen, it involves inter alia somebody somewhere giving up power: politicians or bureaucrats or senior doctors. If the process is to work, the group who must be won over is the politicians. Fortunately they are the least obstructive. They have something to gain by being seen to listen to the voice of the informed citizen. Bureaucrats and senior doctors lose power with no balancing factor. Related to this second point is the role of public participation in building new social institutions and in turn social coherence. (The latter may well be advantageous in the context of the social determinants of health but other than noting that and its potential importance, the point is not taken further here.) There are arguments (Muller 2003) for seeking to build new social institutions at this point in history. In Australia, for example, the recent past and especially the past decade has seen major erosion of some social institutions: the public service has become more politicised; there has been heavy political leaning on the public broadcaster; the independence of the judiciary has been threatened; the structure of the economy has become more neoliberal and the tax base has shrunk with a resultant move to market power and away from democratic government control; and globalisation has seen a shift of power to international organisations, such as the World Trade Organization, and to international controls at the expense of local democratic freedoms.

It would be foolish to suggest that threats to our freedom can be halted by organising a few public consultations on Australian healthcare. There is an argument, however, that to start a trend in that direction could be important. It makes a lot of sense to start the process in health, given the concerns that the public have regarding healthcare at any time, but especially now. There is an interest in the pursuit of social justice in this sector which is perhaps more telling and simply stronger than in many others.

Community consultation about what?

There are all sorts of issues in which and for which the involvement of citizens might come into play. Their involvement can be used for decision making at a national level down to some very local town or village locality. There is no strong argument for ruling out any of these levels in principle. Citizens do need to feel involved. Such feelings are perhaps stronger at a local level but in the author's experience people in Western Australia have had no problem in acting as citizens at the state level. What is more open for debate is the locus of the decisions and the level or specifics of involvement (Mooney 2007).

Perhaps the best way to use citizens is to get them to inform the ethical base of health service decision making, providing – or as a minimum assisting in providing – the values or principles on which to base healthcare delivery. It might stop at this level and the example given below is about setting principles. How to decide what citizens should do or get involved in is not easy, but there are two key guides. First, the issues to be addressed by citizens must be ones in which they want to get involved. They need to be able to claim some ownership of them. If they do not, then they and those seeking their involvement may be wasting their time. Second, but closely related, the issues ought to be ones that citizens have some knowledge of or can obtain adequate knowledge of without too much effort. Citizens are not well placed to form judgments about which medicines to prescribe in particular circumstances for instance, and the chances are they will not want to anyway.

'The legitimacy' of whatever a community consultation comes up with also matters. There are two sides here: the citizens' and the current decision makers'. First, citizens will be quick to be cynical about being consulted if they feel that they are out of their depth technically or they are being used as pawns or as a means to allow decision makers to put a tick in a box saying 'community consulted'. Second, there will be many, particularly those who have the property rights, that is, the power over decision making currently, who will be willing to criticise anything that communities come up with: the matters are too complex for ordinary citizens; citizens really don't want to be involved; these are technical matters; consulting the community is always flawed and biased; whoever leads the process will lead the citizens; and so on. Against this background, the question of legitimacy to decision makers inevitably looms large. Ensuring that citizens are randomly selected, that they are well informed and that they avoid wish-listing by having their preferences constrained within some limited resources helps to reduce criticism of the values they derive. Decision makers are more likely to accept community values if they are about broad value issues than if they get closer to the technical province of, say, medical matters. Such issues as equity, its definition and relative importance are ones that most would concede are the legitimate concern of the public.

Priority setting

The other issue that citizens might legitimately participate in, closely aligned with principles and values, is that of priority setting. Who should set priorities in healthcare remains an issue of debate. Whatever the flaws and problems in involving informed citizens in a priority setting approach, there is no better group to do so if these priorities are about more macro-level issues, such as choosing between different disease groups or between the health of different social or cultural groupings. For more technical matters, such as the mix of employment of different categories of staff, the role of citizens is likely to be less and in some instances minimal or zero. (See Iedema, Sorensen, Jorm & Piper, Chapter 7.)

What does priority setting involve? There are many different approaches to priority setting (Honigsbaum et al 1995) but the one most commonly advocated by economists is 'program budgeting and marginal analysis' that involves:

- giving a picture of what current spending goes to in terms of 'programs' such as client groups (e.g. care of the elderly, mental health, maternity care) or disease groups (cancer, heart, diabetes) or geographical or social groups
- then asking: if, say, $1 million were taken from care of the elderly and transferred to child care would the loss in benefit to the elderly be less than the gain for children? If the answer is yes, then efficiency tells us to make that shift. And then ask the same question with respect to another $1 million.

The idea here is straightforward and rational. Making such comparisons of these 'marginal' changes between programs, hence the name Program Budgeting and Marginal Analysis (PBMA), is difficult in practice since it can involve trading off very different forms of benefit – apples and oranges. But people do in reality trade off apples and oranges and as citizens they can do it in heathcare as well. Olsen & Donaldson (1998) asked a Norwegian community to choose between more hips, more hearts and a helicopter ambulance. The community were able to do so. Such a choice involves trading off quality of life with hips; quantity of life with hearts; and primarily equity with the helicopter ambulance.

Should citizens make choices such these? It is difficult to see who else could. In Australia, priority setting has largely been left to politicians and the Australian Medical Association (AMA). There is nothing 'wrong' with that, at least with respect to politicians. The question is: Can it be better? This is an ethical question. Much that democratically elected politicians decide has by its nature to be determined in some broad mandate at elections where health is considered in a package with education, foreign affairs, tax policy, and so on. Deliberative democracy at least allows something closer to 'grass roots democracy'. It can also capture finer detail than is possible at elections, such as the principles that might underpin healthcare policy.

Another argument for involving citizens directly is that they can act as a countervailing power to bureaucrats and medical organisations such as the AMA in Australia. The former can and do influence policy using their own values, sometimes doing so explicitly, more often implicitly. Such a position is defended on the basis that otherwise there would be a values vacuum. The latter do so by powerful lobbying and they are not neutral. Countering pressure from medical associations is for governments and bureaucrats. One way of doing so is to be able to say: 'Ah the people have spake and what they say is ...'

Having found that the four citizens' juries in WA with which the author has been involved have tended to support greater equity in resource allocation in the state health service (Mooney 2007), particularly Aboriginal health, the author has attempted to use this information in the media to influence public debate. Quoting the voice of the people is certainly more powerful than that of one academic health economist.

Citizens' juries – an example

Public consultation comes in all sorts of shapes and sizes. Citizens' juries are the main focus of discussion here; others are consensus conferences, deliberative polling, focus groups, public meetings and forums, and population surveys of various types. Citizens' juries are preferred because:

- they are randomly selected
- they avoid the self-selection bias of many of the others
- the participants are directed to be and think as citizens
- they meet as a group which inter alia strengthens the community/citizen role
- they have time to reflect and deliberate as a group
- the information base they work with is common, or at least what they are presented with by experts
- they do not have to receive the information passively (they can question the experts and ask for additional information)
- they can be constrained in terms of the resources at their disposal in making their choices, which avoids wish-listing (which other forms of consultation can promote).

Following is an example of one particular citizens' jury. The example is from Australia, although the principles and practice involved can be usefully applied elsewhere. This jury was held in Busselton, southwest Western Australia in October 2005 and was followed by, and the results used to inform, a public health forum that took place on the succeeding two days. That forum involved 260 people including members of the public who were not randomly selected, health service staff, healthcare consumers, local government staff and councillors and other community representatives. Their task was to look at more operational issues, but beyond mentioning that public forum, no more is made of it here.

Citizens' jury – the background

This section explains the background to the citizens' jury, sets out the values and principles they came up with, describes the citizens' evaluations of the process and presents a short conclusion.

A group of citizens was randomly selected from the southwest of Western Australia from the electoral roll (but additionally with two Aboriginal people chosen separately). About 30 of these people expressed interest. These were whittled down to 13. The process ensured a good mix of age, gender and geographical location.

The purpose of the jury was to allow the local health service, the South West Area Health Service (SWAHS), to tap into the community's preferences for the principles and values they wanted to underpin the local health service's decision making.

The jury was brought together for an evening mainly to 'break the ice' and to be given a little more information about what was involved in the jury process. They were asked to consider themselves as being citizens of the southwest – not from Bridgetown or Albany and not bringing their own personal baggage with them. Primarily, however, the evening session involved socialising over a meal.

The jury was also given an example of principles but deliberately not from the health sector as this might have influenced them in their choice of principles. Education was used and principles such as preparation for the workforce, advancing academic standards, and being good citizens were presented and discussed.

On the following morning the citizens were reminded that they were to act as citizens of the southwest. They were told that what they came up with would be used first as the basis of the deliberation at the health forum on the subsequent two days and thereafter as the values foundations on which SWAHS would plan in future. In these two contexts their findings were to be sacrosanct.

They were then presented with information by 'experts' (senior SWAHS staff) on the health of the people in the southwest and relevant demographics, the services currently available, the resources available and their current deployment, safety and quality issues, and the organisational and other constraints that SWAHS faces. They were also given the opportunity to quiz the experts who presented the information.

It was clear that some of these 'experts', in this case bureaucrats, struggled with the idea that citizens' values should count. The CEO championed the idea, which left his fellow bureaucrats having to comply with the process and indeed the values. It is around such issues that a strong champion for citizens' juries is necessary.

Thereafter the jurists were given time to reflect and discuss as a group what principles and values they wanted to underpin the decision making of SWAHS. They then came up with a list of these principles and values, set out below.

Finally, the jury endorsed the principle of involving the community in establishing the principles and values on which SWAHS should base its decision making. They were very much in favour of the principle of informed citizens setting the principles.

The principles and values of decision making in healthcare

Fairness
The principle on which the citizens placed most weight was fairness (equity). They defined this in terms of equal access for equal need, where equal access would involve equal opportunity to use health services. The barriers to using health services were

seen as many and included money, distance and racism. Equal access was seen to arise where people perceived the barriers they faced to be equally high; need was taken to be capacity to benefit (i.e. how much good could be done?) and benefits to disadvantaged people were to be weighted more highly (e.g. higher weighted health gains for Aboriginal people) as a form of positive discrimination.

They had a particular concern for those people who were most disadvantaged, especially the health of Aboriginal people.

At the same time the jury acknowledged that there can be a trade-off or competition between equity and efficiency. They felt that from what they had heard from the experts, the existing balance between the two would be improved if more weight, especially geographically, were placed on efficiency and less on equity.

Efficiency

Efficiency was seen by the jury in two ways: first in terms of doing things as well but more cheaply or doing more with the same resources; and second it was about doing as much good as possible (benefit maximisation) with the resources available.

The citizens were of a view that the second type of efficiency needed more emphasis, that is, there needed to be more consideration given to priority setting across different programs. For example should SWAHS spend more on maternity care even if that meant less on care of the elderly?

With one notable exception they were less inclined to argue for higher priorities and increased spending for certain specific areas than for ensuring that such priority setting was done explicitly. The exception was services for the mentally ill.

Where they would have made savings if these had to be made was through hospital rationalisation. They believed that the existing deployment of resources to and in hospitals and emergency departments was potentially inefficient and asked that SWAHS examine ways to rationalise these. They suggested for example that some of the hospital buildings might be converted into aged care facilities or used to provide services for the mentally ill.

Trust with respect to safety

A third principle or set of principles related to quality, safety and risk management. In this context their strategy could be condensed to what amounted to one of trust. They trusted SWAHS to 'take care of' these issues on behalf of the southwest community.

Prevention

The next principle was prevention. They wanted a higher priority for prevention but sought to emphasise the need to target prevention activities and ensure that health service resources for prevention were then used efficiently and did result in 'value added'. By this they meant that, where other organisations (e.g. the Cancer Council, Heart Foundation) were already involved in prevention, SWAHS should avoid duplication and concentrate on prevention that would not otherwise be pursued.

In discussing health promotion within the context of prevention they saw the objective of such health promotion as being about promoting informed choices on health issues.

Self-sufficiency

This area sends some of its patients to Perth, which is the capital of Western Australia, with major tertiary level hospitals. Given that for some patients there is choice between treating them locally or sending them to Perth, the question arises then as to the extent to which this should occur. Is there a desire for greater self-sufficiency in the southwest? On this principle, the citizens had no strong views but felt that total self-sufficiency did not make sense. They argued simply that the extent of self-sufficiency must and should vary by condition.

Holistic care

The jury expressed concerns about practising medicine and treatment in terms of 'body parts' medicine and saw an increasing role for holistic health. In this context they considered the Aboriginal Community Controlled Health Organisation (ACCHO) type model as being a useful one for all patients and not just Aboriginal people (Mawson et al 2007). This model seeks to reflect the preferences of Aboriginal people for health and in turn health services to be seen as whole of body health and healthcare.

Transparency and accountability

The citizens supported transparency and accountability in decision making in SWAHS. They saw the holding of the citizens' jury as an indication of a willingness on the part of senior management at SWAHS to attempt to be transparent and to boost accountability to the public.

Community values

Finally the jury endorsed the principle of involving the community in establishing the principles and values on which SWAHS should base its decision making. They were very much in favour of the principle of informed citizens setting the principles.

Citizens' evaluation

After the event the participating citizens were mailed a questionnaire asking them to evaluate various aspects of the jury process. Most responded by mail; four were interviewed by phone. There was thus a 100% response. The general response of the citizens to the jury process was one of satisfaction, approval and enthusiasm. More specifically:

- With respect to information most but not all agreed with the decision not to provide advance reading. Nonetheless, overall more information would have been better. It seems that it is with respect to the amount of information where things might be improved rather than with respect to the type of information.
- The time allotted for the jury's deliberations, from 9am to 4pm in the one day, was for some rather too little, for others about right. No one argued that it was too long.
- Several points were made with respect to what was thought to be the best aspect of the whole process, and insofar as anything emerged as a general picture, it seems to have been the opportunity to have been involved in the group process. No picture emerged of what the worst aspect was.

Summing up citizens' juries

The overall conclusion of the organisers was that the citizens' jury had been a success. The participants were able to act as citizens and were comfortable to play this role; they believed they do have a role to play in health service decision making; they were able to reach a consensus on a clear set of values and principles; and they felt the process was enjoyable and worthwhile. Perhaps the key findings beyond that are that they wanted more resources for prevention, more for Aboriginal health and more for the mentally ill. Forgoing spending on hospitals and emergency departments was their way of freeing the resources for SWAHS to be able to pay for these extras which they sought.

It is relevant to note that in the subsequent forum the values and principles that the jury developed were overwhelmingly endorsed by the members of the forum.

Experiences with the four citizens' juries that the author has facilitated in Western Australia suggest that the people on the jury very much like the idea of being given the role of citizens (Mooney 2007). It is worthy of note that they seemed to see this as being rather novel and they embraced the role with great enthusiasm. All the juries were of the view that one of the best aspects of the system was being given the opportunity to sit with other citizens, to be able to express their views in a structured way and to have their voices heard.

Conclusion

The voice of citizens in decision making and priority setting in health is essential because budgets are finite and means must be found to allocate available resources rationally. Community participation in healthcare is advantageous in delivering more efficient healthcare and more broadly in assisting to enhance democracy. For the first, efficiency is more likely to come from allocative efficiency than from operational (i.e. technical) efficiency. It can lead to better allocation of resources in the sense of doing more social good. It can create an environment where there is more debate about the objectives and goals of the system. The sort of community consultation that is likely to prove most fruitful is that which emphasises citizens acting in the role of setting principles and values to underpin healthcare delivery. Here objectives and goals which are too often just assumed or implied can be held up to public scrutiny and if desired changed.

The enhancement of democracy is no small advantage but certainly cannot be achieved if it is only the health sector where citizens' juries are used. At this level there needs to be a more general consideration of the relationship between the voice of the people and the nature of our social institutions. It is here that examination is required of how to manage the plurality of interests and grapple with balancing power in decision making. Democracy can be thick or thin or anywhere in between. Increasingly we are faced with a thinner and thinner version in Australia. Community consultations used honestly and genuinely to allow the voice of the informed people to be heard more is a way to thicken democracy and our democratic institutions, including in healthcare. Managing clinical processes will only be effective if the 'right' healthcare decisions are being made. Healthcare decisions that respond to community needs and preferences are those that this chapter seeks to address.

References

Abelson J, Eyles J 2002 Exploring the Link Between Public Involvement/Citizen Engagement and Quality Healthcare A Review and Analysis of the Current Literature. Online. Available: http://www.hc-sc.gc.ca/hcs-sss/pubs/qual/2003-qual-simces/2003-qual-simces-6_e.html 25 Sept 2007

Anderson E 1993 Value in Ethics and Economics. Harvard University Press, Cambridge

Bell D 2004 Communitarianism. Online. Available: http://plato.stanford.edu/entries/ communitarianism 25 Sept 2007

Boswell J 1990 Community and the Economy. The Theory of Public Cooperation. Routledge, London

Bristol Primary Health and Social Care 2006 Towards a more caring city. Report of the 2006 citizens' jury on the research priorities for Bristol primary health and social care – July 2006. Online. Available: http://www.bristol.ac.uk/hsrc/research/other/citizens/report.pdf 25 Sept 2007

Glasner P 2001 Rights or rituals? Why juries can do more harm than good. Participatory Learning and Action Notes 40: IIED

Honigsbaum F, Richards J, Lockett T 1995 Priority Setting in Action Health Services Management Centre, Birmingham. Radcliffe Medical Press, Oxford

Kashefi E, Mort M 2004 'Grounded Citizens' Juries: A Tool for Health Activism? Health Expectations 7:1–13

Little M 2000 Ethonomics: the ethics of the unaffordable. Archives of Surgery 135:17–21

Mawson F, Madgwick M, Judd J et al 2007 Transition to Governance. Building Capacity in an Indigenous Community. Online. Available: http://www.sprc.unsw.edu.au/ASPC2007/papers/Mawson_211.pdf 1 Dec 2007

McIver S 1998 Healthy debate? An independent evaluation of citizens' juries in health settings. Kings Fund, London

McPherson C B 1977 The Life and Times of Liberal Democracy. Oxford University Press, Oxford

Mooney G 2004 Evidence-based medicine: objectives and values. In: Kristiansen I S, Mooney G (eds) Evidence Based Medicine. In its Place. Routledge, London

Mooney G 2007 Citizens' juries: the basis for health policy whoever wins the election? Online. Available: http://cpd.org.au/article/citizens-juries-basis-for-health-policy 1 Dec 2007

Mooney G, Blackwell S 2004 Whose health service is it anyway? Medical Journal of Australia 180:76–78

Muller J Z 2003 The Mind and the Market. Anchor Books, New York

Olsen J-A, Donaldson C 1998 Helicopters, hearts and hips: Using willingness to pay to set priorities for public sector healthcare programmes. Social Science and Medicine 46:1–12

Robinson J 1972 Consumers' sovereignty in a planned economy. In: Nove A, Nuti D M (eds) Socialist Economics. Penguin, Harmondsworth

Romanow R J 2002 Building on Values: The Future of Healthcare in Canada. Online. Available: http://www.hc-sc.gc.ca/english/care/romanow/hcc0086.html 25 Sept 2007

Sen A 1992 Inequality re-examined. Clarendon Press, Oxford

Taylor C 1989 Sources of the Self. The Making of the Modern Identity. Cambridge University Press, Cambridge

Vuori H 1984 Overview – community participation in primary healthcare: a means or end? IV. International Congress of the World Federation of Public Health Associations. Public Health Review 12:331–339

World Health Organization 1954 Report of the Expert Committee on the Health Education of the Public. Technical Report Series 89. WHO, Geneva

Implications for practice

Roslyn Sorensen & Rick Iedema

Introduction

Each of the foregoing chapters contributes to our understanding of why health services should be managed, what should be managed, and, as importantly, how and by whom. This chapter brings together the main points from the chapter contents to draw out the implications for practice.

Clinical process management is embryonic in its development. When considering how to improve the operation and performance of health services, practitioners naturally look to similar environments for ideas. Many processes used in manufacturing and transportation are regarded as sufficiently similar to those in health for adaptation and use. Hence, the principles and practices of other sectors are being appropriated for processes whose specificity we know still little about. For its part, health in Australia is administered by government departments within a largely bureaucratic model.

Consequently, health shares similarities in its model of administration and in its general environment with other public services departments. Included here are firm managerial hierarchies, service rules and regulations, performance discipline and control, a high level of public scrutiny and rigorous expectations of public accountability.

Yet, even though healthcare has similarities with industry, transportation and the public service generally, it is also unique. Much of the technology of healthcare is centred and dependent on social interaction. Further, those who seek health services are in a vulnerable position and reliant on others to define and act in their best interests. Life-and-death decisions are a matter of routine. Individual careers and reputations are made or lost within a competitive social context of clinical care. Moreover, healthcare is practised within an environment of uncertainty and experimentation yet with high technical, ethical and legal standards. Within this dynamic and often turbulent mix, health service managers and clinicians strive to manage the complexity, diversity and uncertainty inherent in health service delivery to the best of their ability. Knowing the methods to do so is important for their success, understanding how 'health' works, and appreciating what it has in common with other administrations and where it differs, is essential to this endeavour.

A range of policy frameworks set the broad directions of healthcare and the parameters within which objectives are to be achieved. In Australia, the Australian Health Care Agreements (ACHAs) is the major policy instrument that delineates healthcare delivery programs, funding models, improvement strategies and performance evaluation. The managerial model on which health policy and health service administration is based is a useful one in healthcare in setting objectives, striking performance targets, monitoring achievement and ensuring resource efficiency, particularly if applied as intended, that is, at arm's length from those setting the objectives. Operating effectively in this environment requires clinicians and managers not only to understand the political environment of health, but also to acquire a high level of process knowledge and managerial skills to transform the environment of healthcare, as commentators in this book describe. In this chapter we discuss:

- transforming healthcare environments
- transforming healthcare practices
- transforming healthcare outcomes.

In concluding, we identify some 'new vehicles' that may have a place in the transforming process.

Transforming healthcare environments

Re-evaluating healthcare priorities

Health is a system in stress. Effectively managing healthcare centres on whether and how the stress can be removed or ameliorated to transform health into a sustainable, coherent, purposefully managed and productive system for those who are treated by it and those who work in it. While, clearly, a link between achieving health targets and the existence of efficient and effective services to do so is self-evident, how governments mediate the link is an issue. Managing clinical processes, we contend, is an essential activity and skill that links health processes to service effectiveness and to outcomes. In learning to manage the pressures and demands on the system that the foregoing chapters outline, services will need the strategic, operational and communicative space within which to experiment. The investment of public funding in health services and their importance to individual and community wellbeing will always mean that health is a political issue. Governments will always need to manage the politics of health. But governments cannot manage health services; they do not have the knowledge, expertise, understanding or commitment to clinical care to do so. Therefore, removing the micromanagement of health problems and distancing health services from the competition and conflict between governments that underlie much of the over-administration and under-management is essential if practitioners are to redesign a system that can respond appropriately to patient and community needs. Change around the margins will not reinvigorate the system as this book envisages. Those committed to achieving high standards of care in well-managed high-performing health services and those who claim ownership of them are most likely to achieve this transformation, particularly if they drive the innovative methods that illuminate how frontline work is done and how it can best be managed.

'Health' is not produced by professionals alone. It is co-produced by clinical caregivers *and* patients, as well as by services *and* communities. Involving communities in healthcare can help set the parameters within which service direction and funding priorities are made. The power that organised communities can bring to bear on elected officials can be formidable, and as Mooney points out, where local communities are given a voice in how funds are spent, the priorities for funding and the values on which decisions are made will inevitably differ from those of health bureaucrats. Similarly, where patients are given a voice in how services and their outcomes are structured, the principles for deciding on the minutiae of clinical treatment and the processes guiding consumers' involvement in dealing with care preferences and unexpected outcomes will also differ from those favoured by clinicians (Iedema et al 2007).

While governments have the responsibility to manage the gap between service demand and supply, they are not the only stakeholder group who can or should make difficult decisions, such as what healthcare 'good' should be funded over another. Nor are they the only ones with the expertise and interest to do so. Economic policy is not a sufficient strategy to manage health services, because the pressures confronting them are not necessarily or not only economic in nature, even though the repercussions of a failure to manage the pressures almost certainly affect 'the bottom line'. Communities also have a stake. Mooney advances a process of deliberative democracy through which the values of communities can be gauged and incorporated into healthcare decision making and that takes local priorities and values into account. Citizens' juries can counterbalance the power of bureaucrats, medical organisations, and professionals generally, and by doing so, the potential arises to move beyond a concept of performance based solely on measurable quantitative indicators to one based also on qualitative measures that concern communities and reflect their values.

Redesigning health systems

Public health services are funded predominantly by public investment. How this money is spent and whether value is achieved are important questions in assessing service efficiency and effectiveness. While indicative of government commitment, the total amount spent on health is not necessarily an indicator of value. Making the best use of the available resources, however, is. As Leggat demonstrates, operations management techniques can improve overall service productivity and quality, and can be adapted to healthcare. Indeed, operations management principles and practices can play a constructive role in addressing the uncoordinated, fragmented and dislocated nature of health services. Small-scale time-limited cycles of product testing (e.g. the PDSA model also discussed later in this chapter), for instance, are becoming essential models for designing and continually improving 'final healthcare products' as the health system reorganises as a production system. Considering the low levels of quality achieved in healthcare compared with those of other industries, applying operations management techniques may be an urgent task in health as long as they appropriately address concerns around clinical work.

In moving to a production-based approach to healthcare delivery clinical and corporate work must be more meaningfully linked, as Leggat also suggests. Integrating measures of performance is a good starting point, specifically connecting efficiency and effectiveness goals and activities within the organisation. Clinical process management skills are those that will aid clinicians and managers to transform inputs into outputs and outcomes, and the structures to support them. Clinical work is the core business of health services and the core process to be managed. It integrates clinicians, and managers, within the interdependent services that, together, produce healthcare and linking the separate processes that constitute clinical work are important steps in this integration. Skill is required to span the boundaries of fragmented services and to produce and manage knowledge between the diverse caregivers within individual services and between diverse clinical, clinical support and administrative support units to produce meaningful information through which service performance can be managed. A key function for managers, then, is to practically support service integration by establishing information systems capable of providing performance data accessible to managers and clinicians alike, constructing indicators of performance across service modalities that take account of the clinical and managerial interests involved, agreeing the indicators that measure performance and value, and reviewing outcomes. This requires investment not only in information systems, but agreement between key stakeholders about what constitutes performance.

Transforming healthcare means shifting the focus from a traditional conception of healthcare as a craft-based service delivered by individual medical practitioners to one based on a set of coordinated activities delivered by a multiplicity of caregivers with a diverse range of skills and expertise, dislocated over time and space but which must cohere to achieve desired outcomes for patients. Doing so calls on health professionals to collaborate to negotiate and design new healthcare products and to coordinate their activities. This implies reconfiguring the roles and responsibilities of those who provide services and realigning professional attitudes, values and relationships as tasks change in line with changing healthcare needs. This reconfiguring presages the importance of an inquiring, competent and flexible workforce within a co-production conception of healthcare outcomes. It also presages the importance of a workforce clear about the objectives of healthcare and their part in achieving them, about what the organisation expects of them and about their role as members of self-directed multidisciplinary teams.

Transforming healthcare practices

Reshaping the healthcare workforce

Stanton identifies opportunities to strategically use human resource management (HRM) to develop a healthcare workforce capable of responding to this dynamic environment. The importance of good HRM practices becomes clear given evidence of the relationship between a competent healthcare workforce and patient outcomes. The variable results of the broad-based industrial relations approach to health sector reform suggests there is a strong argument for building the capacity of local workforces as the instrument of transformation, rather than to pitch reform initiatives industry wide.

Hence, the dimensions of workforce morale, leadership, skill building and collaborative team-based competencies themselves become a subset of high performance practices as Stanton alludes. Included here will be concrete evidence that members of individual caregiving and managerial professions can move beyond sectional professional allegiances to create the democratic practices inherent in collaborative team-based delivery of care. Such practices imply the capacity to share information and decisions, to balance autonomy and accountability, to systematise, standardise and coordinate care delivered by multidisciplinary teams and to measure, monitor and reshape performance as a collective endeavour.

Meshing the different knowledge bases, values and practices of the disparate professions and specialties that constitute modern day healthcare is important in achieving this level of collectivity. As important is taking into account the changing composition of the workforce through increasing feminisation, casualisation and skill escalation. If the healthcare professionals who deliver care are to 'own' the system, and their part in it, all members of the workforce must be able to practically contribute their ideas and enthusiasm, and hence the capacity of managers to appreciate the value of and accommodate employee participation becomes paramount in motivating people to do so. To exploit these emerging opportunities health service managers must reconceptualise HRM as a key transformational strategy.

Reorganising the processes of care

Health services are transformed by linking skilled people with processes that work. In complex, diverse and dislocated healthcare, organising and coordinating care between myriad entities is a standard requirement. Claridge & Cook outline the tools, processes and rules necessary to assist managers and clinicians in this endeavour. As they describe, clinical pathways are a means through which operations management principles can become embedded in health service delivery, and their capacity to assist managers and clinicians to simultaneously manage the seemingly conflicting objectives of efficiency, effectiveness and safety suggest that devices such as this are central to managing clinical processes. Pathways do so by delineating the sequence of diagnostic and treatment activities which diverse multidisciplinary clinicians engage in for specific case types, and, by extension, pathways contain the domains of clinical and organising performance within which measures can be developed around core clinical services. The scepticism that some clinicians hold for these devices is misplaced. By initiating, negotiating and defending them, clinicians own the processes, and by applying them to care routines that can be readily systematised and standardised, they relieve themselves of unnecessarily burdensome tasks and the need to constantly reinvent care routines for individual patients whose care is predictable, thus releasing them for more complex work.

In tandem with process reorganisation comes the thorny issue of managing behaviour. Claridge & Cook conclude that it is an essential component in complying with organisational expectations in which co-negotiated process agreements become central. This process of negotiating and agreeing can allow autonomy of practice to be balanced with accountability for outcomes where discretionary and non-discretionary tasks are identified as part of pathway-based multidisciplinary teamwork. If this is so, then teams become not only the creators and repositories of final service clinical pathways, but also the definers of behaviour and sanctioners of the rules that accompany them. That is, team members themselves make the rules with which the team complies. This element of clinical process management becomes central when seen in the light of evidence-based practice and incorporating the expert contribution of all team members within the concept of collective shared care.

Spanning care boundaries

As Kerosuo points out, this sharing requires the spanning or even possibly the dismantling of the numerous boundaries that hamper it, especially for people with multiple complex and chronic conditions. As she indicates, people now live longer with conditions from which they would once have died much earlier. Solving organisational problems, therefore, goes hand in hand with appropriately mobilising the advanced medical technologies that increase patient longevity. As discussed earlier, coordinating patient care across numerous geographically dispersed caregivers, each of whom offers seemingly different, separate and independent services that can at times duplicate effort to the detriment of the patient and of the service, is one such problem. Clearly, as patterns of care change in response to changing disease patterns and increasing longevity, so too will clinical practice. Kerosuo's discussion of patient trajectories here is illuminating in exposing the missed steps, duplication and misunderstandings that can occur in unattended and uncoordinated patient care. By becoming familiar with these tools and the opportunities they afford to illuminate patient trajectories, communicative spaces are created through which clinicians can identify the missteps, heal the discontinuities and bring a dimension of convenience and satisfaction to themselves and to their patients that is presently unattainable. Socially, these new communicative spaces facilitate disparate clinicians coming together in loosely connected networks as precursors to more tightly coupled multidisciplinary teams.

Reinventing healthcare teams

As these networks and teams form, pathways of care automatically emerge as clinicians and patients solve the problems of discontinuity that become embedded as future practice. Thus, clinical and patient pathways become the systematised products of multidisciplinary team communication. Their existence may also be evidence of effective team processes as the pathways they construct are the products of accumulated evidence and experience. Hence, teams themselves determine the composition of pathway components, incorporate the expertise and knowledge of their individual members and evaluate the results in a series of evolving steps. In expounding on the place of multidisciplinary team care (MTC), Willis, Dwyer & Dunn assert that such teams are a new direction in healthcare. These authors remind us that 'the organisation of clinical treatment is about dealing with human need and suffering'. Thus, teams can also fulfil a key objective of modern day healthcare: centring the patient in healthcare decisions. Through participative team processes patients and families, as well as health professionals, challenge, discard, revise or update new ways forward, critical in environments of uncertainty and experimentation, but also relevant in regular and routine care.

If disciplinarily diverse members of multidisciplinary teams have the capacity to pool information and share decisions, it follows that if the focus of care changes, for instance as clinical circumstances, caregiver capacities and patient needs that can change over time, leadership can also change. Thus, the traditional doctor, nurse and patient hierarchy becomes an anachronism. Yet, as we know, teams are also constituted by members whose individualism and autonomy is often central to their professional training and mode of practice. Clearly, retraining clinicians with individualist orientations as effective team members is a critical factor in transformed healthcare. As well, a level of flexibility and organisational literacy is required in institutional terms for people who participate in different teams, for instance in horizontal teams within clinical workplaces, or in vertical teams within the wider organisation. Even though these teams will have different roles and functions and ways of operating, some level of consistency is also required and this brings with it a dilemma. On the one hand, some advocate explicit procedures and protocols about how teams function, while on the other, there is a danger that proscribing too closely how teams work may be at variance with the flexible approaches advocated for self-directed teams. Nonetheless, in circumstances where power asymmetries proliferate, parameters are needed to guide member behaviour. The critical aspects here, we believe, are accepting the inclusive, democratic nature of teamwork, understanding its purpose and ensuring that meeting processes are explicit and agreed.

Co-producing care

It is through such shared capacities that care is co-produced. As patients and clinicians discuss options together, reveal values and preferences, decide on treatment and agree on plans of care, they produce a collective care product, and as Iedema, Sorensen, Jorm & Piper note, the view of patients as passive recipients of care defined by others is giving way to one of patients as active co-producers of care assisting to define and design the care product they desire to consumer. The newly coined term 'prosumer' heralds this more proactive stance that is as relevant in health, perhaps more so, as it is in industry. It acknowledges that patients themselves are experts in their condition and care and have valuable information and ideas to contribute. It is reinforced by evidence that active patient participation is strongly associated with better patient outcomes. This modern view of consumers presages a new type of work and a new type of worker – one who can acknowledge limitations, exhibit humility, accept others' lay views as important and embrace others' expertise. It also presages a different kind of system, where the participation of consumers is invited, welcomed and valued.

Reconceptualising programs of care

By participating, the expectations of consumers can be shaped, as can those of health professionals. As Berg, Schellekens & Bergen discuss in relation to care programs, the study of healthcare work, such as that carried out by MTCs, lends itself to understanding not only what needs to be done, but also how it can be done differently, thereby redefining what consumers can expect from the service, as well as service standards and services processes. Thus, as the content of clinical work is systematised and standardised for populations of patients in care programs, so too is the organisation of care, and the inconvenience of ad hoc, stepwise, fragmentary, uncoordinated healthcare planning and delivery for both patients and caregivers becomes a relic of the past. However, as intimated throughout the book, the care of some patients is not routine.

Through 'flexibilisation', reconceptualised care programs avoid the danger of a 'one size fits all' approach. The inbuilt flexibility of this 'mass customisation' approach, that is, producing a customised product within a mass-produced process, satisfies the inherent conflict between autonomy and accountability by allowing clinicians to tailor care to the needs of individual patients while taking advantage of production techniques applied to clinical case types to manage the increasing volume of demands for service, quality, safety and efficiency.

A further advantage of the care program model in the context of our discussion is its capacity to be applied systematically within health services to integrate the multiple streams of care, information systems and associated data-gathering capabilities so as to inform and direct improvement strategies that connect them. To do so, it is imperative that data is produced and available in a format and timeframe appropriate for clinician and clinical manager use, and hence redirecting the central monitoring of performance data in administrative formats, to program monitoring of data in clinical managerial formats. As clinicians are judged on their performance rather than status, the organisational dynamics change. Roles become restructured; responsibilities delegated; clinicians and clinical and lay managers develop new skills sets. Care programs are thus evolving entities that become the vehicle for coalescing and embedding the elements of operations management, workforce skilling, clinical pathway development and MTC.

Transforming healthcare outcomes

Reprioritising quality improvement initiatives

Transforming healthcare organisations and healthcare outcomes is a big task that cannot be done all at once. Warburton proposes the Economic Evaluation Loop (EEL) as a prioritising model. By gathering evidence on which to assess the costs and benefits of a change project before it is fully implemented, and by linking this process with the Plan–Do–Study–Act(ion) (PDSA) model of small scale rapid cycle improvements, each cycle is evaluated before proceeding to the next as the process continues throughout its evolving life. The applicability of the model at the clinical, organisational and policy levels suggests that it is an essential tool for cost effectively managing clinical processes. It is immediately applicable, for instance, in testing the components of care programs that Berg, Schellekens & Bergen propose above and becomes part of the new skills of clinical managers. Through this approach scarce healthcare resources are conserved as patient safety and quality improvement projects are evaluated, supported and prioritised based on sound evidence of value.

Rediscovering quality

This concern for quality improvement is not a recent phenomenon. It has had a long history in health organisations as the end point of clinical work. As Boaden & Harvey point out, however, early attempts to encourage quality activities in medical and nursing professions tended to be insular and limited. The organisational-level strategies now focused on promoting technical quality through developing and disseminating evidence via generic tools that replaced profession-specific approaches are being incorporated into policy that mandate organisational responsibility for quality, for instance clinical governance. But the recent high-profile attention given to quality failures and adverse events is pushing quality improvement initiatives under the generic banner of patient safety. As we have argued, patient safety and risk management activities can be practically incorporated as a subset of overall service quality, because quality improvement strategies should automatically take account of patient safety issues. To do the opposite, to separate patient safety into a separate and discrete strategy, holds a danger that patient safety is seen as an 'add-on' to standard healthcare delivery that can be as easily dropped if the need arises. Thus, not only should quality be seen as a multidimensional concept, it is also an essential ingredient in good healthcare to be built into systems and processes from the beginning. What we argue for, then, is not only the importance of technical organising skills through which clinical care processes can be conceptualised, systematised and standardised, but also the importance of possessing the values through which these ideas are promoted and defended, including, importantly, to those who resist modernising practices.

Reducing the risks to patient safety

Merry reinforces the integral nature of quality and its multiple dimensions and warns that an overemphasis on safety 'add-ons' can actually be detrimental to patient care. Notably, while Merry acknowledges that many healthcare processes are open to systematisation and standardisation, many are not, and clinical experience and judgment remain important skills. The caution he counsels is also important. It further reinforces the new skill of identifying where standardisation and systematisation can be applied, and where flexibility must be retained. A similar caution relates to the use of statistical process control methods, promoted in operations management to measure and manage quality and safety. Knowing where such methods can be applied and where they can't further reinforces the centrality of having an intimate knowledge of in situ clinical processes in understanding where this line should be drawn.

The expectations on clinicians and organisations to manage risk are becoming increasingly mandatory. There is ambiguity, however, about the effectiveness of many of the risk management strategies being pursued, particularly if their intention is to protect caregivers rather than patients. Nonetheless, the capacity to classify errors brings the capacity to manage them, specifically to identify their cause and to eliminate or ameliorate their effect. Evidence is imperative but it is not always available, as Warburton notes, and incident reporting, information sharing, clinical expertise and consensus building all contribute to reducing risk. In this regard, those who work in clinical units are those most likely to know the inherent risks and how to address them. Teams become the crucibles for skill development as clinicians deliberate on specialised safety and quality issues and remediate risk. What this implies is that teams are the bedrock of desirable healthcare cultures; ones that exhibit a capacity to collectively develop techniques and processes of a quality service, a language to discuss them, and the behaviour, knowledge and skill necessary to manage safety, reduce risk, improve quality and conserve resources.

Revamping healthcare policy

Policy must support developing cultures. Policy derives from the macro level, such as the AHCAs already mentioned; it also derives from the micro level to frame systems redesign. In comparing two micro-level policies at different time scales, Jorm, Banks & Twohill show just how far policy development has come in supporting systems redesign. Policy now includes a number of mandatory elements not present in earlier policy that assist to standardise policy development and to reduce the variability of its implementation across local health regions. The explicit use of best evidence, the participation of stakeholders, caregiver accessibility to information and explicit accountability mechanisms are all included here, as are consultation mechanisms, although not yet of the standard of deliberative democracy that Mooney espouses.

But problems remain. The paucity of research activity and insufficient evidence to link organisational factors and medical errors and patient safety, for instance, limit the extent to which policy can and does support practice. Further, the distrust of doctors for policy made by credible organisations suggests that the place of policy in clinical practice change is not yet fully accepted. Where clinicians resist evidence and avoid practice change, they become policymakers themselves by virtue of their unilateral actions. Even if clinicians do accept policy change, there are problems implementing them. Policy overload and the failure of directives to penetrate beyond the professional bureaucracy to practitioners impede the type of safety cultures that Merry espouses. Policies that do penetrate, for instance clinical governance, that seek to encourage self-surveillance of clinicians in practice, in reality serve to increase the extent of external manager surveillance that may be a reaction to clinician (non)acceptance of reform. This takes us back full circle, where imposed micromanagement of health problems might appear to solve immediate, short-term problems, but ultimately fails to address the long-term more intractable problems of transforming stressed public health systems.

Conclusion

If, as Busse & Wismar (2002) maintain, there is a relationship between health status targets and health programs, it follows that by improving health services, health status will also improve. Thus, the mere existence of health services is not the single determining factor for achieving health targets; health services must also produce cost-effective care to have maximum effect. How, then, can health services achieve it? In this concluding section, we synthesise the theory and practice of the foregoing chapters to address questions raised at the outset.

As acknowledged throughout this book, the environment of healthcare is transforming: changing social and demographic trends, increasing consumer expectations, the ageing of the population and a rise in chronic diseases are all leading to greater demands for healthcare in hospitals and in the community. These changes put pressure on a system that is neither able nor designed to cope with them. To do so, health services must transform: the labour force must reorganise, health professionals and managers must restructure roles, responsibilities and skills, and policymakers must support clinical process management. As Chassin (1998) asserts, new vehicles are needed to do so. The types of new vehicles proposed in this book are not intended as 'add-ons' to the present systems, but to replace them. This does not mean doing more things; it does mean doing things differently.

Doing things differently means dismantling the service over-administration that Hunter (1996) discusses, and increasing its management. It means accepting that management is at the core of good health service and embracing it as an essential skill. Decreasing central administration will involve delegating responsibility for decisions about clinical care and clinical systems to where clinical work is actually carried out: in clinical units, specifically to the health professionals and clinical managers who manage them. Thus the balance of power shifts from administrators to health professionals as the power to act shifts. Hence, transforming health services requires administrators to relinquish part of their power to others who may be better placed to negotiate the difficult health service and healthcare decisions that transforming requires. But power and the autonomy it implies incur accountability. Health professionals at all levels must accept that having power to decide on the manner in which health services and healthcare are delivered means being accountable to other stakeholders for their outcomes and including them in decisions that affect them.

The place of managerialism in healthcare

Accountability is a key element in the managerial model criticised as inappropriate for administering public services (Considine 1997b), including for public health services (Currie 1998, Learmonth 1997, Marmor 1998). Even though managerialism may have provided a framework to replace 'a variegated, disordered mix of organisational forms and types' (Considine 1997b:94), the 'managerial autocracy' (Considine 1997b) that accompanies it, that is, managerial authority and a manager's right to manage, is strongly contested. However, the expertise and values of health professionals are neither designed for nor sufficient to manage the organisational complexity of modern health services (Marmor 1998), while, equally, the narrow scope of healthcare managerialisation has resulted in a dismissal by many clinicians of the potential benefits of management. This narrow scope is inherent in the set of commercial principles that were simply transferred from private business to the public sector (Painter 1997). By removing the private sector bias (e.g. of cost containment, service rationalisation and top-down performance surveillance) (Considine 1997a), the benefits of managerial intervention might become more apparent, particularly its application in aiding an understanding of the nature of the organisational problems in the health sector and how they might be resolved. Ham's view (2005) is important in advocating for a planning framework within which the overarching objectives of healthcare are agreed and set. How those objectives are met, however, and the strategies designed and implemented to do so are the responsibility of health service and clinical managers and health professionals to determine. We believe this to be the crux of public health sector managerialism. The dichotomy between 'top' decision makers and 'bottom' decision takers is artificial. Both organisational levels have legitimate interests in reform strategies and their outcomes, and each has complementary knowledge and skills to bring to bear. How these two levels of the organisation practically integrate their interests and activities to benefit the organisation as a whole is the core of this book.

The place of consumers

One such reorientation is the place of consumers in health service priority setting and resource allocation, specifically empowering consumers and communities by bringing them directly into health decision making (Anderson 1996). Consumers and communities are the direct beneficiaries of health services and their opinions, preferences and experiences are therefore central. Further, communities are enthusiastic to be involved and their input is constructive (Davis et al in press). Neither health policymakers nor health professionals necessarily know what is best for the 'system', but as the recipients of care, consumers are well placed to assess and comment. Their contribution becomes essential in balancing and arbitrating among the interests of other stakeholders, and is important for de-emphasising economic policy as the main criterion for priority setting. Thus, to reorient the direction of healthcare, communities will share decisions about health service priorities in their local areas through formal, regular communication forums; these processes will be sufficiently flexible to take differing local conditions and local needs into account; and consumers, health service managers and health professionals together will determine their type, frequency and intended outcomes. Feedback will be given to communities about final priorities and justification made if community recommendations are not incorporated.

Evaluating the effectiveness of these consumer-involvement processes to managing health services and to changing the relationship between decision making and health outcomes is mandatory. Evaluation measures will be both quantitative and qualitative, and they will include process as well as outcome measures, because process measures capture important information about care not directly measured as outcomes (Werner et al forthcoming). Patients' perceptions, lived experience and hence knowledge of service impact are examples. With the rise of the prosumer, the social, interactive essence of healthcare is emphasised, and the moral and practical benefits of initiatives such as open disclosure (Iedema et al 2007) presage a very different healthcare reorientation. The preparedness for clinicians to acknowledge, record and address medical incidents, the capacity of patients to define desired components and standards of service expected, and the organisational capacity to systemically, methodically and practically respond to incidents, for instance, are process measures that signify the capacity for improvement in healthcare outcomes that can be measured, monitored and managed.

The place of performance management

It follows that health services should be reconceptualised as single entities whose systems are interrelated and interdependent, rather than a loose collection of seemingly unrelated activities. Performance, then, becomes a collaborative effort, and designing and implementing integrated performance systems reflects this interconnectedness and encourages organisational cohesion and coherence of purpose. Within the framework of health service objectives, performance domains will emerge within which indicators can be developed to measure performance at the clinical program level that are then rolled up to aggregated measures at the corporate level, rather than the other way around. This sequencing mirrors the shift in power and decision making and recognises clinical units as the locus of healthcare. Informed by Barley & Kunda's studies of work (2001) integrated performance systems are capable of responding to changing healthcare objectives, changing consumer priorities and service expectations. These studies, based on grounded methodologies such as ethnographies, recognise communities of practice as the primary unit of analysis, comprised of practitioners who do similar work. Hence, teams are reinforced as the core organising structure in healthcare, and the diversity of clinical expertise that team members contribute fosters service innovation, improvements in patient care and organisational effectiveness as health services transform (Lemieux-Charles & McGuire 2006).

From the foregoing discussion, and for the purposes of this book, we define the main domains of performance as technical, organisational and social. The technical aspects of care resolve around evidence-based best practice treatment of what works to reduce unwarranted variation. Implementing technical best practice consistently, as noted, is difficult. Some health systems allow for the voluntary uptake of evidence by clinicians while others mandate its use. Neither is ideal. The voluntary nature of clinical governance, for instance, means that uptake is sporadic and idiosyncratic, and while mandating has been successful in some countries, for example in France (Durand-Zaleski et al 1997), the strategy is less successful in countries with more conservative and traditional medical professions that operate independent of state control, such as in Australia (Freddi 1989).

Transforming the technical dimension

In the view of Grol & Grimshaw (1999) implementing technical change is best handled as a project with implementation frameworks built into the organisational infrastructure. Steps that cover developing a proposal; analysing the target setting; linking interventions to needs; anticipated facilitators and obstacles; developing a plan; implementing; and evaluating it are all encompassed within such a framework (Grol & Grimshaw 1999). These steps are essential preconditions to technical change (Durieux et al 2000) but are merely formulas if the accompanying social processes to engage the ownership of users and to negotiate and tailor generalised evidence to local conditions (Gibler et al 2005, Parkers et al 2002) are omitted. The myriad stakeholders in health hold different views of its goals and therefore the activities intended to achieve them. Thus, all stakeholders must experience a process of iterative 'sense making' through which users and potential users are given the opportunity to collectively share their views (Clemmer et al 1999), to agree and disagree on organisational purpose, and ultimately to form a consensus about the direction of change, the strategies to implement it and their place in it.

Transforming the organising dimension

Information on which implementation of technical best practice can proceed is drawn from meaningful data. Clinical data systems provide clinicians with information on which to analyse performance, assess effectiveness, and change care regimes accordingly. Obtaining clinically meaningful data requires reconceptualising how care should and can be organised. This involves devising ways through which care that is delivered by diverse multidisciplinary clinicians often dispersed over time and location can be anticipated, coordinated and executed (Timmermans & Berg 1997). Managers and clinicians both need systems capabilities to organise care around programs comprised of clinical case types through which the sequence of care processes is systematised and the quality of care delivered is standardised. Without systems that coherently interconnect care activity horizontally and vertically, clinical and managerial activity cannot be coordinated efficiently, and clinically and managerially meaningful data cannot be produced and compared. These systems of care organisation are also central to managing clinical processes. They not only integrate the process of multidisciplinary sequencing of evidence-based therapeutic and diagnostic events for specific conditions, associated clinical documentation, risk management, quality of care, health outcome indicators, utilisation review and costing (Hindle & Degeling 2000), they are also an information system capable of producing local evidence for evaluation of care effectiveness that then trigger practice improvement. Revised, they are also a patient communication device providing information about treatment and informed consent.

Transforming the social dimension

It is through social interaction that clinicians and managers 'make sense of' the environment in which they work, and patients of the environment in which they are treated. Collaboration and cooperation, therefore, determine the quality of relationships through which clinical work is carried out in health, specifically between doctors and nurses who treat patients in common, but also between clinicians and managers as they develop the intermediate clinical processes that link the particularities of individual patient care to aggregate organisational performance. Thus, health professionals have an organisational as well as professional responsibility to improve collaboration and the quality of interaction as it relates to patient care. Narrative is the way through which emerging and encoded knowledge about patients, patient care and service organisation is transferred (Barley & Kunda 2001:87), specifically through 'narratively oriented teams'. In writing about bed blockage in a stroke program in the Netherlands, van Wijngaarden et al (2006) describe this process of collective learning through which health professionals consolidate the fragmented goals that each has to healthcare, make knowledge between them explicit, and come to an understanding about how the problems between them can be resolved. Indeed, Benner (2001) insists that healthcare teams take responsibility for this collective learning. As communities of practice (Bate & Robert 2003), these teams create communicative spaces to review and produce shared kinds of knowing and doing. As workplace ethnography shows (Iedema et al 2007), such spaces foster cultures of participation as each person understands that work is co-produced, that everyone has a part in producing it and that each needs to iteratively explore, understand and acknowledge what their part is.

Managing knowledge

Teamwork is thus a process of continual structuring and restructuring done through, to and with both technology and people. Anchored in 'thick communication', such teamwork engenders an 'unselfconsciously conscious' manner in staff that Weick & Roberts (1993) call 'mindful heeding', or 'heedfulness'. Heedful health professionals are attuned to the complex dynamics of patient care as well as to each others' ways of engaging with those dynamics. That is, heedfulness is engendered through ongoing communication and frequent co-presence, and this produces attentiveness to staff's own and colleagues' ways of working and coping. In managing clinical processes, the effective organisation of care is based on this social-communicative capability.

Clinicians must have appropriate skills to communicate with patients and with each other, to negotiate roles and responsibilities, to collectively review evidence of outcomes, to negotiate changed forms of care based on this evidence, and to recognise situations that are challenging for themselves or for colleagues, and that require explanation, exploration, and perhaps debriefing. Clearly, such a capacity implies that boundaries are spanned to manage collective knowledge and knowledge-generation between clinicians, patients and relatives within units, between interdependent clinical and service units and between clinical and administrative domains.

The pivotal role of clinical managers

The workforce that will undertake this transformation may not yet be employed in the health sector, or may not yet have the necessary skills. While the participation of all workforce members is implied in the transforming process, the role of clinical managers is pivotal. Understanding what the organisation expects of them, fulfilling an organisational role and accepting organisational accountability for decisions and outcomes is essential to meeting health service objectives. Hence, clinician expectations must be reshaped in the context of transforming health services to include collaboration and cooperation as standard requirements, sincerely supported, sought and promoted. Thus, as pivots, clinical managers must possess a management and organisational orientation that encompasses a *relational* and a *technical* dimension. Relationally, this orientation presupposes ongoing and co-present communication with frontline staff as the principal means for negotiating the complexities of care and disease, for mediating between macro-organisational demands and micro-organisational constraints, and for building commitment across professional boundaries and levels of seniority. Technically, such an orientation presupposes establishing systems through which clinical care is organised, ensuring such systems are iteratively designed and revisited involving all relevant stakeholders, and developing information support systems through which clinicians, managers, patients and communities know the standard of healthcare provided and through which evidence for improvement is gathered. Developing such a workforce capability triggers human resource strategies to recruit managers and clinicians able to accept that management skills are as important as clinical skills and prepared to extend them. Likewise, it triggers corporate managers to activate organisational support services that practically assist clinical managers and clinicians to establish the managerial, organisational, clinical and social-communicative processes that underpin good care.

Balancing autonomy and accountability

Providing services in and being recompensed by public sector organisations implies that clinicians develop a level of commitment to the organisation and its purpose. Their commitment is crucial as health services transform. Yet clearly there is danger in circumscribing behaviour too closely to conform to organisational requirements as there is in privileging unlimited autonomy. What is desirable is to balance autonomy with accountability; maintaining a level of autonomy through which clinicians and managers can respond flexibly to local conditions and individual capacities while at the same time accepting responsibility and accountability for organisational outcomes. Performance contracting at the service and individual level is a way for both services and clinicians to negotiate roles and responsibilities within the evolving parameters of health service objectives: to agree expected outcomes, to negotiate the level and standard of resources commensurate with performance expectations and to balance discretionary and non-discretionary actions in ways that involve adequate inter- and intra-disciplinary communication. Egol et al (1999) call for hospital pathways that formally recognise the role of clinical managers and that detail procedures about establishing multiprofessional team planning and review processes that can identify and solve problems and resolve conflict. These pathways are intended to 'soften' the boundaries that divide health professionals and managers. Inroads are being made through changed roles such as 'nurse practitioner' and 'hospitalist', although the fear of loss of identity, work conditions and entitlements and the still largely clinical orientation of these roles means that transforming highly segmented, fragmented and professionalised health workforces takes time, effort and skill (Doyal & Cameron 2000).

Summing up

The blunt instruments used at the macro level to change the health system, while powerful, cannot open this 'black box' of professionalised clinical work and health service delivery. Value-laden conceptions of managerial models of public sector administration and isolated micromanagement of contentious issues, such as risk management, miss the system-wide and communication-intensive implications of transforming a health service structured as an interconnected entity. Presently, health is managed as a collection of separate services in which medical activities take precedence, in the absence of recognition that wards, clinical support services and corporate functions connect and impact on service effectiveness. Put another way, patients, nurses, doctors, managers, clinical support staff, allied health professionals, hotel staff, administrators and policy-makers, together, produce healthcare. If health services are to meet the care needs of individual patients and patient populations, health services must be managed as a continuum within which each part in the production process interconnects with the next, and the performance of one is recognised as affected by the performance of the service before it. Without this recognition, 'organisational learning' remains single loop, that is, managing active errors, while the double loop learning needed to illuminate and resolve latent errors is forgone (Argyris & Schön 1978).

Managing the system of health and improving the outcomes of those who are serviced by it and the wellbeing of those who work in it can best be achieved by directing effort at understanding how clinical care is actually produced and creating spaces for staff where such understanding can be discussed, extended, negotiated and maintained. This will not be principally at the level of clinical decision making, where the care of individual patients is paramount, nor will it be at the level of management abstraction where disembodied data on budgets, activity, throughput and complaints is primary. It will take place at the level in between, where clinical managers must make sense of the services within their responsibility, where those who produce care must come together in a meaningful way in multidisciplinary teams to plan, organise, deliver, review and improve it as an interconnected process, and where the participation of patients and families is actively sought as a legitimate and essential part of the planning and healing process. This will mean devising a method through which these objectives can be managed simultaneously at the point at which healthcare is produced: in clinical workplaces. The role of clinical managers becomes pivotal in managing the clinical processes of care and the communication processes that such care presupposes, by connecting the resources, skills, knowledge and experience between these two ends.

Moving forward

Many organisations and individuals around the world undertake research and promote the use of clinical process management. To bring this work together, Berding has compiled a comprehensive list of useful sources and resources on the range of issues, problems and solutions contained in the book that are being pursued internationally (see Resources). This list is intended to make this relevant information available for further research to develop knowledge in the field. In her chapter, Berding lists key organisations, accompanied by a description of what can be accessed on their internet sites. These sources are intended to promote clinical process management as an essential set of skills through which clinicians and managers can manage clinical processes in the health services.

As the process of health service transformation proceeds, there is a need to build such a repository of empirical data on work in various settings that can be used for broad comparative analysis. This book is designed to be a part of this repository. It has advanced a range of theory and practice, and has proposed new ideas and instruments to aid the transformation. It has done so by harnessing and combining the skills and knowledge of social scientists, clinicians and economists to lay out a foundation for developing a workforce capable of managing 21st century health issues.

References

Anderson J M 1996 Empowering patients: Issues and strategies. Social Science & Medicine 43:697–705

Argyris C, Schön D A 1978 Organisational Learning. Addison–Wesley, Reading

Barley S R, Kunda G 2001 Bringing Work Back In. Organization Science 12:76–95

Bate P, Robert G 2003 Knowledge management and communities of practice in the private sector: Lessons for leading the quality revolution in health care. In: Dopson S, Mark A L (eds) 2003 Leading Health Care Organizations. Palgrave Macmillan, Basingstoke and New York, pp 81–99

Benner P 2001 Creating a culture of safety and improvement: A key to reducing medical error. American Journal of Critical Care 10:281–284

Busse R, Wismar M 2002 Health target programmes and health care services – any link? A conceptual and comparative study (Part 1). Health Policy 59:209–221

Chassin M R 1998 The urgent need to improve quality. JAMA 280:1000–1005

Clemmer R P, Spuhler V J, Oniki T A et al 1999 Results of a collaborative quality improvement program on outcomes and costs in a tertiary critical care unit. Critical Care Medicine 27:1768–1774

Considine M 1997a The Corporate Management Framework as Administrative Science: A Critique. Institute of Public Administration Australia, Melbourne

Considine M 1997b Managerialism strikes out. In: Considine M, Painter M (eds) Managerialism: the great debate. Melbourne University Press, Melbourne

Currie G 1998 Managerialism in the health service: partnership or conflict in a management development program. Health Services Management Research 11:192–9

Davis R, Koutantji M, Vincent C in press Patients' willingness to question health care staff on issues related to their medical treatment. Quality and Safety in Health Care

Doyal L, Cameron A 2000 Reshaping the NHS workforce. British Medical Journal 320:1023–1024

Durand-Zaleski I, Colin C, Blum-Boiscard C 1997 An attempt to save money by using mandatory practice guidelines in France. British Medical Journal 313:943–946

Durieux P, Nizard R, Ravaud P et al 2000 A clinical decision support system for prevention of venous thromboembolism: effect on physician behaviour. JAMA 283:2816–21

Egol A, Fromm R, Guntupalli K et al 1999 Guidelines for intensive care unit admission, discharge and triage. Critical Care Medicine 27:633–638

Freddi G 1989 Problems of organisational rationality in health systems: political controls and policy options. In: Freddi G, Bjorkman J W (eds) Controlling Medical Professionals. Sage Publications, London

Gibler W, Cannon C, Blomkalns A et al 2005 Practical Implementation of the Guidelines for Unstable Angina/Non-St-Segment Evaluation Myocardian Infarction in the Emergency Department. Circulation 111:2699–2710

Grol R, Grimshaw J 1999 Evidence based implementation of evidence based medicine. Joint Commission Journal on Quality Improvement 25:503–13

Ham C 2005 From targets to standards: but not just yet. British Medical Journal 330:106–107

Hindle D, Degeling P 2000 Managing Clinical Production Systems. The Centre for Hospital Management and Information Systems Research, Sydney

Hunter D J 1996 The changing roles of health care personnel in health and health care management. Social Science & Medicine 43:799–808

Iedema R, Mallock N, Sorensen R et al 2007 Final Report: Evaluation of the National Open Disclosure Program. University of Technology, Sydney

Learmonth M 1997 Managerialism and public attitudes towards UK NHS managers. Journal of Management in Medicine 11:214–21

Lemieux-Charles L, McGuire W L 2006 What Do We Know about Health Care Team Effectiveness? A Review of the Literature. Medical Care Research and Review 63:263–300

Marmor T 1998 Hope and hyperbole: the rhetoric and reality of managerial reform in health care. Journal of Health Services & Research Policy 3:62–4

Painter M 1997 Public Management: Fad or Fallacy? In: Considine M, Painter M (eds) Managerialism: the great debate. Melbourne University Press Melbourne

Parkers J, Hyde C, Deeks J et al 2002 Teaching critical appraisal skills in health care settings [Cochrane review]. The Cochrane Library

Timmermans S, Berg M 1997 Standardization in Action: Achieving Local Universality through Medical Protocols. Social Studies of Science 27:273–305

van Wijngaarden J D H, de Hont A A, Huijsman R 2006 Learning to cross boundaries: The integration of a health network to deliver seamless care. Health Policy 79:203–213

Weick K E, Roberts K H 1993 Collective mind in organizations: Heedful interrelating on flight decks. Administrative Science Quarterly 38:357–381

Werner R M, Bradlow E T, Asch D A forthcoming Does Hospital Performance on Process Measures Directly Measure High Quality Care or Is it a Marker of Unmeasured Care? Health Services Research

Moving forward

Friederike Berding

Introduction

This chapter is designed as a repository of information and useful resources for further research about the major themes of clinical process management presented in the previous chapters. Included here is information regarding:

- pathways
- clinical governance
- quality management/improvement/assurance
- patient safety
- risk management
- evidence-based practice
- guidelines
- performance measurement
- multidisciplinary teamwork
- evidence-based design.

Based on internet research, the chapter provides details about the work of government, academic and provider organisations researching clinical process management and the information provided on their websites.

Resources available from international organisations are presented first. Then the emphasis shifts to organisations in Anglo-American countries including Australia, the UK, the US, Canada and New Zealand. Europe follows including Denmark, France, Germany, Ireland, the Netherlands and Spain. With regard to structure of information under the individual countries, government departments and organisations are presented first, followed by non-governmental organisations and associations.

Resources and information on clinical process management in Asian, African and South American countries such as Argentina, Japan, Malaysia, Singapore, India, China and South Africa are presented based on organisation websites. Where information has been given for international websites, it has been indicated where English text is available or where sites in English are under construction.

International organisations

AGREE Research Trust (ART)

www.agreetrust.org

The AGREE (Appraisal of Guidelines Research and Evaluation) Research Trust (ART) is an international collaboration providing a framework for assessing the quality and effectiveness of clinical practice guidelines. Material relating to the AGREE Instruments such as a training manual and a user guide is available on the website.

Cochrane Collaboration

www.cochrane.org

The Cochrane Collaboration is an international not-for-profit organisation producing systematic reviews of healthcare interventions. The website contains up-to-date information about the effects of healthcare and evidence-based healthcare databases.

Guidelines International Network

www.g-i-n.net

The Guidelines International Network (G-I-N) is an international association of organisations seeking to improve the quality of healthcare by promoting systematic development of clinical practice guidelines and their application into practice. The website links a large amount of web-based information on clinical practice guidelines. The members' section provides access to a database of published guidelines and related details and to tools for producing and implementing evidence-based guidelines. The public sections contain instruments for developing evidence-based guidelines, guidelines and related publications on specific health topics and links for further guideline information.

International Society for Quality in Healthcare (ISQua)

www.isqua.org

The International Society for Quality in Healthcare (ISQua) is a not-for-profit, independent organisation providing services to support excellence in healthcare delivery and continuous improvement of quality and safety of care. It serves as an international multidisciplinary forum designed to share expertise. The website provides information about the organisation's official journal (*International Journal for Quality in Healthcare*) and international conferences and seminars offering the possibility to download selected presentations, poster and abstracts. An extensive list of links to other relevant organisations is also available.

Joint Commission International (JCI)

www.jointcommissioninternational.org

Joint Commission International (JCI) is dedicated to continuously improving the safety and quality of healthcare service through providing education and consultation services and international accreditation.

Joint Commission International Centre for Patient Safety (ICPS)
www.jcipatientsafety.org

The Joint Commission International Centre for Patient Safety (ICPS), a joint initiative of Joint Commission and Joint Commission Resources (JHCR), works collaboratively with other organisations and agencies to continuously improve patient safety in all healthcare settings providing patient safety solutions to healthcare organisations. On the website, the section Patient Safety Practices is an online resource for healthcare professionals and the public. It contains over 900 links to patient safety websites, with tips, tools and resources for addressing patient safety problems. In addition, further information such as abstracts of current literature on patient safety and a sample outline for a patient's safety plan as well as a range of website links are provided.

World Health Organization (WHO)
www.who.int/management/quality/en/

The World Health Organization (WHO) provides on its website the section 'Management of quality care' that deals extensively with topics relevant to quality and safety in health services, including quality assurance, standards, accreditation, user satisfaction, patient safety, and monitoring and evaluation of quality of care.

Various documents produced by the WHO and others containing concepts and issues as well as tools and guidelines are available for download and give comprehensive information on the topics mentioned above.

World Alliance for Patient Safety
www.who.int/patientsafety/en/

The World Alliance for Patient Safety was created by WHO to facilitate the development of patient safety policy and practice as well as the improvement of quality of care worldwide. As a basis for international collaboration and action, the alliance provides on its website information about its activities and research projects, patient safety news of member countries and related events, and solutions for patient safety including extensive information and guidelines. An information centre gives a clear overview of articles, reports and documents that can be downloaded while the Patient Safety Journal library provides access to abstracts of a collection of scientific journal articles that are related to patient safety.

Anglo-American organisations

Australia – government

Department of Health and Ageing (DoHA)
www.health.gov.au

The Australian Department of Health and Ageing (DoHA) publishes on its website a range of statistical information relevant to the safety and quality of Australia's healthcare system and provides links to other Australian and international health-related organisations and resources.

Australian Institute of Health and Welfare (AIHW)
www.aihw.gov.au

The website of the Australian Institute of Health and Welfare (AIHW) provides information and statistics in various areas of health and welfare. The website is clearly divided in subject areas. In particular, the section 'Safety and quality of healthcare' is valuable in providing a comprehensive collection of healthcare safety and quality statistical information from various Australian and international sources that can be downloaded from the website or found through links. Links to other Australian statistical information on safety and quality of healthcare and a comprehensive list of other Australian organisations that provide data and information with a short description and an overview over main reports and data are also available.

Australian Commission for Safety and Quality in Healthcare (ACSQHC)

www.safetyandquality.org

The Australian Commission for Safety and Quality in Healthcare (ACSQHC) aims to develop a national strategic framework and associated work program to improve safety and quality in healthcare. It provides a Measurement for Improvement Toolkit which provides a set of practical methods to measure the safety and quality of clinical healthcare services and can be accessed online. The website also contains a valuable knowledge portal that enables users to search for information on safety and quality in healthcare. It provides collections of links to freely available internet resources, for example to databases, online journals and books, clinical guidelines, pathways and protocols and information for health consumers and about evidence-based practice resources.

National Health and Medical Research Council (NHMRC)

www.nhmrc.gov.au

The National Health and Medical Research Council (NHMRC) is an expert body promoting the development and maintenance of public and individual health standards. In the publications sections of the website, reports, fact sheets, forms and guidelines are available. For example with regard to clinical practice guidelines, the website contains a comprehensive range of general as well as specialist information for researchers, clinicians and other health professionals.

National Institute of Clinical Studies (NICS)

www.nicsl.com.au

The National Institute of Clinical Studies (NICS), an institute of the NHMRC, is Australia's national agency for improving healthcare by helping to close gaps between evidence and clinical practice. The website provides reports that include statistical information on aspects of current healthcare practice, related to best practice information and guidelines implementation resource sheets.

Centre for Research Excellence in Patient Safety (CRE-PS)

www.crepatientsafety.org.au

The Centre for Research Excellence in Patient Safety (CRE-PS) is dedicated to developing national research capability and capacity that in turn improves patient safety. It conducts and promotes research to improve quality, safety, efficiency and effectiveness of healthcare focusing on using data to monitor quality of care, improving information transfer and patient safety, and reducing medication errors. The website contains information on projects undertaken in these areas including projects on performance reporting, quality indicators, team coordination and clinical pathways. Moreover, information about various seminars carried out by CRE-PS, a list of references in part with the option of accessing the full text and the newsletter *Australian Patient Safety Bulletin* are available.

Australian Resource Centre for Healthcare Innovations (ARCHI)

www.archi.net.au

The Australian Resource Centre for Healthcare Innovations (ARCHI) is the knowledge sharing hub for Australian health professionals and health service managers who are working to deliver better patient journeys. More than just a source of information,

ARCHI is a dynamic hub that actively supports the learning process for health professionals. ARCHI supports 'communities of practice' – promoting discussion and sharing tools and resources.

New South Wales

Department of Health

www.health.nsw.gov.au

The New South Wales Department of Health has published information on sentinel events reported by its healthcare facilities. Other recent publications include information relevant to the quality and safety of healthcare that can be accessed through the website.

Clinical Excellence Commission (CEC)

www.cec.health.nsw.gov.au

The Clinical Excellence Commission (CEC) is part of the NSW Patient Safety and Clinical Quality Program. On its website, the CEC provides information about a range of projects and programs currently undertaken by the CEC, for example in the field of quality system assessment, patient safety, leadership and performance indicators. Toolkits for assistance and reports concerning, for example, patient access, clinical quality and its assessment and patient safety are also available online.

Queensland

Queensland Health

www.health.qld.gov.au

Queensland Health has published statistics related to the safety and quality of healthcare in various reports on its website.

Victoria

Department of Human Services

www.dhs.vic.gov.au

The Victorian Department of Human Services has published reports on the activity and performance of its public hospitals.

Victorian Quality Council

www.health.vic.gov.au/qualitycouncil

The Victorian Quality Council was established as an expert strategic advisory group to lead the safety and quality agenda for Victorian healthcare services. The website provides access to publications and resources including safety and quality tools, guidelines, reports, information on workshops and presentations, newsletters and a selection of articles as well as links to related websites.

Australia – non-government

The Australian Council on Healthcare Standards (ACHS)

www.achs.org.au

The Australian Council on Healthcare Standards (ACHS) is an independent, not-for-profit organisation, supporting the improvement of the quality of healthcare in Australia through continuous review of performance, assessment and accreditation. The website contains reports based on clinical indicators reported by healthcare organisations participating in the ACHS's programs.

Australian Patient Safety Foundation (APSF)

www.apsf.net.au

The Australian Patient Safety Foundation (APSF) is a not-for-profit independent organisation dedicated to the advancement of patient safety. Resources available from the website include a list of published articles on patient safety.

The Joanna Briggs Institute

www.joannabriggs.edu.au

The Joanna Briggs Institute (JBI) is an international collaboration promoting health-care that is based on the best available evidence. The website provides access to best practice information sheets on various topics such as the reduction of medication errors, technical reports, the newsletter *The Bulletin*, a comprehensive list of protocols providing information on projects and a links page which is clearly divided into interest-based categories. Furthermore, it contains an online journal and publication collection and databases; however, these are mostly restricted to members' access.

United Kingdom – government

Department of Health (DH)

www.dh.gov.uk

The Department of Health (DH) supports, funds and sets the overall strategic direction for the NHS and social care organisations.

National Health Service (NHS)

www.nhs.uk

> NHS in Northern Ireland: www.n-i.nhs.uk
> NHS in Scotland: www.show.scot.nhs.uk
> NHS in Wales: www.wales.nhs.uk

National Library for Health

www.library.nhs.uk

This website offers access to databases, for example pathways databases, and the organisations creating and using them.

National Patient Safety Agency (NPSA)

www.npsa.nhs.uk

The National Patient Safety Agency (NPSA) has been created to improve patient safety by reducing medical errors and incidents occurring in the NHS. The website is divided into three sections.

Within the *Patient Safety Division*, the NPSA collects and analyses data on patient safety incidents and disseminates advice and solutions on identified issues using three formats (patient safety alert, safer practice notice, patient safety information). Moreover, the website provides tools such as a guide to safer patient care, risk assessment guides or a root cause analysis toolkit as well as information on teamwork and a monthly published patient safety bulletin.

The National Clinical Assessment Service promotes patient safety by providing advice for dealing with performance concerns. The website contains comprehensive information such as toolkits, a resource directory and various publications (reports, case analyses).

The National Research Ethics Service (www.nres.npsa.nhs.uk) promotes and facilitates ethical research to maintain a review system that protects the safety, dignity and wellbeing of research participants. The website provides information on the development of the service and related online resources.

saferhealthcare

www.saferhealthcare.org.uk

saferhealthcare is an online resource to improve patient safety in healthcare settings providing case studies, tools, reviews, news and comments. The website is structured around topics containing information (papers, reports, articles) on issues such as the importance of safety, leadership skills and teamwork, providing analytical tools and theoretical information as well as examples of practice in healthcare settings and the implementation of safety improvement. An area called workspace is available that allows individuals and organisations to keep track of their data in safety improvement work.

NHS Institute for Innovation and Improvement

www.institute.nhs.uk

The NHS Institute for Innovation and Improvement supports the NHS by developing and disseminating new ways of working, new technology and leadership. It has replaced the NHS Modernisation Agency, the NHS University and the NHS Leadership Centre. At the website, the section Quality and Value, which supports the improvement of operating performance, is particularly helpful. It contains extensive information, for example case studies, reviews, presentations, articles and tools, in areas such as lean thinking, experience-based design and indicator development and measurement.

The Improvement Network (TIN)

www.tin.nhs.uk

The Improvement Network (TIN) is involved in improving services for the benefit of patients, service users and caregivers. The website provides information on the development of leadership towards more patient orientation and tools and techniques for service improvement.

Scotland

Integrated Care Pathway Users Scotland (ICPUS)

www.icpus.ukprofessionals.com

www.icpuc.org.uk

The Integrated Care Pathway Users Scotland (ICPUS) is an established network using integrated care pathways in many different clinical areas. The ICPUS website provides presentations held on ICPUS events and it gives extensive information on integrated care pathways such as an overview of integrated care pathways, details about their background, use, benefits, advantages and disadvantages. In addition, a forum allows users to view and add details in specific areas of integrated care pathways design and implementation. After subscribing, users can contact other healthcare professionals to share and discuss problems, experiences and solutions. The website also contains a list of links to useful websites of related events, journal articles and organisations.

NHS Quality Improvement Scotland (NHS QIS)

www.nhshealthquality.org

NHS Quality Improvement Scotland (NHS QIS) is an organisation that works to improve the quality of care and treatment delivered by health services. It also acts as an umbrella for the Scottish Health Council (SHC) and the Scottish Medicines Consortium (SMC). NHS QIS provides advice and guidance on effective clinical practice to improve health services. By setting clinical and non-clinical standards of care and reviewing and monitoring the performance of NHS services, the organisation promotes patient safety. Moreover, NHS QIS develops, supports and implements clinical governance through the Clinical Governance and Patient Safety Support Unit. With allocated funds to NHS boards and in collaboration with NHS Education for Scotland (NES) and Glasgow Caledonian University, a national clinical governance and risk management education program has been provided since September 2006. Details about the key features of the complete work program of the unit/organisation can be found on the website.

Scottish Intercollegiate Guidelines Network (SIGN)

www.sign.ac.uk/patients

The Scottish Intercollegiate Guidelines Network (SIGN) outlines how patients are involved in guidelines development.

United Kingdom – non-government

Healthcare Commission

www.healthcarecommission.org.uk

The Healthcare Commission is an independent body, set up to promote and drive improvement in the quality of healthcare and public health by ensuring that healthcare services are meeting standard areas such as safety, cleanliness and waiting times. The commission assesses the performance of healthcare organisations, awards annual performance ratings for the NHS and coordinates reviews of healthcare by others.

National Institute of Clinical Excellence (NICE)

www.nice.org.uk

The National Institute for Health and Clinical Excellence (NICE) is the independent organisation responsible for providing national guidance on the promotion of good health and the prevention and treatment of ill health. NICE publishes on its website a simple guide explaining decisions about guidance at NICE that can be viewed and downloaded. Information on the three areas of health in which NICE produces guidance, public health, health technologies and clinical practice, is presented. In the field of clinical practice, the Centre for Clinical Practice develops clinical guidelines (based on the best available evidence) on the appropriate treatment and care of people with specific diseases and conditions. The website also contains implementation tools and a section outlines the opportunities available for patient, carer and public involvement in the development of NICE guidance.

OpenClinical

www.openclinical.org

OpenClinical is a not-for-profit organisation that helps to promote healthcare knowledge management applications. The OpenClinical website supports the learning about and tracking developments on advanced knowledge management technologies for healthcare such as point-of-care decision support systems, guidelines and clinical workflow.

United States – government

US Department of Health and Human Services (HHS)

www.hhs.gov

The US Department of Health and Human Services (HHS) is the US government's principal agency for health protection and human services provision. The department covers a wide spectrum of activities that are mainly carried out by the corresponding public health service agencies.

Agency of Healthcare Research and Quality (AHRQ)

www.ahrq.gov

www.innovations.ahrq.gov

The Agency of Healthcare Research and Quality (AHRQ), as one of the HHS agencies, sponsors, conducts, and disseminates research to provide evidence-based information in order to improve healthcare outcomes as well as quality, safety and effectiveness of healthcare. The website gives extensive information about AHRQ and its work areas. The sections with clinical information (e.g. evidence-based practice, outcomes and effectiveness, technology assessment, clinical practice guidelines) and quality and patient safety (e.g. measuring healthcare quality, medical errors and patient safety) are especially valuable when searching clinical process management. Reports, programs, research and analyses in the according fields as well as their outcomes and findings are published on the website. Links to related or sponsored organisations such as the NQMC and the NGC are also provided. A Healthcare Innovations Exchange features new innovation profiles and quality tools on patient-centered care.

National Quality Measures Clearinghouse (NQMC)

www.qualitymeasures.ahrq.gov

The National Quality Measures Clearinghouse (NQMC) is a database and website for information on specific evidence-based healthcare quality measures and measure sets. Sponsored by AHRQ, NQMC promotes access to obtain detailed information on quality measures.

National Guideline Clearinghouse (NGC)

www.guideline.gov

The National Guideline Clearinghouse (NGC) is a public resource for objective, detailed information on clinical practice guidelines and their implementation and use provided by the AHRQ. The websites is a database of evidence-based clinical practice guidelines and related documents which users can access and browse for free online to find summaries and full-text guidelines.

Patient Safety Network (PSNet)

http://psnet.ahrq.gov/

The Patient Safety Network (PSNet) is a web-based resource. Featuring continuously updated information on patient safety including news, resources and links to important research, the website provides searching and browsing capability.

United States – non-government

American Society for Healthcare Risk Management (ASHRM)

www.ashrm.org

The American Society for Healthcare Risk Management (ASHRM) is a personal membership group of the American Hospital Association that promotes risk management strategies and professional leadership. The website provides an extensive collection of resources including articles and newsletters focussing on insurance, patient safety, quality of care and open disclosure.

Consumers Advancing Patient Safety (CAPS)

www.patientsafety.org

Consumers Advancing Patient Safety (CAPS) is a consumer-led not-for-profit organisation formed to be a collective voice for individuals, families and healers who wish to prevent harm in healthcare encounters through partnership and collaboration. CAPS is committed to exploring and contributing the wisdom and experience that consumers can offer to patient safety research, education of both consumers and providers, reporting of bad outcomes and near misses, development and implementation of solutions that can prevent harm, and policymaking that will help create healthcare systems that are safe, compassionate and just.

Institute for Healthcare Improvement (IHI)

(Dr Donald Berwick)

www.ihi.org

The Institute for Healthcare Improvement (IHI) is a not-for-profit organisation supporting the improvement of patient care throughout the world. The website is structured around topics such as improvement of patient safety. Each topic area contains information for improvement including tools, links, literature and proposed changes for organisations. Furthermore, a separate section disseminates information on IHI programs, success stories and headlines. A comprehensive selection of white papers presents problems and respective ideas, changes and methods for improvement. The website also contains a workspace area designed to allow people to keep track of their improvement work by collecting data on key measures and applying tools for measurement and evaluation.

Institute of Medicine (IOM)

www.iom.edu

The Institute of Medicine (IOM) is a private not-for-profit organisation that provides objective, evidence-based advice to policymakers, health professionals, the private sector and the public. The website provides information divided by topics. In particular the section on healthcare and quality is valuable. It contains information about current projects and reports addressing healthcare services and the quality of care. All reports of the IOM are available for free online reading.

Joint Commission

www.jointcommission.org

The US-based agency of Joint Commission aims to improve the safety and quality of care by providing accreditation and related services. While the accreditation standards themselves are not published, the website offers information about the standards as well as a large number of resources about patient safety and performance measurement, and public policy reports.

National Patient Safety Foundation (NPSF)

www.npsf.org

The National Patient Safety Foundation (NPSF) is an independent not-for-profit organisation focussing on the enhancement of patient safety. The websites contains a resource centre that provides extensive information about patient safety including definitions, fact sheets, brochures, articles, government documents, newsletters and links to video streaming on the web. A discussion forum is also available as well as a list of links to other patient safety and related organisations.

Picker Institute

www.pickereurope.org

www.pickerinstitute.org

The Picker Institute is an independent, not-for-profit research and development institute that measures patient experiences using surveys and other methods to gain feedback on the quality of healthcare and uses this to improve services. Research evidence is used to promote innovative, intelligent approaches to meeting patients' needs. The institute aims to make the views of patients and citizens count throughout health policy and practice.

Canada – government

Health Canada

www.hc-sc.gc.ca

Health Canada is the federal department responsible for helping Canadians maintain and improve their health. The website contains information on all aspects of the Canadian public health system including downloadable reports and publications.

Canada – non-government

Canadian Patient Safety Institute (CPSI)

www.patientsafetyinstitute.ca

The Canadian Patient Safety Institute (CPSI) is an independent not-for-profit corporation that performs a coordinating and leadership role across health sectors raising awareness about patient safety and promoting effective strategies and leading practices for improvement.

Canadian Council on Health Services Accreditation (CCHSA)

www.cchsa.ca

The Canadian Council on Health Services Accreditation (CCHSA) assists health service organisations to examine and improve the quality of care and service. With regard to patient safety, the website provides comprehensive resources including analyses, surveys, projects and analysis tools and techniques as well as access to Health Accreditation Reports and Accreditation Standard newsletters. In addition, a database allows searches of leading practices and processes by themes such as governance, patient safety, quality improvement and best practice or standards including information management, leadership and partnerships.

Canadian Health Services Research Foundation (CHSRF)

www.chsrf.ca

The Canadian Health Services Research Foundation (CHSRF) is an independent, not-for-profit corporation supporting evidence-informed management. The website contains information in areas such as patient safety, teamwork, leadership, performance and quality of care. A special section called 'Managing for quality and safety' advises about research, resources, such as reviews and reports, and events related to managing the safe delivery of high-quality services in health. A list of links to organisations and initiatives involved in quality and safety is also available. Recognising the large impact nursing care has on quality of care and patient safety, the section 'Nursing leadership, organisation and policy' addresses these issues further and provides information on news and resources.

New Zealand – government

New Zealand Ministry of Health

www.moh.govt.nz

The New Zealand Ministry of Health publishes a large range of documents on different health issues that can be accessed via the website. Access to evidence-based health information from international online databases and electronic datasets for selected services is provided.

New Zealand – non-government

New Zealand Guidelines Group (NZGG)

www.nzgg.org.nz

New Zealand Guidelines Group (NZGG) aims to ensure delivery of high-quality health and disability services through cultural change based on evidence and effectiveness. The website offers a variety of resources on evidence for consumers.

Quality Health New Zealand

www.qualityhealth.org.nz

Quality Health New Zealand was established by the health sector to help improve the standards and performance of health and disability services.

Europe

Europe-wide organisations

ECRI Europe

www.ecri.org.uk

ECRI Europe is an independent not-for-profit health services research agency, providing independent research data. Its mission is to improve the safety, quality and cost-effectiveness of healthcare. The focus is on healthcare technology, healthcare risk and quality management and healthcare environmental management. It has been active in patient safety and has databases of information and regular newsletters.

European Pathway Association (E-P-A)

www.e-p-a.org

This association is an international network of researchers, managers and clinicians as well as academic and supporting institutions who want to support the development, implementation and evaluation of clinical/care pathways and share knowledge on this healthcare management concept. The website provides extensive information about the concept and methodology (history, definition) of care pathways. In order to obtain more information on this association and the concept as well as recent literature overviews, interested readers can get in touch with board members and other contact people as well as join the association for free. A report on the E-P-A activities can be downloaded from the website. The website also provides a reference list.

European Society for Quality in Healthcare (ESQH)

www.esqh.net

Based in Limerick, Ireland, ESQH is a not-for-profit organisation dedicated to the improvement of quality in European healthcare.

Denmark

DSI Danish Institute for Health Services Research

http://www.dsi.dk/engelsk.html

DSI Danish Institute for Health Services Research is an independent not-for-profit research institute. It provides research, communication and consultancy services for and with the health sector.

France

Haute Autorité de Santé (HAS) (French National Authority for Health)
www.has-sante.fr

This authority was established by the French Government although it is not a government body but rather an independent public body with financial autonomy that aims to improve the quality of patient care. The website may be viewed in English or French.

Germany

German Coalition for Patient Safety
www.aktionsbuendnis-patientensicherheit.de

The German Coalition for Patient Safety is sponsored by Germany's Federal Ministry of Health. Some English text is available.

Ärztliches Zentrum für Qualität in der Medizin (AEZQ) (Agency for Quality in Medicine) (AQuMed)
www.aezq.de/english

The Agency for Quality in Medicine (AQuMed) is a not-for-profit organisation initiating and organising health quality programs. The AQuMed website provides links to the specific websites of the programs such as:

International Guideline Databases
http://www.leitlinien.de/leitlinienanbieter/fremdsprachig_en/view

This website provides a collection of links to international guideline databases and organisations producing guidelines.

German Patient Information Clearinghouse (GPIC)
http://www.patienten-information.de/content/english

The German Patient Information Clearinghouse (GPIC) offers a free gateway to reliable consumer and patient information in German (there is an introduction in English).

National Program for Disease Management Guidelines
http://www.versorgungsleitlinien.de/english

The program was set up to provide evidence-based medical guidance for disease management programs. Guidelines are only available in German but some reports are in English.

Institut für Qualität und Wirtschaftlichkeit im Gesundheitswesen (IQWiG) (German Institute for Quality and Efficiency in Healthcare)
http://www.gesundheitsinformation.de/homepage.2.en.html

This is the health information site of the German Institute for Quality and Efficiency in Healthcare, an independent, not-for-government and not-for-profit foundation that has been created to support evidence-based decision making in German healthcare services.

Ireland

Health Information and Quality Authority

www.hiqa.ie

The Health Information and Quality Authority is an independent authority set up to help drive continuous improvement in Ireland's health and social care services.

Health Intelligence

www.ich.ie

Health Intelligence is responsible for capturing and utilising knowledge to improve health outcomes in Ireland. The website contains information on the activities and priorities of Health Intelligence within the Irish health service.

The Netherlands

Dutch Platform Patient Safety

www.platformpatientveiligheid.nl/english.php

English text is not yet available. The English version of this website was 'under construction' at the time of printing.

Netwerk Klinische Paden (Belgian Dutch Clinical Pathway Network)

www.nkp.be

The Belgian Dutch Clinical Pathway Network presents on its website the fields in which it is active including clinical pathways and related concepts such as patient safety, quality control, multidisciplinary teamwork, operations management and evidence-based medicine. The network provides education in these areas and supports projects on pathways and multicentre research projects and benchmarking as well as research and international collaboration. While only network members have access to a section with all details on all projects, there is a range of publications about the fields mentioned above such as general information, examples and literature of clinical pathways and a list of links to other resources.

Dutch Institute for Healthcare Improvement (CBO)

www.cbo.nl/english

The Dutch Institute for Healthcare Improvement develops instruments and methods for quality improvement and care, such as evidence-based guidelines, visitation (external peer review) systems, as well as programs for improving patient flow and patient safety. A range of guidelines is available in English.

Netherlands Institute for Accreditation of Hospitals (NIAZ)

www.niaz.nl/en

Through accreditation, the Netherlands Institute for Accreditation of Hospitals (NIAZ), a not-for-profit institution set up by hospital organisations and the Netherlands Order of Medical Specialists, aims to stimulate hospitals to improve the quality of the organisation of healthcare and in quality assurance.

Spain

Fundación Avedis Donabedian (FAD)

www.fadq.org

The Fundación Avedis Donabedian (FAD) is a not-for-profit organisation that acts as an accreditation partner of Joint Commission International for Spain. The website provides information in Spanish about patient safety and common models of quality management as well as links to articles, related organisations and journal websites.

Spanish Society for Quality in Healthcare
www.calidadasistencial.es/ing/index.php

The Spanish Society for Quality in Healthcare is a merger between scientific organisations aiming to drive the continuous improvement of quality in healthcare. The website contains references, bibliographic information and links to organisations and institutions related to quality management, patient safety and risk management.

Asia

Japan

Japan Council for Quality Healthcare
jcqhc.or.jp

English text is not yet available. The English version of this website was under construction at the time of printing.

Malaysia

Public Health Department, Ministry of Health Malaysia
www.dph.gov.my

Description of services not available on site.

Malaysian Society for Quality in Health
www.msqh.com.my

The Malaysian Society for Quality in Health is an independent, not-for-profit organisation working actively in participation with healthcare professionals to ensure safety and continuous quality improvement in health.

Singapore

Ministry of Health
www.moh.gov.sg

The Ministry of Health Singapore presents clinical practice guidelines for a wide range of healthcare topics.

India

National Accreditation Board for Hospitals & Healthcare Providers (NABH)
www.qcin.org

As part of the Quality Council of India, the National Accreditation Board for Hospitals & Healthcare Providers (NABH) was set up to establish and operate accreditation programs for healthcare organisations in India.

China

Peking University Centre for Evidence-Based Medicine and Clinical Research
pkuebm.bjmu.edu.cn

The Peking University Centre for Evidence-Based Medicine and Clinical Research is a multidisciplinary centre that strives to promote medical research that helps to improve clinical practice and healthcare services and application of research findings to patients' care and policymaking, with an ultimate goal of continuously increasing the quality and efficiency of healthcare services.

(South) Africa

Cohsasa: The Council for Health Service Accreditation of Southern Africa (Cohsasa)
www.cohsasa.co.za

The Council for Health Service Accreditation of Southern Africa (Cohsasa) assists a range of healthcare facilities to meet and maintain quality standards by enabling healthcare professionals to measure themselves against these standards.

Department of Health
www.doh.gov.za

The Department of Health's website provides a range of statistics, fact sheets and guidelines.

South America

Argentina

Institute for Clinical Effectiveness and Health Policy (IECS)
www.iecs.org.ar

The Institute for Clinical Effectiveness (IECS) is an independent, not-for-profit organisation, created by professionals from the medical and social sciences devoted to research, education and technical support with the main goal of improving efficiency, equity, and quality of healthcare systems and policies in Argentina.

Index

Printed in Dunstable, United Kingdom

85047109R00161